CHRONIC DISEASE
EPIDEMIOLOGY
AND CONTROL

SECOND EDITION

Edited by: ROSS C. BROWNSON • PATRICK L. REMINGTON • JAMES R. DAVIS

AMERICAN PUBLIC HEALTH ASSOCIATION

American Public Health Association
1015 Fifteenth St., NW
Washington, DC 20005-2605

Mohammad N Akhter, MD, MPH
Executive Director

8M   11/98
Printed and bound in the United States of America.

Cover Design: Jane Perini, JEP Graphics, Potomac, MD
Typestting: Wolf Publications, Inc., Frederick, MD
Set in: ITC Garamond
Printing and Binding: United Book Press

ISBN 0-87553-237-3
Library of Congress Catalog Card Number: 98-74062

CONTENTS

MAJOR CHRONIC DISEASES

PREFACE

Since the publication of the first edition of *Chronic Disease Epidemiology and Control* in 1993, public health practitioners have encountered many new challenges and opportunities in their prevention efforts. For example, changes in how health care is delivered, particularly the growth of managed care, are altering the day-to-day roles of many public health agencies. Similarly, new information technologies, including the rapid evolution of microcomputers, software, and the Internet, offer exciting possibilities.

The need for public health involvement in chronic disease control is reflected in the large number of Year 2010 Health Objectives, at both national and state levels that address chronic disease issues. To meet this demand, public health professionals must become knowledgeable in the science and practice of chronic disease control. To enhance the technical capacity for delivering effective programs, there has been a critical need for a book that addresses the broad range of issues related to chronic disease control.

The purpose of this book remains the same as that of the first edition—to provide practical information on chronic disease epidemiology, prevention, and control. The book is intended to support a broad range of chronic disease control activities, and it is designed to serve as a quick reference guide for practicing health professionals who need to locate critical background information for public and professional education and for developing appropriate interventions.

This book is intended for several audiences. First, it can be useful to professionals involved in the practice and teaching of chronic disease epidemiology, prevention, and control at all levels. In state health agencies, the book can be helpful to staff involved in primary and secondary prevention of chronic diseases, including epidemiologists, physicians, nurses, health educators, and health promotion specialists. In local health agencies, administrators, physicians, nurses, health educators, and sanitarians should find it of value. In academic institutions, it can provide helpful background information on chronic diseases for students taking beginning and advanced public health courses. Although the book is intended primarily for a North American audience, there is literature drawn from all parts of the world, and we believe that much of the information covered will be applicable in any developed or developing country.

The authors of the various chapters in this book were selected for both their scientific expertise and their practical experience in carrying out chronic disease control programs at the community level.

The new edition includes 16 chapters and is organized into three major sections: (1) Public Health Approaches to Chronic Disease Control, (2) Selected Lifestyle Risk Factors, and (3) Major Chronic Diseases. In the new edition, we reflect feedback we have received informally from colleagues, suggestions from a survey of readers conducted in 1996, and input from the APHA Publications Board. Earlier chapters has been updated and two new chapters (ie, physical inactivity, diet and nutrition) have been added.

Chapter 1 of this book provides a historical review of chronic disease control, a brief explanation of the current status of chronic disease control programs, and a discussion of the prospects and challenges for chronic disease control during the next decade and beyond. Chapters 2 and 3 briefly review the methods used in chronic disease epidemiology and chronic disease surveillance. Chapter 4 provides an overview of chronic disease control intervention methods, providing a theoretical grounding for interventions that address the diseases and risk factors discussed in later chapters. It also summarizes some of the important features of successful interventions and provides practical examples. Many of the concepts and resources discussed in Chapters 1 through 4 should assist readers in developing a more in-depth understanding of the remaining chapters in the book.

In section two, Chapters 5 through 10 focus on modifiable risk factors to chronic diseases. The chapters in this section examine the important areas of tobacco use, alcohol use, physical inactivity, diet and nutrition, high blood pressure, and high blood cholesterol.

The final section of the book describes major chronic diseases— cardiovascular disease, cancer, chronic lung diseases, diabetes, arthritis and other musculoskeletal diseases, and neurologic disorders.

A standard format has been used for all chapters that focus on specific risk factors and chronic diseases, to allow the reader quick and easy access to information. Each chapter begins with a brief introduction, reviewing the significance of the chronic condition and the underlying biological or physiological process of disease. The next section addresses descriptive epidemiology by examining high-risk groups (including minority populations), geographic variation, and trends over time. The third section describes the best available estimates of the magnitude of specific risk factors and their contributions to each disease or condition. An additional section discusses prevention and control measures. When available, specific examples of practical and effective public health interventions are reviewed, as well as recommendations for future research and demonstration. A bibliography and list of resources are also included to facilitate access to additional information.

This book is not intended to provide a complete and final review of chronic disease epidemiology and control. Because the field is so broad, with overlapping issues, any division of the topic becomes somewhat arbitrary. There are literally thousands of different chronic diseases. We have chosen to focus on those that account for a large proportion of morbidity and mortality in the adult population and to emphasize risk factors that can be modified through public health interventions.

Future research will continue to expand our understanding of chronic disease epidemiology and control. Epidemiologic studies will identify new risk factors and quantify their effects. Intervention studies underway will expand the array of interventions available for public health practitioners.

Chronic disease epidemiology and control is a rapidly expanding field. There is a clear and increasing need for public health professionals with knowledge and expertise in chronic disease control. We hope this book will become a useful resource for health professionals as they are called on to meet new challenges.

RCB
PLR
JRD

ACKNOWLEDGMENTS

Many individuals and organizations made the revised edition of this book possible. Original input and support were provided by the Association of State and Territorial Chronic Disease Program Directors and, in particular, James Marks, David Momrow, Randy Schwartz, and Fran Wheeler. Several individuals reviewed chapters or contributed information: Amy Eyler, Sarah Landis, Marian Minor, F. Javier Nieto, and Michael Pratt. We are grateful to Brenda Brooks, Tracey Cannon, and Heidi Mosher, who assisted in technical editing, graphics, and clerical support. We are thankful to Ellen Meyer, Director of Publications at APHA. We also appreciate the guidance from our liaisons with the APHA Publications Board, Walter Jakubowski and Hugh McKinnon.

RCB
PLR
JRD

FOREWORD

In this century, the United States has seen an immense shift in the causes of death and disability. In 1900, the major causes of death were infectious diseases such as pneumonia, tuberculosis, and diarrhea. Today, chronic diseases such as heart disease, cancer, stroke, and diabetes account for more than 70% of deaths in the United States annually.

Advances in epidemiology and disease control have shown that much of the death and disability caused by these chronic conditions is preventable through a broad range of actions:

• Modifying personal risk factors through smoking prevention and cessation, improved dietary habits, and increased physical activity;
• Expanding the use of early detection practices such as mammography and Pap testing;
• Implementing comprehensive, high-quality school health education programs; and
• Achieving more healthful environmental and social policies such as the use of automobile air bags, better nutrition guidelines, and comprehensive clean indoor air regulations.

Lester Breslow, MD, MPH
Jeffrey P. Koplan, MD, MPH

State-of-the-art technologies in chronic disease control have not been applied systematically in the public health arena, especially at the local health department level. In many cases, activity at the local level has been severely limited to only a few interventions, such as hypertension screening.

The challenge to the public health system is to incorporate known methods of chronic disease control into regular programs. This is critical to achieving the health objectives for the Year 2000 and those in development for 2010.[1,2] Without strong programs aimed at these areas, health departments run the risk of becoming increasingly irrelevant to the major health issues of our time. To develop effective chronic disease control programs, the public health system must make a commitment to provide adequately trained personnel and funding for public health agencies to address the leading causes of death and disability.

This book will support that endeavor by aiding in planning, public education, professional education, policy development, program evaluation, teaching, and grant writing. The first edition of *Chronic Disease Epidemiology and Control* served as an essential tool for the people who are responsible for reducing the enormous burden of chronic diseases. We anticipate this new edition will be even more useful.

REFERENCES

1. Public Health Service. *Healthy People 2000: National Health Promotion and Disease Prevention Objectives.* Washington, DC: US Dept of Health and Human Services; 1991. DHHS publication PHS 91-50212.
2. Health People 2010 Website. http://web.health.gov/healthypeople/

CONTRIBUTORS

Barbara E. Ainsworth, PhD, MPH, FACSM
Department of Epidemiology and Biostatistics and Department of Exercise Science
School of Public Health
University of South Carolina
Columbia, South Carolina
(*Physical Inactivity*)

Michael C. R. Alavanja, DrPH
Division of Cancer Epidemiology and Genetics
National Cancer Institute
Rockville, Maryland
(*Cancer*)

Robert F. Anda, MD, MS
National Center for Chronic Disease and Health Promotion
Centers for Disease Control and Prevention
Atlanta, Georgia
(*Cholesterol*)

Henry A. Anderson, MD
Wisconsin Department of Health and Social Services
Division of Health
Madison, Wisconsin
(*Chronic Lung Diseases*)

Dileep G. Bal, MD, MPH
Cancer Control Branch
California Department of Health Services
Sacramento, California
(*Cancer*)

Donald B. Bishop, PhD
Center for Health Promotion
Minnesota Department of Health
St. Paul, Minnesota
(*Diabetes*)

Lester Breslow, MD, MPH
School of Public Health
University of California at Los Angeles
Los Angeles, California
(*Foreword*)

Carol A. Brownson, MSPH
Program in Occupational Therapy
Washington University School of Medicine
St. Louis, Missouri
(*Cardiovascular Disease*)

Ross C. Brownson, PhD
Department of Community Health and Prevention Research Center
School of Public Health
Saint Louis University
St. Louis, Missouri
(*Preface, Methods in Chronic Disease Epidemiology, Cancer*)

James R. Davis, PhD
Psychology Department
University of Missouri-Columbia
Columbia, Missouri
(*Preface, Intervention Methods for
Chronic Disease*)

Mary C. Dufour, MD, MPH
National Institute on Alcohol Abuse
and Alcoholism
National Institutes of Health
Bethesda, Maryland
(*Alcohol Use*)

Linda J. Dusenbury, MS, RN
Physical Activity and Health Initiative
California Department of Health
Services
Sacramento, California
(*Cardiovascular Disease*)

Susan B. Foerster, MPH, RD
Nutrition & Cancer Prevention
California Department of Health
Services
Sacramento, California
(*Diet and Nutrition*)

Gary M. Franklin, MD, MPH
School of Public Health and Commu-
nity Medicine
University of Washington
Seattle, Washington
(*Chronic Neurologic Disorders*)

Gary A. Giovino, PhD
Office on Smoking and Health
National Center for Chronic Disease
Prevention and Health Promotion
Centers for Disease Control and
Prevention
Atlanta, Georgia
(*Tobacco Use*)

Jay M. Goldring, PhD
Colgate-Palmolive Company
Piscataway, New Jersey
(*Chronic Lung Diseases*)

Richard A. Goodman, MD, MPH
Epidemiology Program Office
Centers for Disease Control and
Prevention
Atlanta, Georgia
(*Chronic Disease Surveillance*)

Russell P. Harris, MD, MPH
Department of Medicine
School of Medicine
University of North Carolina
Chapel Hill, North Carolina
(*Methods in Chronic Disease Epide-
miology*)

Marc C. Hochberg, MD, MPH
Division of Rheumatology and
Clinical Immunology, Department
of Medicine and Department of
Epidemiology
University of Maryland School of
Medicine
Baltimore, Maryland
(*Arthritis and Other Musculoskeletal
Diseases*)

David S. James, MD
Division of Pulmonary and Critical
  Care Medicine
Department of Medicine
University of New Mexico School of
  Medicine
Albuquerque, New Mexico
(*Chronic Lung Diseases*)

Jeffrey P. Koplan, MD, MPH
Centers for Disease Control and
  Prevention
Atlanta, Georgia
(*Foreword, Current Issues and
  Challenges in Chronic Disease
  Control*)

Lawrence H. Kushi, ScD
Division of Epidemiology
School of Public Health
University of Minnesota
Minneapolis, Minnesota
(*Diet and Nutrition*)

Darwin R. Labarthe, MD, PhD
University of Texas Health Center at
  Houston
School of Public Health
Houston, Texas
(*High Blood Pressure*)

R. Brick Lancaster, MA, CHES
National Center for Chronic Disease
  Prevention and Health Promotion
Centers for Disease Control and
  Prevention
Atlanta, Georgia
(*Intervention Methods for Chronic
  Disease Control*)

Caroline A. Macera, PhD, FACSM
Division of Nutrition and Physical
  Activity
National Center for Chronic Disease
  Prevention and Health Promotion
Centers for Disease Control and
  Prevention
Atlanta, Georgia
(*Physical Inactivity*)

James S. Marks, MD, MPH
National Center for Chronic Disease
  Prevention and Health Promotion
Centers for Disease Control and
  Prevention
Atlanta, Georgia
(*Current Issues and Challenges in
  Chronic Disease Control*)

Patrick E. McBride, MD, MPH
Departments of Medicine—Cardiol-
  ogy and Family Medicine
University of Wisconsin School of
  Medicine
Madison, Wisconsin
(*Cholesterol*)

Matthew T. McKenna, MD, MPH
National Center for Chronic Disease
  Prevention and Health Promotion
Centers for Disease Control and
  Prevention
Atlanta, Georgia
(*Current Issues and Challenges in
  Chronic Disease Control*)

Lorene M. Nelson, PhD
Department of Health Research and
Policy
Stanford University School of Medi-
cine
Stanford, California
(*Chronic Neurologic Disorders*)

Craig J. Newschaffer, PhD
Jefferson Medical College
Thomas Jefferson University
Philadelphia, Pennsylvania
(*Cardiovascular Disease*)

Thomas E. Novotny, MD, MPH
Office of Global Health
Centers for Disease Control and
Prevention
Health, Nutrition, Population Pro-
gram
World Bank Group
Washington, D. C.
(*Tobacco Use*)

John S. Reif, DVM, MSc
Department of Environmental Health
Colorado State University
Fort Collins, Colorado
(*Cancer*)

Patrick L. Remington, MD, MPH
Department of Preventive Medicine
University of Wisconsin School of
Medicine
Madison, Wisconsin
(*Preface, Chronic Disease Surveil-
lance*)

Edward J. Roccella, PhD, MPH
National High Blood Pressure
Education Program
National Heart, Lung, and Blood
Institute
Bethesda, Maryland
(*High Blood Pressure*)

Jon S. Roesler, MS
Center for Health Promotion
Minnesota Department of Health
St. Paul, Minnesota
(*Diabetes*)

David A. Savitz, PhD
Department of Epidemiology
School of Public Health
University of North Carolina
Chapel Hill, North Carolina
(*Methods in Chronic Disease Epide-
miology*)

Randy Schwartz, MSPH
Division of Community and Family
Health
Maine Bureau of Health
Augusta, Maine
(*Intervention Methods for Chronic
Disease*)

Jean C. Scott, RN, DrPH
Division of Rheumatology and
Clinical Immunology, Department
of Medicine and Department of
Epidemiology
University of Maryland School of
Medicine
Baltimore, Maryland
(*Arthritis and Other Musculoskeletal
Diseases*)

William R. Taylor, MD, MPH
Georgia Department of Medical
   Assistance
Atlanta, Georgia
(*Current Issues and Challenges in
   Chronic Disease Control*)

Fran Wheeler, PhD
Prevention Center
School of Public Health
University of South Carolina
Columbia, South Carolina
(*Intervention Methods for Chronic
   Disease*)

Bruce R. Zimmerman, MD
Division of Endocrinology
Mayo Clinic
Rochester, Minnesota
(*Diabetes*)

CHAPTER 1

CURRENT ISSUES AND CHALLENGES IN CHRONIC DISEASE CONTROL

The accomplishments of public health have contributed greatly to the decrease in mortality rates and change in the patterns of death and disease in the United States. Infant mortality has fallen from 150 deaths per 1000 live births in 1900 to 7.5 per 1000 in 1995. Life expectancy from birth has risen from 47 years in 1900 to almost 76 years in 1995—an increase of more than two days for every week that has passed since the beginning of this century.[1] Despite the marked reductions in overall mortality, disparities remain among certain subpopulations in the United States—most notably people of low socioeconomic status and Blacks.

The leading causes of death have changed in this century from infectious diseases to chronic diseases. In 1900, the three leading causes of death were pneumonia and influenza; tuberculosis; and gastritis, enteritis, and colitis. These diseases accounted for nearly one-third of all deaths (Table 1.1).[2] Today, heart disease, malignant neoplasms, and cerebrovascular diseases (stroke) are the three leading causes of death, accounting for almost two-thirds of all deaths (Table 1.2).[1] Reflecting these changes in the leading causes of mortality, the primary emphasis of public health efforts has begun to shift from microbiologic investigation of communicable diseases to a focus on the role of behavioral and environmental risk factors and methods for preventing disease, disability, and death in a population.

In 1988, the Institute of Medicine published a report, *The Future of Public Health*, which described the mission of public health as assuring conditions in which people can be healthy.[3] The distinctive roles of public health agencies in this mission are to assess the health needs of the community,to develop comprehen-

Matthew T. McKenna, MD, MPH
William R. Taylor, MD, MPH
James S. Marks, MD, MPH
Jeffrey P. Koplan, MD, MPH

Table 1.1—Death Rates and Percent of Total Deaths for the 10 Leading Causes of Death in the United States, 1900

Cause of Death	Death Rate per 100,000	Percent of Total Deaths
All causes	1719	100.0
Pneumonia and influenza	202	11.8
Tuberculosis	194	11.3
Gastritis, enteritis, colitis	143	8.3
Heart diseases	137	8.0
Symptoms, senility, ill-defined conditions	118	6.8
Vascular lesions affecting central nervous system	107	6.2
Chronic nephritis and renal sclerosis	81	4.7
Unintentional injuries	72	4.2
Malignant neoplasms	64	3.7
Diptheria	40	2.3
All other causes		32.6

Note: Data compiled from National Office of Vital Statistics.[2]

sive public health policies, and to assure that the services necessary to achieve this goal are being provided to the community.

Comprehensive national legislation for the United States to address health care reform was proposed and vigorously debated in the early 1990s. Recent market-oriented reform in health care delivery, principally in the form of managed care, has begun to displace traditional fee-for-service medicine as the primary mode of financing the delivery of medical services. Managed care generally promotes a more "population-based" approach to improving the health of enrolled patients, and hence offers

health departments new opportunities as well as challenges.[4] To fulfill the general mission outlined by the Institute of Medicine report and to contend with the changing circumstances of health care delivery, public health practitioners need to accept an expanded role in developing and implementing effective community-based prevention programs and in mobilizing social support for control of chronic diseases.

DEFINITION OF CHRONIC DISEASE

Chronic diseases have been referred to as chronic illnesses, noncommunicable diseases, and

Table 1.2—Death Rates and Percent of Total Deaths for the 10 Leading Causes of Death in the United States, 1995

Cause of Death	Death Rate per 100,000	Percent of Total Deaths
All causes	880	100.0
Diseases of heart	281	32.0
Malignant neoplasms	204	23.2
Cerebrovascular diseases	60	6.8
Chronic obstructive pulmo- nary diseases	40	4.5
Accidents	34	3.9
Pneumonia and influenza	32	3.6
Diabetes mellitus	23	2.6
Human immunodeficiency virus infection	16	1.8
Suicide	12	1.3
Chronic liver disease and cirrhosis	10	1.1
All other causes		19.2

Note: Data compiled from National Center for Health Statistics.[1]

degenerative diseases. They are generally characterized by uncertain etiology, multiple risk factors, a long latency period, a prolonged course of illness, noncontagious origin, functional impairment or disability, and incurability.

In more general terms, a chronic disease can be defined as a disease that has a prolonged course, that does not resolve spontaneously, and for which a complete cure is rarely achieved. Although this definition of chronic disease encompasses a wide range of diverse disease processes, it provides a practical framework for their control.

The causes of many chronic diseases remain obscure, but epide-miologists have identified risk factors for many of the leading chronic diseases (Table 1.3). It is clear from Table 1.3 that control of a single risk factor, such as cigarette smoking, can often reduce the risk of many chronic diseases. The complexity of chronic disease control is also apparent in Table 1.3 and in later chapters. For example, a single disease designation, such as cancer, may actually consist of hundreds of different diseases, each with separate risk factors. In addition to the many modifiable risk factors, many genetic and physiological factors increase the risk of chronic diseases.[5-7]

The extended time frame associated with the development and

Table 1.3—Interrelationships between Various Chronic Diseases and Modifiable Risk Factors, United States

	Cardiovascular Disease	Cancer	Chronic Lung Disease	Diabetes	Cirrhosis	Musculoskeletal Diseases	Neurologic Disorders
Tobacco use	+	+	+			+	?
Alcohol use	+	+			+	+	+
High cholesterol	+						+
High blood pressure	+						?
Diet	+	+		+		+	+
Physical inactivity	+	+		+		+	+
Obesity	+	+		+		+	+
Stress	?	?					
Environmental tobacco smoke	?	+	+				
Occupation	?	+	+		?	+	?
Pollution	+	+	+				
Low socioeconomic status	+	+	+	+	+	+	

Note: + = established risk factor; ? = possible risk factor duration of chronic diseases implies, almost by definition, that rapid changes in disease trends are difficult. Therefore, interventions aimed at preventing and controlling chronic disease must be implemented with a persistent, long-term perspective.

GOALS OF CHRONIC DISEASE CONTROL

The goals of chronic disease control are to reduce the incidence of disease through prevention, delay the onset of disability, alleviate the severity of disease, and prolong the individual's life.[8] Verbrugge has suggested that chronic disease prevalence and disability will increase as life expectancy increases and the lethal outcomes of disease are controlled.[9] On the other hand, Fries has suggested that life expect-

ancy is relatively limited. Hence, the proportion of people who will live to very old ages (ie, older than 85 years) will not increase.[10] Besides the assumption that the human life span is fixed, the Fries model also assumes that the onset of chronic diseases and disabilities can be delayed or compressed into a shorter time span before death and that senescence can be modified. Therefore, chronic disease could occupy a smaller portion of a person's life span, and the need for medical care in later life could decrease.[10]

These alternate hypotheses give rise to two models of the future chronic disease burden (Figure 1.1). In the first model, the average age at onset of chronic conditions remains unchanged, whereas mortality is delayed and chronic conditions occupy a greater proportion of

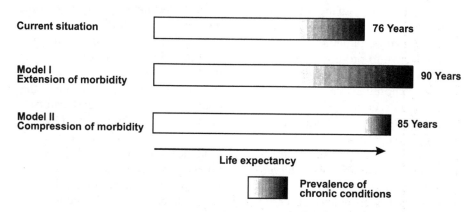

Figure 1.1—Alternative models of extension or compression of morbidity as life expectancy is extended.

extended life. The second model predicts an extension of vigorous life and a compression of morbidity. Whichever model proves more accurate, preventing disability from chronic diseases should be a prime goal of public health efforts. Chronic disease control should focus on morbidity as well as mortality; it should emphasize postponement of occurrence rather than cure, and it should have the goal of improving the quality of life.[11]

A strategic objective for chronic disease control is to change the public's perception of chronic diseases and their complications from one of inevitability to one of preventability. A reduction in chronic disease burden may best be achieved by altering factors that place a person at higher risk for chronic diseases, such as tobacco use, lack of physical activity, and poor nutrition. Unfortunately, changing a person's fundamental and ingrained behaviors can be difficult. It may be more effective to promote the adoption of healthy behaviors through comprehensive health education in school and other efforts to change behavior in children and young people.[12] However, there is empirical evidence that successful implementation of effective interventions can result in timely reductions in the impact of chronic diseases.[13] For example, smoking cessation in middle aged men is associated with

a 40% decline in the risk of death from coronary artery heart disease within just one year.[14]

CONTROL

The distinction between treatment of disease and promotion of health or early detection of disease has been recognized since early times. In classical Greek mythology, Asklepios and his two daughters, Panacea and Hygeia, were deities of medicine and health. Panacea represented the treatment of people who were ill, and Hygeia embodied living wisely and preserving health. Today, Panacea could represent the usual activities of the medical care system, and Hygeia could embody disease prevention and health promotion.

Accepting that chronic diseases are not an inevitable consequence of aging is the first step toward chronic disease control. Understanding the natural history of a disease provides the heuristic framework for the design of prevention methods. Without preventive intervention, the course of a chronic disease can be viewed as a continuum from the disease-free state to asymptomatic biological change, clinical illness, impairment and disability, and ultimately death.[15] Although this simple linear model illustrates the basic concept of chronic disease progression, the physical and social

6

manifestations of chronic diseases result from the simultaneous and complex interaction of several diseases at different stages on this continuum.

Prevention and control are interrelated, and the two terms are often used interchangeably. Prevention suggests that an intervention occurs before the onset of a disease or early in the course of a disease, whereas control efforts may occur later in the disease course and reinforce prevention efforts in a population. The precise boundary between prevention and control is not distinct, however.

A commonly used scheme classifies prevention as primary, secondary, or tertiary, according to where it is applied along the disease continuum (Figure 1.2). Primary prevention reduces disease incidence; secondary prevention decreases the duration and severity of disease through early detection and treatment before signs and symptoms occur; and tertiary prevention reduces complications of the existing disease.[16]

Primary prevention is directed to susceptible people before they develop a particular chronic disease. These preventive interventions reduce the incidence of disease and, consequently, its sequelae. The causes or risk factors for a disease must be established for primary prevention to be feasible. Examples of primary prevention interventions

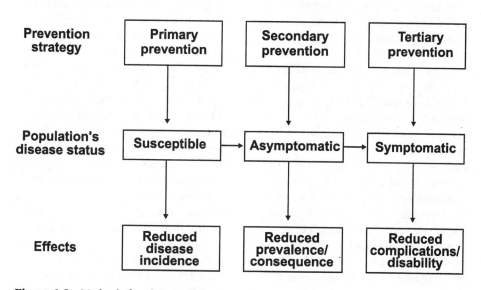

Figure 1.2—Methods for chronic disease prevention and control.

include smoking prevention and cessation programs, dietary recommendations to reduce the consumption of saturated fat, and promotion of physical activity.

Secondary prevention is directed to people who are asymptomatic but who have developed biologic changes resulting from the disease. Strategies for secondary prevention may be referred to as "disease control," because the goal is to reduce the consequences of the disease. Secondary prevention generally does not reduce the incidence of disease but instead detects the condition at an earlier, more treatable stage. Screening for cervical and breast cancers are examples of secondary prevention. Screening programs are recommended only under certain conditions: if the natural history of the disease permits early detection; if a screening test is available to accurately detect the disease at an early stage; if treatment at early stages can alter the consequences of the disease; and if the screening test is acceptable to the populations at highest risk for the disease.

Tertiary prevention is directed at preventing disability in people who have symptomatic disease. Strategies for tertiary prevention may be to prevent the progression of a disease and its complications or to provide rehabilitation. For example, eye examinations for people with

diabetes can detect retinopathy early when this condition can be promptly treated, preventing progression to blindness. Although the public health system has less frequently focused on developing strategies for tertiary prevention, issues such as quality of life, the cost of long-term health care, and the aging population's demand for health care services make prevention of disabilities an emerging priority for chronic disease control.

POTENTIAL AND EFFECTIVENESS

In the United States during 1990, heart disease, cancer, and cerebrovascular disease were the three most common causes listed on death certificates; these diseases accounted for almost two-thirds of all deaths. In 1993, McGinnis and Foege reported on their reclassification of all deaths during 1990 according to the contributing factors that actually caused these deaths.[17] They estimated that smoking, diet and physical activity patterns, and alcohol use were the actual causes of about 40% of all deaths.[17] Clearly, interventions aimed at changing the impact of these underlying factors on health status have the potential to prevent disability and death due to chronic diseases. Thus, the potential for prevention remains high. Public health agencies need to expand programs in chronic disease prevention and health promotion and to develop more effective strategies to help people adopt healthier lifestyles.

The urgent care required for treatment of people with acute illness will always remain a priority in health care. However, additional investments can be productive in maintaining health and preventing chronic diseases. Growing evidence documents the cost-effectiveness of these interventions to control chronic disease. For example, clinical trials have shown that counseling by physicians can have a powerful influence on cessation rates for tobacco smokers.[18] A recent assessment of the cost-effectiveness of 500 medical interventions showed that physician counseling against smoking is very cost-effective in comparison to other accepted medical practices (Table 1.4).[19] Similarly, dietary interventions to reduce levels of serum cholesterol have been shown to be at least as cost-effective as coronary artery bypass surgery. Optimal chronic disease control will require shifting the focus from episodic care for acute illnesses to emphasis on a continuum of services across a variety of settings. (More detailed descriptions of strategies for intervention are provided in Chapter 4.)

PRIORITIES AND STRATEGIES

The current priorities and strategies for chronic disease control are the result of a complex relationship between government agencies, managed care organizations, and other medical provider groups and voluntary health organizations. Government health agencies fund and conduct health education and research, develop policies, establish standards, provide financing for medical care, deliver medical services to the poor, and monitor the health status of the population. Voluntary health agencies fund research, provide public and professional education, stimulate social and legislative changes, and create visibility for prevention and treatment through their large cadre of volunteers. The medical care sector delivers services, provides preventive medicine through primary care, and establishes professional guidelines that improve the quality of services.

In 1979, *Healthy People: The Surgeon General's Report on Health Promotion and Disease Prevention* set the direction for chronic disease control.[20] This report concluded that further improvements in health were most likely to be achieved through disease prevention and health promotion rather than through increased medical care services and health expenditures. After a review of age-specific risks for mortality, actions were recommended in five priority areas: smoking, high blood pressure, alcohol consumption, nutrition, and physical activity. These conclusions were recently substanti-

Table 1.4—Estimates per Year of Life Saved for Selected Medical, Life-Saving Interventions

Intervention Category	Description	Cost/Life-Year Saved
Smoking cessation advice	Smoking cessation advice for men age 50-54	$ 990
	Smoking cessation advice for men age 45-49	$ 1 100
	Smoking cessation advice for men age 35-39	$ 1 400
	Smoking cessation advice for women age 50-54	$ 1 700
	Smoking cessation advice for women age 45-49	$ 1 900
	Smoking cessation advice for women age 35-39	$ 2 900
Cholesterol treatment	Low-cholesterol diet for men age 60 and > 180 mg/dL	$ 12 000
	Low-cholesterol diet for men age 30	$ 19 000
	Lovastatin for men age 45-54, no heart disease and ≥300 mg/dL	$ 34 000
	Lovastatin for women age 45-54, no heart disease and cholesterol ≥ 300 mg/dL	$ 1 200 00
Coronary artery bypass graft surgery (CABG)	Left main coronary artery bypass graft surgery (vs medical management)	$ 5 600
	3-vessel coronary artery bypass graft surgery (vs medical management)	$ 12 000
	2-vessel coronary artery bypass graft surgery (vs medical management)	$ 28 000
Other - Prevention	Mammography every 3 years for women 60-65	$ 2 700
	Annual mammography and breast exam for women age 40-49	$ 62 000
	Annual (vs every 2 years) cervical cancer screening for women age 30-39	$ 4 100
	Hypertension screening for men age 45-54	$ 5 200

Note: Adapted from Tengs *et al.*[19]

ated for coronary artery heart disease in a study where simulation models were used to analyze the determinants of the 30% decline in mortality from this disease in the United States between 1980 and 1990.[21] The authors in this study concluded that at least 50% of the decline was attributable to reductions in risk factors for persons with and without coronary artery heart disease.

Incorporating the concepts of age-specific risks and their preventability, Breslow and Somers advocated a philosophical reorientation in personal health care to emphasize prevention.[22] This lifetime health-monitoring program incorporates scientific knowledge into specific health goals and professional services for each of 10 age groups, and the authors recommended that these preventive services should be covered by medical care insurance policies.

Standard guidelines for preventive services also have been established. The US Preventive Services Task Force published an updated version of its *Guide to Clinical Preventive Services* in 1996.[23] This report recognized that primary prevention has a profound potential for improving health. It also recognized that the role of primary care providers should be enlarged from diagnosis and treatment of illness to include counseling patients about their risk behaviors and the need to accept greater responsibility for their own health. A companion book to the task force report has also been published. This work outlines specific strategies for implementing the recommended interventions in the clinical setting.[24]

HEALTH CARE AND ACCESS

The control and prevention of chronic disease are inextricably linked with issues of the current and future cost of health care. In 1996, the estimated costs of health care in the United States exceeded one trillion dollars.[25] This cost was more than 13% of the gross domestic product, up from slightly more than 7% in 1970, and represents an annual expenditure of almost $3900 per person. Chronic diseases consume more than 60% of the total health care dollars in the United States.[26] These expenditures can be expected to grow substantially because of the inevitable increase in the number of elderly residents that will result from the aging of the "baby boom" generation.

A second major factor driving health care costs is that medical care inflation has consistently out paced general inflation. A predominant dynamic contributing to this situation has been the inefficiencies inherent in the traditional fee-for-service reimbursement system in the United States. This system economically rewards providers and hospitals for performing more diagnostic and therapeutic procedures. The ascendancy of managed care has at its base the desire to incorporate incentives to contain costs.[27] Decreases in expenditures can result from improved efficiency or from limitations in the services provided. These limitations can be achieved by reductions in the quality of existing services, or reductions of services that provide little or no health benefit. Done well, managed care will improve efficiency of delivery of quality effective services and reduce those services that are of little benefit. This requires a level of analysis and information and system control that are not yet demonstrated but are not unreasonable to expect.

The third engine of growth in health care costs is technological advancement. Medical conditions have been increasingly managed with more expensive and intensive tests and interventions that add costs. Some of these advancements undoubtedly lead to substantial improvements in outcomes, but many only provide minimal benefits over older technologies, frequently at much higher costs.[28] Overall health presumably improves with technological progress although total health care costs increase as well. Until recently, most of the growth in costs has been largely attributable to medical care inflation and technological development.[29] However, between the years 2010 and 2030, the aging of the population will contribute more to overall cost increases than it has in the preceding 80 years.[30]

Major challenges for chronic disease control specialists will be to develop a consensus on national health goals and to generate better information for making decisions about resource allocation for programs and services. The emergence of managed care as the principal force in the restructuring of medical practice also provides major challenges for public health practitioners involved in the prevention and

control of chronic diseases. A common component of managed care plans are reimbursement mechanisms that result in financial risk being shared by the provider and the insurer for the costs of care. This situation contrasts with traditional fee-for-service reimbursement, in which all the costs for care were historically billed to the insurer, who then passed the expense on to the payer of insurance premiums. In the United States, these payers have usually been employers who provide health coverage to their workers as a benefit, or the government that provides coverage to certain subgroups of the poor (eg, blind, disabled, parents with dependent children) under Medicaid and to older adults through Medicare.

Estimates indicate that over 50 million people in the United States (about 20% of the population) are enrolled in managed care plans and that 40% to 65% of the population will be enrolled in such plans within the next 5 years.[30] In addition to the emergence of managed care as the dominant system for providing privately financed medical care, publicly funded programs such as Medicare and Medicaid have provided incentives for recipients to switch into managed care plans. Many health departments previously used funds from direct patient services to support activities such as surveillance and health education programs as well as uncompensated services for the poor and uninsured. However, such clinical services are increasingly being contracted to managed care organizations, and the result is lost revenues for public agencies. Even when public facilities retain services as participants in a managed care plan, the lower reimbursement rates result in less surplus funds to support educational programs or to provide uncompensated care.[31]

Despite the fiscal challenges posed by health care reforms, interaction between health departments and managed care organizations appears to offer great opportunities to facilitate the implementation of chronic disease prevention programs for at least two reasons.

First, managed care organizations have traditionally emphasized population oriented, prevention services.[32] As a result, they frequently possess well-developed systems to measure internal performance, which focuses on the provision of preventive care.[4] In addition, a set of health indicators called the Health Plan Employer Data Information Set (HEDIS) was developed jointly by managed care organizations, purchasers, and consumers to evaluate the quality of health services provided to enrolled members.[33] Of the 16 indicators of effectiveness of care in a recent version of HEDIS (version 3.0), 7 involve the provision of

primary or secondary preventative services for chronic diseases. These indicators include screening for breast and cervical cancer, treatment with a beta blocker after a myocardial infarction, appropriate use of medications for patients with asthma, retinal examinations for patients with diabetes, counseling for smoking cessation, and assessment of health status for senior citizens. The information systems required to monitor the delivery of these services could be coordinated with other public health surveillance activities to augment the availability of information about the incidence and prevalence of chronic conditions in the community.[34]

Second, managed care organizations are responsible for defined populations, and hence they can efficiently deliver health promotion and preventive services directly to clients and systematically encourage contracted providers.[4] However, annual turnover from one managed care plan to another is high, particularly for Medicaid populations. Consequently, there is little direct financial incentive for any individual plan to launch expensive health promotion or prevention programs that may only provide benefits far in the future when the recipients of the current services are unlikely to be clients. Nevertheless, disease prevention and early detection are usually viewed positively by the public, and managed care organizations frequently advertise the efficient provision of quality preventive services to attract new enrollees. Public health agencies can provide unique expertise to managed care plans in areas such as health promotion, surveillance and information systems, and prioritization of prevention strategies.

Activities to promote prevention of chronic disease (eg, water fluoridation and installation of walking trails in public parks) have traditionally been funded through public revenues. Such activities deserve support from managed care organizations because they effectively prevent conditions that would be expensive to treat in the medical setting. Public agencies should explore the development of partnership arrangements with the managed care organizations in their area to coordinate a community, as well as clinical, programs for preventing chronic disease in all the members of the community.[4] Such a community-based approach with a long-term perspective could benefit each of the managed care organizations because all citizens are potential clients.

Despite the promise offered in the current expansion of prevention-oriented managed care organizations, burgeoning health care costs in the United States have resulted in growing numbers of uninsured people. Approximately 15% of Americans, about 40 million people, do not have health insurance.[35] The number of uninsured persons has grown by more than 35% since 1980. Traditionally, health care insurance has been provided to workers and their families as an employment benefit. However, the proportion of working persons with employment-based health insurance coverage has decreased steadily since the late 1980s, so that in the mid-1990s, 57% of uninsured individuals are in families with an adult who works. More than 10 million persons in families earning incomes below the federal poverty level have no health insurance and do not qualify for Medicaid.[36]

Local government agencies such as health departments and public hospitals are frequently responsible for providing care to uninsured persons in the United States. The need to provide direct clinical services to growing numbers of uninsured persons will continue to present a daunting challenge to health departments and specialists in chronic disease. The increasing size of the pool of uninsured persons has the potential to actually increase the overall expenditures on health care because these persons do not have ready access to preventive services. Therefore, they are more likely to develop conditions that could require more costly, acute care interventions. General improvements in access to all health care services will be necessary if the full potential of chronic disease prevention and control is to be realized.

CURRENT CHALLENGES IN CHRONIC DISEASE CONTROL

Information on Chronic Diseases

An epidemiologic surveillance system for monitoring trends in chronic diseases is an essential part of chronic disease control. The system is needed for three key reasons: (1) to identify groups of people who are at risk of chronic disease or who experience fewer benefits from interventions; (2) to measure the effect of program interventions; and (3) to identify newly emerging chronic diseases. Reliable and geographically specific data on the burden from chronic diseases and risk factors are lacking for most communities in the United States.[33] Also, data are clearly inadequate to assess the status of many socioeconomically disadvantaged groups.[37]

Although mortality data are a major source of information for measuring the impact of chronic diseases, measures of morbidity and quality of life are more relevant for estimating the total burden from chronic diseases. Two approaches that combine the number of years of life lost from premature death with the loss of health from disease and disability are the quality-adjusted life-year (QALY), which is often used in cost-effectiveness analyses, and the disability-adjusted life-year (DALY).[38] The DALY was initially presented in the *World Development Report*, which was issued by the World Bank in 1993.[39] Both of these measures express disability as a proportion of healthy life-years, based on the severity and duration of non-fatal health conditions. A detailed analysis using the DALY found that 50% of the burden of disease in developed countries such as the United States arises from the disabilities associated with predominantly non-fatal conditions (eg, arthritis) and that 75% of this disability burden results from chronic diseases.[40] Traditionally, many health care priorities have been developed only on the basis of diseases that cause the most deaths. These results suggest that control of chronic diseases can be optimally pursued as a high priority only when there are better measures of the incidence and prevalence of chronic diseases, their effects on independent living, their costs, and the effectiveness of control measures.

Applied Research

Applied research has provided a strong scientific base for many public health interventions. Often, the most important research issue is not the efficacy of the prevention technology itself but the effectiveness of the application of the intervention to the general population and the adaptation of the technology to population subgroups at highest risk. Research in this area reflects the need to increase the benefits that can be realized from prevention by bringing it into more widespread use in the community and in the health care system. Public health professionals should continue to move from developing the scientific base of prevention to implementing and evaluating public health programs for the control of chronic diseases.

Reducing Disparities in Special Populations

Death rates remain elevated among socioeconomically disadvantaged groups and some minority populations, particularly Blacks. In the United States in 1995, total mortality rates for Blacks compared to Whites were 55% higher for women and 65% higher for men in 1995.[2] An analysis of the National Health and Nutrition Examination Survey (NHANES) Epidemiologic Follow-up Study explored the strength of the relationship between income and mortality for both Blacks and Whites.[41] The investigators found that the proportion of total mortality attributable to poverty for black men and women were 38% and 27%, respectively. The proportion of total mortality attributable to poverty for White men and women were 19%

and 11%, respectively. Another analysis of the same data revealed that 38% of the excess mortality for Blacks could be accounted for by differences in family income, and another 31% of the difference was explained by well-established risk factors, such as smoking, high cholesterol levels, and physical inactivity.[42]

The association between poverty and higher rates of morbidity, disability, and mortality has been observed since the 12th century. Possible explanations for these higher rates include not only the disproportionate burden of established risk factors associated with poverty but also a constellation of conditions, such as inadequate or crowded housing, poor education, substandard medical care, and exposure to a hazardous environment. In the United States, the additional legacy of racial discrimination further exacerbates the disparities in social status and health for minorities.[43] In disadvantaged populations, increased susceptibility to diseases may also result from stressful life events, social and cultural changes, and behaviors that have been adopted to cope with stress.[44] For example, several studies have shown that elevated blood pressure is associated with experiences of racial discrimination.[45] In addition, members of racial minorities and persons with lower socioeconomic status appear to receive less intensive medical care, even when there is equivalent financing for services, such as in the Medicare system.[46]

Social and Health Policies

Increasing evidence indicates that individual behaviors affect a person's risk of developing chronic diseases. People must assume greater responsibility for their health, but it is important that supportive social norms and health policies facilitate healthy behaviors. Reinforcing messages from many sources must be available, and their implementation should address a broad range of health issues. For example, strong laws to control smoking in public places and regulations to require adequate food labeling may help in prevention efforts directed at a variety of diseases. An excellent example of the synergistic effect of health policies with health promotion campaigns has been the implementation of the California Tobacco Tax and Health Promotion Act.[47] This legislation combined a $0.25 increase in the tax assessment on each pack of cigarettes sold in the state of California with a requirement that 20% of the revenues from the tax be used for health education programs to reduce tobacco use. A statistical time-trend analysis indicated that the tax and the educational campaign each independently contributed to a total reduction in cigarette sales of 1 billion packs of cigarettes from 1990 through 1992. About 80% of this reduction was attributed to the increase in the tax assessment. (More details on the potential of coordinating social and legal policy with health promotion messages to prevent chronic diseases are presented in Chapter 4.)

Communication of Health Risk

Mobilizing support for policies designed to prevent chronic disease and disability will require accurate communication of health risks and the benefits of healthy behaviors. The perceived threat from a health risk may be exaggerated when exposure to the risk is considered involuntary, as in environmental exposure to hazardous wastes; when effects of the risk are unknown or unfamiliar; or when exposure to the risk is associated with dramatic and immediate consequences, as in an airplane crash. Often, this tendency to exaggerate a risk is aided by intense media coverage of the event. Unfortunately, the reverse is true for voluntary or familiar exposures and those that have delayed or long-term consequences. For example, the health risk associated with smoking is underestimated by society because (1) smoking tobacco is considered to be an individual's choice, (2) it has been an accepted social behavior, and (3) it leads to disease only after years of exposure.

Disability as a Consequence of Chronic Disease

Effective interventions need to be developed to reduce the prevalence of disability and to help people with disabilities to adapt and become self-sufficient. Disability is defined as a limiting health condition that interferes with the performance of socially defined activities and roles such as work.[49] Disability results from the complex interaction be-

tween the level of impairment or actual anatomically determined functional limitation and a person's expected roles and tasks in the social environment. In the United States in 1994, more than 39 million people reported a limitation in activity due to a chronic condition (Table 1.5).[49] Limitations in activity are more common among older adults, women, and persons in low-income groups. With the aging of the

Table 1.5—Distribution of Activity Limitation Due to Chronic Conditions, United States, 1994

Category	With Activity Limitation[a]		With Limitation in Major Activity[b]	
	Number, thousands	%	Number, thousands	%
All persons	39 059	15.0	26 796	10.3
Age group				
Under 18	4 711	6.7	3 448	4.9
18-44	11 094	10.3	7 708	7.1
45-64	11 407	22.6	8 628	17.1
65 and over	11 847	38.2	7 013	22.6
Sex				
Male	18 206	14.4	12 811	10.1
Female	20 853	15.7	13 985	10.5
Family income				
Under $10 000	6 544	28.0	4 924	21.1
$10 000-$19 999	7 877	21.1	5 573	15.0
$20 000-$34 999	8 007	14.8	5 465	10.1
$35 000 and over	9 448	9.4	5 806	5.8

[a] Includes major activities such as working, keeping house, going to school, or living independently, and other activities such as civic, church, or recreational activities.
[b] Includes major activities such as working, keeping house, going to school, or living independently.
Note: Data compiled from Adams and Marano.[49]

population and the increase in the prevalence of disability with age, chronic disease control will become more important.[50]

High-Risk and Population-Based Approaches

Interventions for chronic disease control can be divided into those targeted to high-risk populations and those targeted to the general population. A general population-based approach has several advantages. The common risk factors for chronic diseases are usually present in a large proportion of the population. Most of the cases of chronic disease arise from the intermediate- and low-risk groups, and, therefore, small changes in risk in the intermediate-risk group will result in a greater overall disease reduction than will greater changes in the high-risk group.[51] Furthermore, changing the behavior of an entire population through social marketing and reinforcing social norms often is easier than changing the behavior of a high-risk population. A targeted high-risk approach requires the correct classification of people at high risk. The efficiency of this approach depends on the cost of identifying the high-risk group and the effectiveness of the intervention.

An intervention to reduce cholesterol levels illustrates the differences between population-based and high-risk approaches. During the period 1988 to1991, the mean cholesterol level for adults (ages 20 to 74 years) in the United States was 205 mg/dL. Cholesterol levels were high ($\geq$240 mg/dL) in 20% of this population, and 31% of the population had a borderline-high level (200–239 mg/dL). The objective in the population-based cholesterol program is to reduce the mean cholesterol level by decreasing the cholesterol levels of all people, including those with normal, moderate, and high levels. The population-based approach supports individuals' efforts to change their diets by increasing their knowledge and skills and by changing their environment. This effort is accomplished by providing nutrition information, labeling foods, developing healthier food products, creating a social context of positive reinforcement and by encouraging changes in food preparation in restaurants and by food services. In contrast, a high-risk approach attempts to reduce cholesterol levels only in those persons who have elevated cholesterol.[52]

In practice, population-based and high-risk approaches are often combined. People in the population at large are encouraged to reduce their level of risk, and those in the high-risk population receive a more intensive intervention through the traditional medical care system. Often, the community milieu created by the population-based intervention will help those at high risk to initiate and maintain behavioral changes. Major challenges for chronic disease control specialists are to develop better tools for identifying those at high risk and to develop population-specific interventions that can be integrated into a comprehensive, population-based program. For directors of population-based programs, the challenge is to harness the energies and interests of the many community organizations whose policies can affect the health decisions of the community. Interventions must include consistent, reinforcing messages in both the health care setting and nontraditional settings, such as schools, community organizations, and work sites.

Genetic Testing

During the last decade, advancement in the ability of medical science to diagnose inherited diseases has been unprecedented, and the Human Genome Project, which has the goal of mapping the entire human genetic sequence, will further accelerate the availability of numerous tests aimed at identifying specific genes and their function. Many chronic diseases appear to have both genetic and environmental risk factors (eg, hypertension, atherosclerosis, and breast cancer). Genetic tests can identify people who may be susceptible to development of many of these conditions. In some

genetic disorders, a single-point mutation can confer life-threatening consequences (eg, sickle cell anemia or cystic fibrosis), but the interpretation of the newer tests is very complex and requires integration of data from multiple sources. Although many of these discoveries have the ultimate goal of facilitating prevention, accurate diagnosis, and effective treatment, there is limited knowledge about how most of the results should be used in the context of current public health practice.[5]

In the near future, the public health impact of any particular genetic test will probably be limited compared with those of population-based health promotion programs. Current information suggests that the proportion of burden associated with any chronic disease attributable to a specific gene function is limited. However, the long-term potential for this technology is profound. The identification of increased susceptibility to chronic diseases through genetic testing has the potential to affect virtually everyone and can improve the efficiency of preventive measures by facilitating the targeting of interventions. Additionally, the ability to track high-risk genetic patterns through families raises issues analogous to the classic public health activity of tracing contacts to persons with infectious diseases such as tuberculosis, infection with the human immunodeficiency virus, or sexually transmitted diseases. On the basis of their experience with these disease control programs, public health officials clearly have much to offer in the development of policies on issues such as the confidentiality of test results and the potential for difficulties in obtaining employment and insurance for those with a high risk for developing conditions that are costly to treat.[53]

FUTURE DIRECTIONS

The changing demographic profile of the United States population has already begun to transform the private and public health care systems. Population projections for the United States indicate that the proportion of persons 65 years of age and older will increase from 12% in 1995 to more than 20% by the year 2050.[54] The proportion of persons aged 35 through 64 years will increase until the year 2015 and then will begin a steady decline. Both the prevalence of chronic conditions and associated restrictions of activity increase with age (Table 1.5). Older adults and persons with chronic diseases also use the medical care system more often than others and account for a disproportionate share of health care costs.[26] In addition, the relative proportions of minority groups, who experience a disproportionate share of the burden of chronic disease because of

poverty and discrimination, are increasing in many areas. These demographic trends are fundamentally unalterable. However, appropriate responses to these forces will require continuing dynamism in the health care delivery system and new strategies for preventing chronic diseases and disabilities in older adults and among the poor. These efforts should be enhanced by comprehensive, evidence-based *Guidelines for Community Preventive Services*, currently under development.[55]

A better understanding of the psychological and social factors that affect behavior and of the relationship between behavior and chronic disease is necessary if the public health system is to fulfill its new role. The exploding cost of acute care medical services has prompted rapid transformation in the structure of financing and the delivery of medical services. During this transition the number of persons without health care insurance coverage has increased. However, the cost-saving potential of chronic disease control and health promotion can only be realized if disease prevention is established as a major priority and access to medical and preventive health services is made widely available.[11]

Current preventive strategies have targeted diseases and risk factors that cause the greatest mortality, and successful programs have resulted in increased life expectancy. Additional preventive strategies that incorporate considerations of patient satisfaction, as well as emerging technologies such as genetic testing, need to be developed to reduce disability and improve the quality of life associated with chronic diseases and aging. Measures of morbidity and quality of life such as QALYs and DALYs will serve as important outcomes for programs that address chronic disease control and the prevention of disabilities.[38]

Our current level of knowledge about chronic diseases and their risk factors is sufficient to significantly reduce morbidity and mortality. This book outlines that knowledge and challenges the public and private health system to control chronic diseases in the United States.

REFERENCES

1. National Center for Health Statistics. Births and Deaths: United States, 1995. *Month Vital Stat Rep.* 1996; vol 45(3) (suppl 2). DHHS publication 96-1120; October 4, 1996.

2. National Office of Vital Statistics. *Vital Statistics—Special Reports, National Summaries, 1950.* Washington, DC: US Dept of Health, Education & Welfare; 1954.

3. Committee for the Study of the Future of Public Health. *The Future of Public Health.* Washington, DC: National Academy Press; 1988.

4. Centers for Disease Control and Prevention. Prevention and managed care: opportunities for managed care organizations, purchasers of health care, and public health agencies. *MMWR* 1995;44(No. RR-14):1–12.

5. Khoury MJ etal. From genes to public health: the applications of genetic technology in disease prevention. *Am J Public Health.* 1996;86:1717–1722.

6. Wallace RB, Everett GD. Prevention of chronic illness. In: Last JM, Wallace RB, eds. *Maxcy-Rosenau-Last Textbook of Public Health and Preventive Medicine.* 13th ed. Norwalk, Conn: Appleton & Lange; 1992: 805–810.

7. Primer on allergic and immunologic diseases—3rd ed. *JAMA.* 1992;268:2785–2996 (entire issue).

8. Doll R. Preventive medicine: the objectives. In: *The Value of Preventive Medicine. Proceedings from the Ciba Foundation Symposium.* London: Pitman; 1985:3–21.

9. Verbrugge LM. Recent, present, and future health of American adults. *Ann Rev Public Health.* 1989;10:333–361.

10. Fries JF. Aging, natural death, and the compression of morbid-

ity. *N Engl J Med.* 1980;303:130–135.

11. Fries JF, Koop CE, Beadle CE, et al. Reducing health care costs by reducing the need and demand for medical services. *N Engl J Med.* 1996;329:321–325.

12. Tolsma DD, Koplan JP. Health behaviors and health promotion. In: Last JM, Wallace RB, eds. *Maxcy–Rosenau–Last Textbook of Public Health and Preventive Medicine.* 13th ed. Norwalk, Conn: Appleton & Lange; 1992:701–714.

13. Berkelman RL, Buehler JW. Public health surveillance of non-infectious chronic diseases: the potential to detect rapid changes in disease burden. *Int J Epidemiol.* 1990;19:628–635.

14. Ockene JK, Kuller LH, Svendsen KH. Meilahn E. The relationship of smoking cessation to coronary heart disease and lung cancer in the Multiple Risk Factor Intervention Trial (MRFIT). *Am J Public Health.* 1990;80:954–958.

15. Centers for Disease Control. *Positioning for Prevention: An Analytical Framework and Background Document for Chronic Disease Activities.* Atlanta, Ga: US Dept of Health and Human Services; 1986.

16. Last JM, ed. *A Dictionary of Epidemiology.* 3rd ed. New York, NY: Oxford University Press; 1995:130.

17. McGinnis JM, Foege WH. Actual causes of death in the United States. *JAMA.* 1993;270:2207–2212.

18. Kottke TE, Battista RN, DeFriese GH, et al. Attributes of successful smoking cessation interventions in medical practice: a meta-analysis of 39 controlled trials. *JAMA.* 1988;259:2882–2889.

19. Tengs TO, Adams ME, Pliskin JS et al. Five-hundred life-saving interventions and their cost-effectiveness. Risk Analysis. 1995;15:369–390.

20. Office of the Assistant Secretary for Health and the Surgeon General. *Healthy People: The Surgeon General's Report on Health Promotion and Disease Prevention.* Washington, DC: US Dept of Health, Education & Welfare; 1979. DHEW publication PHS 79-55071.

21. Hunink MGM, Goldman L, Tosteson ANA, et al. The recent decline in mortality from coronary heart disease, 1980–1990: the effect of secular trends in risk factors and treatment. *JAMA* 1997;277:535–542.

22. Breslow L, Somers AR. The lifetime health-monitoring program, a practical approach to preventive medicine. *N Engl J Med.* 1977;296:601-608.

23. U.S. Preventive Services Task Force. *Guide to Clinical Preventive Services,* 2nd ed. Baltimore, Md: Williams and Wilkins; 1996.

24. Woolf SH, Jonas S, Lawrence RS. *Health Promotion and Disease Prevention in Clinical Practice.* Baltimore, Md: Williams and Wilkins; 1996.

25. Congressional Budget Office. *The Economic Budget Outlook, 1998–2007.* Washingtion, DC: US Govt Printing Office, 1997:126.

26. Hoffman C, Rice D, Sung HY. Persons with chronic conditions: their prevalence and costs. *JAMA.* 1996;276:1473–1479.

27. Berwick DM. Payment by capitation and the quality of care. *N Engl J Med.* 1995;335:1227–1231.

28. Lubitz J, Beebe J, Baker C. Longevity and medicare expenditures. *N Engl J Med.* 1995;332:999–1003.

29. Grimes D. Technology follies. *JAMA.* 1993;269:3030–3033.

30. Brook RH, Kamberg CJ, McGlynn EA. Health care reform and quality. *JAMA.* 1996;276:476–480.

31. Weissman J. Uncompensated hospital care: Will it be there if we need it? *JAMA.* 1996;276:823–828.

32. Thompson RS, Taplin SH, McAfee TA, Mandelson MT, Smith AE. Primary and secondary prevention services in clinical practice. *JAMA.* 1995;273:1130–1135.

33. National Committee for Quality Assurance. *HEDIS 3.0.* Washington, DC: National Committee for Quality Assurance; 1996.

34. Pollock AM, Rice DP. Monitoring health care in the United States— A challenging task. *Public Health Rep.*1997;112:108–110.

35. Rovner J. The health care system evolves. *Lancet.* 1996;348:1001–1002.

36. Fronstin P. The decline in health insurance and labor market trends. Stat Bull Metropol Insurance Co. 1996;77:28–36.

37. Lee PR, Moss N, Krieger N. Measuring social inequalities in health. *Public Health Rep.* 1995:302–305.

38. Goerdt A, Koplan JP, Robine JM, Thuriaux MC, Van Ginneken. Non-fatal health outcomes: concepts, instruments and indicators. In: Murray CJL, Lopez AD, eds. *The Global Burden of Disease.* Cambridge, Ma: Harvard University Press; 1996:99–116.

39. The World Bank. *World Development Report 1993: Investing in Health.* New York, NY: Oxford University Press; 1993.

40. Murray CJL, Lopez AD. Global and regional descriptive epidemiology of disability: incidence, prevalence, health expectancies and years lived with disability. In: Murray CJL, Lopez AD, eds. *The Global Burden of Disease.* Cambridge, Ma: Harvard Univ Press; 1996:201–246.

41. Hahn RA, Eaker E, Barker ND, Teutsch SM, Sosniak W, Krieger N. Poverty and death in the

United States-1973–1991. *Epidemiology*. 1995;6:490–497.

42. Otten MW, Teutsch SM, Williamson DF, Marks JS. The effect of known risk factors on Black adults in the United States. *JAMA*. 1990;263:845–850.

43. Geiger HJ. Race and health care —An American dilemma? *N Engl J Med*. 1996;335:815–816.

44. Geronimus AT, Bound J, Waidmann TA, Hillemeier MM, Burns P. Excess mortality among blacks and whites in the United States. *N Engl J Med*. 1996;335:1552–1558.

45. Krieger N, Sidney S. Racial discrimination and blood pressure: the CARDIA study of young black and white males. *Am J Public Health*. 1996;86:1370–1378.

46. Gornick ME, Eggers PW, Reilly TW, et al. Effects of race and income on mortality and use of services among medicare beneficiaries. *N Engl J Med*. 1996;335:791–799.

47. Hut T, Sung HY, Keeler TE. Reducing cigarette consumption in California: tobacco taxes vs. an anti-smoking media campaign. *Am J Public Health*. 1995;85:1218–1222.

48. Committee on a National Agenda for the Prevention of Disabilities. *Disability in America: Toward a National Agenda for Prevention*. Washington, DC: National Academy Press; 1991.

49. Adams PF, Marano MA. Current estimates from the National Health Interview Survey, 1994. *Vital Health Stat*. (Series 10, No.193) 1995; DHHS publication PHS 96-1521.

50. Boult C, Altmann M, Gilbertson D, Yu C, Kane RL. Decreasing disability in the 21st century: the future effects of controlling six fatal and nonfatal conditions. *Am J Public Health*. 1996;86:1388–1393.

51. Rose G. The strategy of preventive medicine. New York, NY: Oxford University Press; 1992.

52. Expert Panel on Detection, Evaluation, and Treatment of High Blood Cholesterol in Adults. Summary of the second report of the National Cholesterol Education Program expert panel on detection, evaluation, and treatment of high blood cholesterol in adults. *JAMA*. 1993;269:3015–3023.

53. Pokorski RJ. Genetic information and insurance. *Nature*. 1995;376:13–14.

54. Day JC. Projections of the population of the United States, by age, sex, and race: 1995 to 2050. In: *US Bureau of the Census Current Population Reports*. Series P-25, No. 1130. Washington, DC: US Govt Printing Office; 1996.

55. Pappaioanou M, Evans C. Developing a guide to commu-

nity preventive services: a U.S. Public Health Service initiative. *J Public Health Manag Pract* 1998;4:48–54.

SUGGESTED READING

Centers for Disease Control. *Chronic Disease in Minority Populations.* Atlanta, Ga: US Dept of Health and Human Services, Public Health Service, 1994.

U.S. Preventive Services Task Force. *Guide to Clinical Preventive Services,* 2nd ed. Baltimore, Md: Williams and Wilkins; 1996.

Rose G. *The Strategy of Preventive Medicine.* New York, NY: Oxford University Press; 1992.

Rothenberg RB, Koplan JP. Chronic disease in the 1990s. *Annu Rev Public Health.* 1990;11:267–296.

Woolf SH, Jonas S, Lawrence RS. *Health Promotion and Disease Prevention in Clinical Practice.* Baltimore, Md: Williams and Wilkins; 1996.

2

METHODS IN CHRONIC DISEASE EPIDEMIOLOGY

The methods used to identify the causes of chronic disease have evolved markedly over the past 20 years, particularly in the areas of epidemiologic concepts and quantitative methods,[1] statistical methods,[2] case-control studies,[3] and clinical epidemiology.[4,5] The increasing complexity of methods in chronic disease epidemiology and biostatistics has made it more challenging for public health practitioners to conduct and interpret ongoing research.

In this chapter, we describe the basic concepts of chronic disease epidemiology in order to help practitioners to improve their communication with researchers and to apply their epidemiologic knowledge more effectively in the populations they serve. Some of the concepts in this chapter also lay the foundation for later chapters.

David A. Savitz, PhD
Russell P. Harris, MD, MPH
Ross C. Brownson, PhD

This chapter is not designed as a substitute for more detailed presentations of epidemiologic principles. Readers interested in a more comprehensive presentation of methods in chronic disease epidemiology are referred to Hennekens and Buring,[6] Kelsey et al,[7] Lilienfeld and Stolley,[8] and Gordis.[9]

THE SCOPE OF METHODS IN CHRONIC DISEASE EPIDEMIOLOGY

For diseases of known infectious origin, such as AIDS, measles, and influenza, the presence of a single, known, necessary cause (eg, the microorganism) helps to focus epidemiologic research and intervention strategies. In contrast, the wide variety of chronic diseases lack such unifying causal agents (see also the discussion in Chapter 1). As a result, the methods of study and, ultimately, the methods of disease control differ between infectious and chronic diseases.

The persistence of chronic diseases also influences the methods of epidemiologic study. Because the causal process is prolonged and typically complex, many modest influences, rather than a single predominant cause, often affect the probability of developing disease. The prolonged duration of these diseases, which often includes a presymptomatic phase, provides numerous overlapping opportunities for intervention. For most chronic diseases, the large number of modest risk factors and the diverse opportunities for intervention make their control difficult and typically require a multifaceted approach.

Because disease is the end result of a continuum, it is sometimes difficult to determine whether "disease" is even present at all. For example, the large increase in mammography over the late 1980s and 1990s has led to a large increase in the incidence of a pathologic lesion known as "ductal carcinoma in situ" (DCIS). Although DCIS is not invasive breast cancer, and although probably no more than 50% of women with DCIS will develop invasive breast cancer, DCIS is often treated the same way as invasive cancer, that is, by mastectomy. Many women with DCIS consider themselves to have "breast cancer." Similarly, many men with "prostate cancer" actually have a pathologic lesion that would never have pro-

gressed to clinical disease. In general, as our ability to detect earlier and earlier stages of the disease process improves, the point at which disease truly begins becomes increasingly unclear.[10]

Another important consideration for chronic disease is the meaning of "control" or what it is we are trying to prevent. Chronic disease often affects the quality of life long before it affects the duration of life, if it affects duration at all. People with diabetes, for example, do have higher mortality, but only many years after diagnosis. In the interim, however, they may suffer blindness, kidney failure, painful feet ulcers, leg amputation, or premature heart disease, all as a direct result of having diabetes. Thus, "controlling" diabetes implies not only decreasing mortality from this disease but also decreasing the detrimental effects on quality of life that occur rather than focusing solely on prolonging life. Both disease-specific and general measures of quality of life have been developed and validated,[11] and these measures are being used increasingly to describe the course ("natural history") of disease as well as the effect of various methods of control.

There is a need to pay careful attention to methodologic principles in many areas of the study and control of chronic disease. The need for clarity of terminology and thought is enhanced by the advancements that have been made and the expansion of options for tackling chronic disease through public health measures. In this chapter, we provide some basic terms and concepts common in epidemiologic literature on the etiology (ie, causes) and control of chronic diseases.

AN ILLUSTRATION: BREAST CANCER ETIOLOGY AND CONTROL

To understand methodologic principles, it may be useful to view them from the perspective of a particular goal. Assume that as a public health professional, you are responsible for chronic disease control in a defined population, such as a county or state. Your concern is with breast cancer, a common and life-threatening disease. Furthermore, assume that you have been mandated to describe the patterns of breast cancer occurrence in your region, to identify opportunities for control, and to recommend a strategy for public health programs. You should ask a series of questions, which would apply to a large extent to many other chronic diseases.

1. How much breast cancer is occurring?

This is addressed through measures of disease occurrence: incidence rate, cumulative incidence, and prevalence. Both incidence rate and cumulative incidence indicate the risk of newly acquiring the

disease, whereas prevalence is the number of people who have the disease at a point in time. Mortality rates are often used when incidence rates are unavailable.

2. How does the occurrence of disease vary within your population?

This question is addressed by comparing the risk or incidence of disease among people within the population who have some characteristic (eg, older age) with those who do not have the characteristic. To do this, we use measures of association—rate ratio or risk ratio (ie, relative risk)—and difference measures.

3. How does the burden of breast cancer in your area compare with that in other areas?

In calculating statistics that quantify the disease burden in your area and in other areas, consider the potential for distortion due to such factors as differing age, sex, and race in your population. To avoid distortion, you may need to divide measures of disease occurrence into categories to make them age-, sex-, or race-specific, or standardize them to make the populations comparable.

4. What types of investigations are done to study the etiology and control of breast cancer?

The structure and logic of prospective cohort, case-control, historical cohort, and intervention studies are critical to evaluating the quality of evidence they provide.

5. How do we evaluate whether the study results are valid?

Validity implies the absence of bias—that is, systematic errors that result in incorrect conclusions about associations. The extent to which studies are demonstrably free of bias lends credibility to their results and conclusions. Three biases are commonly considered: (1) confounding, in which other contributors to disease are mixed with the one of interest; (2) selection bias, in which the subjects who are enrolled in the study give a distorted measure of the association; and (3) information bias, in which errors in classification of subjects bias the study results.

6. How do we assess whether associations between potential etiologic factors and breast cancer are causal?

Well-known criteria for causality can be used, but, ultimately, subjective judgments must be made.

7. How much morbidity and mortality might be prevented by interventions?

Although interventions such as education and screening programs often seem valuable, many have little effect on the number of people who suffer from the disease. Therefore, we need to evaluate the effects of intervention programs and use those results to design new and better programs for controlling chronic diseases. Even when there are strong theoretical reasons to expect benefit,

a determination is needed that the intervention reduces mortality or improves quality of life when applied in a real setting. Every intervention, even those that reduce the burden of disease, have a "down side" both through undesired consequences and by consuming resources. Calculating the proportion of a disease that is attributable to a particular risk factor may help to quantify the effect of its reduction or elimination (ie, the population attributable risk).

8. Why should action not be taken on the basis of an individual epidemiologic study?

In this era in which public and media interest in epidemiology is intense, the reasons for not taking action based on an individual epidemiologic study, even if carefully designed, successfully conducted, and properly analyzed and interpreted, need to be emphasized. Obviously, such studies contribute, in some cases very substantially, to providing the basis for public health decisions, but individual studies do not constitute a strong basis for action.

9. How do we assess a series of epidemiologic studies and integrate the evidence to make decisions?

Since a single study is fallible, a series of related studies must provide the necessary evidence for decision makers. Having several studies with the same result, especially if they are well-done randomized controlled trials, bolsters this evidence. Such methods as meta-analysis, which quantify a set of study results, are sometimes useful to help answer this question. Expert panels may be established to evaluate risks and benefits of alternative policies, but recommendations made through this process also need to be critically evaluated.[12,13] Careful evaluation of epidemiologic research findings is required to fully appreciate the social, economic, and health consequences of clinical and public health policy decisions.

In the remainder of this chapter, we will examine these questions in greater detail, using breast cancer and other examples to illustrate methodology.

1. How much disease is occurring?

Several measures are used to quantify the magnitude of disease occurrence, each one valid for a slightly different purpose. *Incidence* (or incidence rate) refers to the number of new cases over a defined time period divided by the "person-time experience of the population"— that is, the number of persons multiplied by the period over which they were monitored; this is often called "person-years." However, in practice, the incidence rate is typically used to describe the number of new cases that develop in a year in a specified population.[7] For

example, if 500 women develop breast cancer in a year in a population of 342 000, the incidence rate would be 146 per 100 000 population. For many chronic diseases, such as coronary heart disease and diabetes, mortality rates are calculated because incidence data are unavailable.

Cumulative incidence is defined as the probability or risk of developing a disease over a defined time period. It ranges from 0 to 1 and indicates the probability that the disease will develop in a population that is monitored over a set period. For example, according to 1988 to 1990 data from the National Cancer Institute,[14] a woman's lifetime risk of developing breast cancer is 0.122, or about 1 in 8. Thus, we can estimate that a girl born today has a 12.2% chance of eventually being diagnosed with breast cancer, although such estimates ignore any competing causes of mortality and are based on the somewhat unrealistic assumption that the present incidence rates will persist over time.

Prevalence also is measured as a proportion—that is, existing cases of disease divided by total population— but the occurrence of disease is measured at a point in time rather than over some interval. At the time of a disease survey, prevalence is defined as the number of existing cases divided by the population count. The prevalence of disease is influenced by the incidence (more new cases yield more existent cases) and persistence of the disease (rapid recovery or rapid death reduces the number of affected individuals at any point in time). For breast cancer, for example, the prevalence greatly exceeds the annual incidence, because most women diagnosed with breast cancer survive for at least 5 years.

Because it is influenced by survival and recovery, prevalence is less valuable than incidence for identifying etiologic factors. For assessing public health needs, however, prevalence may be exactly the measure of interest. For example, women diagnosed with breast cancer are at higher risk of a second breast cancer. Therefore, a prevalence estimate of the number of breast cancer survivors in a given area may be useful in targeting limited public health resources to women in high-risk groups.

2. How does the occurrence of disease vary within the population?

Data from the Surveillance, Epidemiology, and End Results (SEER) program of the National Cancer Institute provide breast cancer incidence rates for women of various ages. From 1987 to 1991, for example, the incidence rate for women aged 30 through 34 years was 25.6 cases per 100 000 person-years.[15] The comparable incidence

rate for women aged 70 through 74 years was 450.3 cases per 100 000 person-years. Having determined the incidence rate in each of the two groups we wish to compare, our next challenge is to determine how that comparison should be summarized.

The ratio of the incidence rate in one group to that in another is referred to as a *rate ratio*. Likewise, the ratio of the cumulative incidence or risk in two groups is termed the *risk ratio* or *relative risk*. Considering the incidence rate in younger women as the reference, we can calculate the rate ratio for women aged 70 through 74 compared with women aged 30 through 34 as 450.3/25.6 = 17.6. Thus, we can say that women in the older age group have an incidence rate 17.6 times that in the younger age group: Breast cancer is predominantly a disease of older women.

One advantage of such ratio measures is the ease of intuitive understanding (ie, disease occurrence is increased over 15-fold among the elderly). Also, this ratio is independent of the absolute incidence rates in the two groups and therefore is directly interpretable: There is a strong association between age and breast cancer. Diseases that differ greatly in frequency can be discussed in similar terms: For example, cigarette smoking increases the risk of lung cancer in women approximately 11-fold and approximately doubles the risk of coronary heart disease in women (Table 2.1).

An alternative to the ratio measure is the *rate difference*, calculated by subtracting the rates from one another. For example, the rate difference between women aged 70 through 74 and women aged 30 through 34 is calculated as follows: 450.3 - 25.6 = 424.7 cases per 100 000 person-years. This difference indicates how much, in absolute rather than relative terms, the disease rates differ in these populations. The advantage of this measure is that the actual amount by which the disease has increased in one group as opposed to another has public health importance beyond the ratio of the two rates. For example, a doubling or even tripling of the incidence or mortality rate may not indicate an important public health problem if the baseline rate is extremely low. The increment in disease burden from doubling a very

small number would be a very small number. The difference in incidence rates, however, provides direct information about the public health effects of a particular exposure. A large difference indicates an important problem, regardless of the size of the baseline rate.

As shown in Table 2.1, the relative risk due to smoking is much greater for lung cancer than for coronary heart disease. However, the rate difference for heart disease (the rate in smokers minus the rate in nonsmokers) for the period 1982 through 1986 is actually greater than the rate difference for lung cancer, because the baseline mortality rate of heart disease is so much greater than that for lung cancer. The public health impact due to increasing heart disease risk twofold is similar to the impact of increasing lung cancer risk 10-fold. Both ratio and difference measures contribute to our understanding of the effect of an exposure on disease occurrence, and both measures should be examined when the data permit.

Table 2.1—Smoking-Related Rate Ratio (Relative Risk) and Rate Difference Estimates for Coronary Heart Disease and Lung Cancer Among Women, United States, 1982–1986[a]

| Disease | Mortality Rate | | Rate Ratio (a/b) | Rate Difference (a - b) |
	Smokers (a)	Nonsmokers (b)		
Lung cancer	131	11	11.9	120
Coronary heart disease	275	153	1.8	122

[a]*Note*: Based on prospective study data from the American Cancer Society's Cancer Prevention Study II.

3. How does the burden of disease in one area compare with that in other areas?

Many local, state, and federal health agencies now calculate incidence rates for various conditions. Likewise, mortality rates (which can be viewed as incidence rates of death) are also published, often for such geographic areas as counties or cities. Public health officials have a natural interest in comparing incidence or mortality rates from other areas with their own to determine which areas have a greater problem.

Although such comparisons are important and sometimes revealing, two potential problems should be kept in mind. The first is the problem of precision: How statistically precise is the calculation of an incidence rate? When rates are calculated for small areas such as a county, the numerator of the incidence rate will be small (for most counties). If only a few cases are detected a year early or a year late, the incidence rate calculated for a particular year may appear much higher or much lower than it is on average over a longer period.

For example, the *incidence rate* for breast cancer calculated from SEER data for 1987 through 1991 is 110 new cases per 100 000 women.[15] A county with 25 000 women would be expected to have about 27 new cases each year (27/25 000 = 110 cases per 100 000). If only four cases were diagnosed too late to be counted for a particular year, the rate would decrease to 23 cases that year (23/25 000 = 92 cases/100 000), yielding an incidence rate ratio of 92/110 or 0.84. If only six cases from the next year were diagnosed a bit early, the rate would appear to increase dramatically to 33 cases per year (33/25 000 = 132 cases/100 000 women), for an incidence rate ratio of 1.20 and an apparent 20% increase in breast cancer incidence.

Thus, rates calculated from cases diagnosed in a single year from an area with a small population are subject to a large amount of variation from year to year and are said to be imprecise. For this reason, one should calculate rates from cases diagnosed over several years to increase the number of cases in the numerator of the incidence rate, thereby increasing the precision of the calculated rate (eg, the SEER rate given above was calculated from cases diagnosed over a 5-year period).

The second major problem with comparing incidence rates among several areas is the comparability of their overall populations. As we have shown earlier, older women have a much higher incidence rate of breast cancer than do younger women, and we can expect a county with more older women to have a higher overall incidence rate of breast cancer than a county with more young women. Yet there would be no special "exposure" (in the sense of some exogenous agent) causing the increased occurrence of breast cancer. How then could we compare the rates in one area with those in another area, accounting for the differing ages, to determine whether some other factors are influencing the rate of breast cancer?

We have two options. First, *age-specific rates* can be calculated. That is, incidence rates may be given only for people in a specific age range. If the incidence rate of breast cancer for women aged 50 through 59 years is much greater in one area than in another, the difference could not have been caused by differences in age distributions between the two groups. A drawback with such calculations is that the problem of precision may be worsened: Fewer cases are diagnosed (therefore, the numerator for the incidence rate is smaller) in a narrow age range than in the entire population. Such age-specific calculations typically require cases diagnosed over longer time periods or from larger populations.

A second way to ease comparison of incidence rates is to adjust the rate to a standard population. This, in effect, combines many age-specific rates into a single *age-adjusted rate*. For example, the breast cancer incidence rate given in the previous example (110 cases per 100 000

women) is age-adjusted to the 1970 US standard population. This means that statistical adjustments were made to the initial calculations to provide the rate that would be expected in the area's population if it had the same age distribution as did the US population in 1970. Rates adjusted to the same standard population can be compared directly: They refer to rates calculated for populations with the same age structure.

4. What types of investigations are done to study disease etiology and control?

Randomized controlled trials (RCT) are considered the most scientifically rigorous type of epidemiologic study. In an RCT, subjects are randomly assigned to either receive or not receive a preventive or therapeutic procedure, such as a clinical smoking cessation intervention or a new drug. The disease course or mortality patterns are then followed over time to assess the effectiveness of the preventive or therapeutic procedure. It is through such RCTs that we have learned of the benefit of screening for breast cancer in women aged 50 years and older.[16]

In contrast to RCTs, which are considered experimental studies, epidemiologists commonly rely on observational studies. In observational studies, the risk factor or disease process is allowed to take its course without intervention from the researcher.

The observational study that is closest to an experiment is the *prospective cohort design*. In this approach, exposed and unexposed subjects are identified and then observed over time for the development of disease. Unlike a true experiment, however, the exposures are observed rather than randomly assigned. Exposures are implicitly "assigned" based on physician recommendations (eg, x-ray use), genetic heritage (eg, family history of breast cancer), or individual behavior (eg, dietary fat intake). Having obtained measures of disease occurrence (incidence rates or cumulative incidence) for both exposed and unexposed groups, the influence of exposure can be quantified as either the ratio of exposed to unexposed (the relative risk) or the difference between exposed and unexposed (the rate difference) as discussed on pages 32–33.

The primary advantage of a true prospective study over other observational designs is the opportunity to actively and intensively measure the exposures of interest prior to the period of disease induction. For example, instead of having subjects recall dietary fat intake over many years, intake could be calculated more accurately if periodic direct measurements were made. For rare diseases and those with a prolonged period between exposure and the manifestation of adverse effects (typical of chronic diseases), however, true prospective studies must be extremely large and prolonged and, therefore, are very expensive.

One way to overcome these problems is to study exposures that occurred in the past and to monitor disease either up to the present or into the future. The ability to conduct these *historical cohort studies* depends on the availability of exposure records that can be linked to disease outcomes. For example, in a study of the effect of radiation exposure used to treat mastitis and the subsequent rate of breast cancer occurrence, Shore and colleagues[17] were able to identify a roster of exposed and unexposed subjects through medical records. When no adequate exposure records exist, investigators have no alternative but to gather the data themselves.

Another design selects study subjects on the basis of their health outcomes; this design intentionally oversamples subjects who have developed the disease of interest. In these *case-control studies*, researchers identify a sample of subjects with the disease, or case patients (often, all available case patients), and a sample of people without the disease (control subjects) from the same population that yielded the case patients. The historical exposures that may have influenced disease risk are ascertained for all subjects, and the frequency of exposure among case patients is compared with that among control subjects. Such studies cannot yield incidence rates or cumulative incidence, because the population at risk is not comprehensively defined; the control subjects are typically a sample of that source population, but the sampling fraction is unknown. An estimate of the ratio of incidence rates or risks can be obtained, however, by calculating the ratio of the odds of exposure among cases (the number exposed divided by the number not exposed) to the odds of exposure among controls, referred to as the *odds ratio*. The odds ratio is intended to approximate the relative risk. No estimate of the risk difference can be obtained from a case-control study.

The obvious advantages of case-control studies are the relative speed with which they can be conducted, because the latent period is all in the past, and the small number of subjects who have to be enrolled. In contrast to a cohort study, in which many subjects who never develop the disease must be monitored, a case-control study includes only a small but adequate fraction of the nondiseased population. The principal weakness is the study's vulnerability to some forms of bias that arise from the fact that the disease has usually occurred before risk factor information was ascertained.

The strengths and limitations of prospective and case-control studies are summarized in Table 2.2.

Disease control strategies are often tested in "quasi-experimental intervention studies," in which a program (eg, education program, screening program, new treatment regimen) is systematically offered to a population and the effect on health is measured. One key objective of such a study is to draw specific conclusions about the intervention. If the health of the population receiving the intervention improves, the investigators must demonstrate that a similar population that did not receive the intervention did not improve. This implies that to clearly interpret the results, such studies require comparison groups, which, unfortunately, are often lacking.

Comparison groups vary in their appropriateness for disease intervention studies. Least convincing are comparisons with national data or populations in other studies. Previous data on the same population are most appropriate if the disease can be shown to have been stable for a long period and if there are no other reasons for a change in disease incidence. The best control groups are those that can be shown to be similar to the intervention population and from which disease information is collected concurrently.

Despite certain limitations, quasi-experimental studies, such as some

Table 2.2—Summary of Strengths and Limitations of Prospective Cohort and Case-Control Studies

Study Type	Strengths	Limitations
Prospective cohort	Opportunity to measure risk factors before disease occurs Can study multiple disease outcomes Can yield incidence rates as well as relative risk estimates	Often expensive Requires large number of subjects Requires long follow-up period
Case-control	Useful for rare diseases Relatively inexpensive Relatively quick results	Possible bias in measuring risk factors after disease has occurred Possible bias in selecting control group Identified cases may not represent all cases

community-wide education programs, have shown that low-cost interventions can significantly improve the population's health.[18]

5. How do we evaluate whether the study results are valid?

The most useful framework in which to consider potential errors in epidemiologic studies is to ask why the calculated measure of association, such as relative risk, may not accurately reflect the causal impact of exposure on disease. If we obtain an odds ratio or relative risk of 2.0, why are we not fully confident that introducing exposure will truly double the risk of disease or that removing it will cut the risk in half?

One reason is the possibility for confounding, in which the influence of one exposure is mixed with the effect of another. This arises when a risk factor for the disease of interest is also associated with the exposure of interest. For example, people who drink alcohol are also more likely to drink coffee. When a study is conducted to examine alcohol use and breast cancer, the possible confounding role of coffee and caffeine must be taken into consideration. The estimated effect of alcohol on breast cancer will be confounded by caffeine intake if (1) caffeine and alcohol use are correlated and (2) caffeine use independently influences the risk of breast cancer.

In an experiment or randomized controlled trial, these potential confounders can be balanced among the study groups through the design of the study and the random manner in which the exposure is assigned. Conversely, in an observational study, potential confounders must be measured and adjusted statistically. The strategy involves creating groups that are similar with respect to the potential confounder and examining the impact of the exposure of interest within each of those groups. For example, we could measure caffeine consumption and create strata of nonconsumers, low caffeine consumers, and high caffeine consumers and assess the role of alcohol use on breast cancer within each of those strata. As long as the potential confounder can be measured, the adjustments will be effective; however, some potential confounders, such as psychological stress, health consciousness, or dietary intake, may be difficult to measure, or we simply may be unaware of the risk factors that should be considered for adjustment.

A different source of bias or distortion comes from *selection bias*, or the way subjects enter or are retained in the study. A faulty sampling mechanism, caused by such problems as nonresponse or refusal to participate, could produce a sample that has a higher or lower disease risk. Note that the only kind of sampling distortion that matters is the selection that influences disease risk. Similarly, in a case-control study, the selected case patients should reflect the exposure distribu-tion of all case patients of interest, and the selected control subjects should reflect exposure in the overall population that produced the cases. The potential for a poorly constituted control group is a major threat to the validity of case-control studies. For example, when we choose control subjects from a hospital, health problems that lead to their hospital-ization may be associated with the exposure of interest. Similarly, when we choose control subjects by telephone screening, omitting households without telephones could introduce a bias.

Another category of bias that can occur in epidemiologic studies is the result of errors in classification of exposure or disease; this is referred to as *information bias*. Although efforts should be made to minimize such bias, errors in classification of exposure are unavoidable. Past exposures such as dietary intake, alcohol use, or physical activity are impossible to measure perfectly, even if we know what aspect of such exposures was the most relevant to disease causation. In many instances, the errors in expo-sure classification can be assumed to be similar for those who do and do not develop disease. This situation, referred to as *nondifferential misclassification* of exposure, results in a predictable bias in which the measure of association (such as odds ratio or relative risk) will be biased toward the null value of no association (1.0 for ratio measures, 0 for difference measures). This means that virtually all reported associations between exposure and disease will be diluted to some degree or missed entirely.

When the patterns of misclassification are different for the study groups, this is referred to as *differential misclassification*. This can occur when exposure is classified differently for diseased and nondiseased subjects or when disease is classified differently for exposed and unexposed subjects. Now the distortion in the measure of association can be in either direction (exaggerated or understated), depending on the precise pattern of error. A particular worry in case-control studies is the possibility of *recall bias*, which is a particular type of differential misclassification. Recall bias exists when the recall of exposure information is different for case patients than for control subjects, presumably because the illness experience of the case patients has in some way altered their memory or reporting of past events. Intuitively, one might expect case patients to overreport exposures that did not occur in an effort to explain their illness. Also, studies suggest that case patients may report accurately (presumably because their memory search is more thorough), whereas control subjects tend to underreport past exposures.[19] In

either situation, the reported exposures of case patients are artificially greater than the reported exposures of control subjects, and the relative risk is falsely elevated.

6. How do we assess whether associations between potential etiologic factors and disease are causal?

Any intervention program or public health action is based on the presumption that the associations found in epidemiologic studies are causal rather than arising through bias or for some other spurious reason. Unfortunately, in most instances in observational epidemiology, there is no opportunity to absolutely prove that an association is causal. Nonetheless, some principles are helpful when one must make this judgment.

The Bradford Hill criteria[20] are often cited as a checklist for causality in epidemiologic studies. These criteria have value but only as general guidelines. Most of Hill's nine criteria relate to particular cases of refuting biases or drawing on nonepidemiologic evidence:

1. Strength of association: Stronger associations are less likely to be the result of some subtle confounding or bias, presuming that major distorting influences would be more readily recognized than small ones.

2. Consistency of association: The association is observed across diverse populations and circumstances, making a particular bias unlikely to explain a series of such observations.

3. *Specificity of association*: The exposure causes one rather than many diseases, and the disease is associated with one rather than many exposures, suggesting that the association is not the result of bias. This is the weakest of the criteria for chronic diseases and might well be eliminated since we now know that many, perhaps most, exposures that influence one health outcome affect others (eg, tobacco, radiation, diet) and that virtually all diseases have multiple causes.

4. *Temporality*: The exposure must precede the disease. This is the only absolute criterion for causality.

5. *Biologic gradient*: A dose-response curve, in which the risk of disease increases with increasing exposure, indicates that an association probably is not the result of a confounder or other bias. This criterion is generally valid, but the absence of a perfect dose-response pattern does not negate the possibility of a causal explanation, because true thresholds or ceilings of effects may exist. Conversely, the presence of a dose-response gradient may be the result of a strong confounder that closely tracks the exposure.

6. *Plausibility*: Evidence from other disciplines suggests the agent is biologically capable of influencing the disease. This is useful supportive evidence when it is available, but the lack of advancements in the other biological sciences should not be used to negate an epidemiologic observation.

7. *Coherence*: The evidence should not be contradictory to the known biology and natural history of the disease (similar to the plausibility criterion).

8. *Experimental evidence*: When attainable, experimental evidence for causality—obtained by removing or randomly assigning exposure—is very strong because both known and unknown confounders are controlled when exposure is randomly allocated.

9. *Analogy*: When other similar agents have been established as causes of disease, then the credibility of theories regarding a new disease operating in a similar manner is enhanced. This is the epidemiologic counterpart to plausibility; however, the supportive evidence comes from other areas of epidemiology rather than from other disciplines.

In practice, the establishment of evidence for causality is largely through the elimination of noncausal explanations for an observed association. Consider, for example, the evidence that alcohol use may increase the risk of breast cancer. A series of further studies might confirm that this relationship is valid and not a result of confounding or other biases such as detection bias (in which disease is more thoroughly diagnosed among alcohol users) or nonresponse bias. By whittling away alternative explanations, the hypothesis that asserts alcohol use causes breast cancer becomes increasingly credible. It is the job of critics to propose and test noncausal explanations, so that when the association has withstood a series of such challenges, the case for causality is strengthened. The danger of formalizing the process of declaring causality on the basis of a checklist or any other mechanistic process is that it can only lead to endless debates about the degree of certainty and can impede needed public health actions. Those who argue that causality must be established with absolute certainty before interventions can begin fail to appreciate that their two alternatives—action and inaction—each have risks and benefits. Decisions must therefore be based on evidence that exposure causes diseases and must take into account the costs of intervention, the potential for the intervention to produce adverse side effects, and the potential costs of failing to act.

For example, the tobacco companies have argued, until recently, that the association between smoking and disease is uncertain. In a technical sense, we will always have some degree of uncertainty, especially with no definitive data from large numbers of subjects randomly assigned

to be smokers and nonsmokers. We have no doubt, however, that the evidence indicates a need to intervene, because smoking has no clear health benefits and scientists have exhausted all reasonable noncausal explanations for the strong associations observed between smoking and a number of diseases. Nonetheless, as tobacco companies continue to convince some individuals that the evidence for causality is not definitive, they create enough controversy to distract some policy makers from supporting needed interventions. Establishing causality is an important goal for epidemiologic research, but absolute proof is not needed to justify action.

7. How much morbidity and mortality might be prevented by interventions?

Some epidemiologic measures are particularly useful in evaluating the potential benefits of intervention. When presented with an array of potential causal factors for disease, we need to evaluate how much might be gained by reducing or eliminating each of the hazards. Relative risk estimates indicate how strongly exposure and disease are associated, but they do not indicate directly the benefits that could be gained through modifying the exposure.

The *attributable risk* is a measure of how much of the disease burden could be eliminated if the exposure were eliminated. The attributable risk represents the proportion of disease among exposed people that actually results from the exposure. This issue might arise in a court case in which an exposed individual claims that the agent to which he or she was exposed caused the disease. Note that we are presuming that the associations reflect causality for the purposes of estimation. The attributable risk among exposed individuals is calculated as follows:

$$\frac{\text{relative risk} - 1}{\text{relative risk}}$$

Thus, a relative risk of 2.0 (risk is doubled by exposure) yields an attributable proportion among exposed people of 0.5. This suggests a 50% chance that the disease resulted from the exposure in this study population.

Of still greater potential value is the incorporation of information on how common the exposure is. Although some exposures exert a powerful influence on individuals (ie, a large relative risk), they are so rare that their public health impact is minimal. Conversely, some exposures have a modest impact but are so widespread that their elimination could have great benefit. To answer the question, "What proportion of disease in the total population is a result of the exposure?" the population attributable risk or etiologic fraction is used. The *population attributable risk* is calculated as follows:

$$\frac{Pe\,(\text{relative risk} -1)}{1 + Pe\,(\text{relative risk} -1)}$$

where Pe represents the proportion of the population that is exposed. Assuming that the relative risk of lung cancer due to cigarette smoking is 15 and that 30% of the population are smokers, the population attributable risk is 0.81 or 81%. This would suggest that 81% of the lung cancer burden in the population is caused by cigarette smoking and could be eliminated if the exposure were eliminated. Because of the effects of interactions between various risk factors, population attributable risk estimates for a given disease can sometimes add up to more than 100%. Although population attributable risk estimates provide a useful estimate of the public health burden, they may be unrealistic as absolute goals, because only rarely can a risk factor be completely eliminated.

Interactions among exposures, also known as *effect modification*, in the causation of disease are of particular importance in fully understanding etiology. Effect modification occurs when the effect of one exposure on disease risk is modified by the presence of another exposure. In the purest form, which is rarely observed, each of two exposures alone may have no effect on disease, but when the two are combined, a synergism occurs causing an increase in disease. Conversely, two exposures that each can influence disease risk independently may be antagonistic, so that in combination they have a smaller effect on disease risk.

In epidemiologic studies, *interaction* is measured as a combined effect of exposures that is larger than would be expected by simply adding the effects of the two separate exposures. Interaction is most easily detected by comparing the disease risk in groups with all combinations of exposure to the group exposed to neither agent. For example, cigarette smoking and asbestos exposure have been demonstrated to multiply the risk of lung cancer (Table 2.3). The risk of lung cancer among nonsmokers who are exposed to asbestos (relative risk = 5.2) is approximately half that of smokers who are not exposed to asbestos (relative risk = 10.8). However, a multiplicative effect is observed among smokers who are exposed to asbestos (relative risk = 53.2).

This measure of interaction has direct implications for developing intervention and prevention programs. If two factors interact, then the benefit of removing a given exposure will be greater if the other exposure is also present. For example, eliminating smoking has even more benefit for a group of workers exposed to asbestos than for workers who are not exposed to asbestos.

Obviously, many factors enter into decisions about interventions, including certainty of causality, amenability to intervention, and social and political issues. However, in the traditional role of epidemiology as the basic science of public health, quantitative considerations of preventable disease can help us make a rational choice. How can we predict what benefits one or more of these interventions might yield in the community? This is where estimates of population attributable risk may be particularly useful. If one considers the earlier example of smoking and lung cancer, it is apparent that lung cancer incidence could be reduced by more than 80% if cigarette smoking were eliminated.

Table 2.3—Relative Risk Estimates for Lung Cancer Associated with Smoking and Asbestos Exposure Among Insulation Workers[a]

	Relative Risk Estimate	
Smoking Category	**No Asbestos Exposure**	**Asbestos Exposure**
Nonsmoker	1.0	5.2
Smoker	10.8	53.2

[a]*Note*: Adapted from Saracci.[21]

8. Why should action not be taken on the basis of a single epidemiologic study?

As scientists and administrators committed to improving the public's health, there is a natural tendency to scrutinize the epidemiologic litera-ture for new findings that would serve as the basis for prevention or intervention programs. In fact, application to public health practice is a principal motive for conducting such research. Adding to this inclina-tion to intervene may be claims from investigators regarding the critical importance of their findings, media interpretation of the findings as the basis for immediate action, and even community support for responding to the striking new research findings with new or modified programs, or elimination of existing programs. Appreciation of epidemiologic methods applied to chronic disease prevention and control leads to the inevitable conclusion that a single epidemiologic study is never suffi-cient for making such decisions. Well-designed and carefully con-ducted research adds evidence to assist in setting policy, but the stakes are so high in economic terms and public credibility that cautious interpretation of research findings that have not been replicated is required.

We have already discussed the validity of epidemiologic research and criteria for causality, but a more direct consideration of why a single study is insufficient for action should be helpful. Breast cancer had rarely been considered a disease that might be affected by environmental pollutants, in contrast, for example, to lung or bladder cancer. However, a paper published in 1993 by Wolff and colleagues[22] changed that perception. This study, which was well designed, carefully conducted, and certainly worthy of publication, reported that pesticide residues from dichlorodiphenyltrichloroethane (DDT) in the blood were positively associated with the risk of breast cancer, with relative risks on the order of 3.0. Media interest was high, and the notion that a common, life-threatening disease could be related in part to environmental agents was both terrifying and promising of the potential for intervention. Though these exposures had been accrued over a lifetime, if found to be related to breast cancer, interventions to reduce body burden would be worthy of consideration. For other reasons, largely based on adverse effects on wildlife, DDT was banned over 20 years ago.

How could a study be "good epidemiology," published in a reputable journal, generate substantial media and public interest, and yet not be worthy of any action on the part of public health practitioners?

First, despite the talents of the investigators and quality of the resulting study, its findings may simply be wrong or misleading. That is, for reasons discussed earlier, even within the population studied, there may well be no causal association between DDT residues and breast cancer. One critical concern is whether the measured levels of DDT residues were affected by early stages of breast cancer rather than the reverse. Also, potential confounding by lactation was examined but produced rather anomalous results, and the number of cases available for analysis was small.

Second, even if valid for the population under study, the generalizability of the findings has to be examined. Can results from women in the New York area be applied to other populations with different exposure histories, different ethnic backgrounds, and different risk factor profiles? Though we look for universal explanations for disease, and occasionally find strong causal factors that account for most of the disease in most populations (eg, smoking and lung cancer), these successes are rare. More often, there are a multitude of interacting factors that must be considered for findings from one population to apply to another.

Finally, even if valid and generalizable, thus making a contribution to public health decision making, what action should be taken for an agent that was banned long ago? At the

margins, in evaluating costs and benefits, this research would (if valid) add to the evidence of health harm from exposure, but in this case, there is not a clear decision to be made. If we had two comparably effective pesticides, one of which was associated with health harm and one was not, such evidence might tip the balance. Public health decisions must integrate the full array of considerations regarding risks and benefits of different courses of action, as discussed below.

9. How do we assess a series of epidemiologic studies and integrate the evidence to make decisions?

Several important methods and tools are available to epidemiologists and practitioners to assist in determining when public health action is warranted. It is often necessary to utilize these because exposure-disease relationships in chronic disease epidemiology typically show relatively weak associations, in which the relative risk estimate is not too deviant from the null value of 1.0. Most accepted risk factors for breast cancer are associated with relative risks of less than 5.0, and often less than 3.0, considered by some to be weak.[23] The closer a relative risk estimate comes to unity, the more likely that it can be explained by methodologic limitations such as confounding, misclassification, and other sources of bias.

Yet, as noted earlier in the description of population attributable risk, even when a risk factor is weak, if highly prevalent in the population, the public health impact can be large. Therefore, we have great interest in determining when even relatively weak associations provide the basis for public health intervention, which can only come from a series of well-designed studies.

Although it is tempting to intervene rather than conduct yet more studies in the face of a serious health problem, in the long run, evaluation of all major interventions is essential. To conduct such an evaluation, investigators must study a comparison group and rule out other factors as the cause of any observed change. The diagnosis of breast cancer in a prominent local citizen, for example, could be the main cause of increased breast cancer screening, rather than a community education program. In programs that combine several interventions, investigators may be able to determine which intervention(s) actually produced the health benefits and whether the results of an evaluation are generalizable to a different population. The debate continues, for example, as to whether the results of studies of reduced serum cholesterol in men can be applied to women. Thus, determining whether a proposed intervention will actually bring about more good than harm can be difficult.

It is important to note that even ostensibly useful interventions may not have positive effects and that almost all programs may have unintended negative effects. An education program to increase breast cancer screening, for example, could have no effect on women who need screening, yet it could raise anxiety among younger women at low risk who do not need screening. The usefulness of a particular screening test is based on several characteristics, including its accuracy, reproducibility, sensitivity, and specificity, as discussed in detail by Morrison.[24]

This section provides an overview of three related methods that have proven useful in assimilating large bodies of evidence in chronic disease epidemiology. In turn, the summarized evidence can be useful in shaping public health interventions and policies. Because this consideration is necessarily brief, readers are referred to other sources for more detail.

Meta-analysis

Meta-analysis is a quantitative approach that provides a systematic, organized, and structured way of integrating the findings of individual studies.[25,26] Over the past two decades, meta-analysis has been increasingly used to synthesize the findings of multiple independent studies. Petitti[26] describes four steps in undertaking a meta-analysis.

1. Identify relevant studies.
Relevant studies must first be identified for inclusion in the meta-analysis. These can be identified through computerized sources such as MEDLINE, review articles, other journal articles, doctoral dissertations, and personal communications with other researchers.

2. Inclusion/exclusion criteria.
Explicit criteria distinguish a meta-analysis from a qualitative literature review. Criteria for inclusion should specify the study designs to be included; the years of publication or of data collection; the languages in which the articles are written (eg, English only or English plus other specified languages); the minimum sample size and the extent of follow-up; the treatments and/or exposures; the manner in which the exposures, treatment, and outcomes were measured; and the completeness of information. Study quality should also be considered. As a minimum, studies should be excluded whose quality falls below some specified rating criteria. Rating scales may be developed to assess the quality of the included studies, though the basis for rating can be controversial and it may be preferable to consider the actual study attributes rather than a summary quality score.

3. Data abstraction. In this step, important features of each study are abstracted such as design, number of participants, and key findings. The abstraction summary should produce findings that are reliable, valid, and free of bias. Blinding of abstractors and re-abstraction of a sample of studies by multiple abstractors may be beneficial.

4. Statistical analysis and exploration of heterogeneity. The data are combined to produce a summary estimate of the measure of association along with confidence intervals, as described in detail elsewhere.[26–28] Data are also examined to determine if the effect across studies was homogeneous and if not, the reasons for heterogeneity.

Meta-analysis is most useful for combining the results of multiple, small, randomized controlled trials whose results are generally consistent yet imprecision is a problem in each individual trial. The method is less useful in situations where trials have found truly heterogeneous results through different methods or because the relationship of interest varies across populations. Partly for that reason, one must be careful not to be overwhelmed by the impressively large numbers that can be accrued in a meta-analysis. While the improved precision is a strength, one must also consider the validity of combining results across studies and whether the estimated size of the effect is large enough to warrant action.

Risk Assessment

Quantitative risk assessment is a widely used term for a systematic approach to characterizing the risks posed to individuals and populations by environmental pollutants and other potentially adverse exposures.[29,30] Risk assessment has been described as a "bridge" between science and policy making.[31] In the United States, its use is either explicitly or implicitly required by a number of federal statutes, and its application worldwide is increasing. There has been considerable debate over the US risk assessment policies, and the most widely recognized difficulties in risk assessment are due to extrapolation-related uncertainties (ie, extrapolating low-dose effects from higher exposure levels). Risk assessment has become an established process through which expert scientific input is provided to agencies that regulate environmental or occupational exposures. A landmark publication in the field of risk assessment is the 1983 report of the National Research Council, sometimes called the "Red Book" because of its cover.[32]

Four key steps in risk assessment are hazard identification, risk characterization, exposure assessment, and risk estimation.[29] An important aspect of risk assessment is that it frequently results in classification schemes that take into account uncertainties about exposure-disease relationships. For example, the US Environmental Protection Agency[33] has developed a five tier scheme for classifying potential and proven cancer-causing agents that includes the following: (1) group A, carcinogenic to humans, (2) group B, probably carcinogenic to humans, (3) group C, possibly carcinogenic to humans, (4) group D, not classifiable as to human carcinogenicity, and (5) group E, evidence of noncarcinogenicity for humans.

Expert Panels and Consensus Conferences

Most government agencies, in both executive and legislative branches, as well as voluntary health organizations such as the American Cancer Society, utilize expert panels when examining epidemiologic studies and their relevance to health policies and interventions.[34] Ideally, the goal of expert panels is to provide peer review by scientific experts of the quality of the science and scientific interpretations that underlie public health recommendations, regulations, and policy decisions. When conducted well, peer review can provide an important set of checks and balances for the regulatory process. Optimally, the expert review process has the following common properties: experts are sought in epidemiology and related disciplines (eg, clinical medicine, biomedical sciences, biostatistics, economics, ethics); panels typically consist of 8 to 15 members and meet in person to review scientific data; written guidance is provided to panel members; panel members should not have financial or professional conflicts of interest; draft findings from expert panels are frequently released for public review and comment prior to final recommendations. One of the successful outcomes of expert panels has been the production of guidelines for public health and medical care. A recent example is the publication of the second edition of the *Guide to Clinical Preventive Services*.[35] This document is a careful review of the scientific evidence for and against hundreds of preventive services (eg, childhood immunizations, tobacco cessation counseling). Its production was overseen by a 10-member expert advisory committee. A related effort is presently underway to develop a *Guide to Community Preventive Services*.[36]

Consensus conferences are a related mechanism that are commonly used to review epidemiologic evidence. The National Institutes of Health (NIH) have used consensus conferences since 1977 to resolve controversial issues in medicine and public health. To date, the NIH has conducted 120 such conferences.[37] For example, a highly publicized consensus conference on breast cancer screening was recently held to determine whether mammography screening for women ages 40 to 49 years reduces breast cancer mortality.[37]

There is one important difference between expert panels such as the US Preventive Services Task Force and a Consensus Development Panel such as the one for breast cancer screening for women in their 40's. Expert panels can take time to develop their recommendations, while the Consensus Development Panel must make its decision within a 2 1/2 day conference, risking some sacrifice of careful judgment for speed.

Both expert panels and consensus development panels work best when they publish along with their recommendations the rationale for their recommendation and the process used to arrive at that rationale. In considering the recommendations of such panels, one should examine the extent to which they are evidence-based, or instead rely on "expert" opinion. Evidence-based recommendations should be given much greater weight.

CONCLUSIONS

In this chapter, we have discussed the issues that help to determine whether associations are causal, the role of intervention research in disease control, and uses of epidemiologic evidence to make public health decisions. We have also outlined several types of epidemiologic study designs and the biases that can complicate interpretation of

Table 2.4—Key Concepts in Chronic Disease Epidemiology

Term	Definition
Incidence rate	$\dfrac{\text{Number of new events in a specified time period}}{\text{Number of persons exposed to risk during this period}}$
Relative risk	$\dfrac{\text{Risk of disease or death in the exposed population}}{\text{Risk of disease or death in the unexposed population}}$
Population attributable risk	Proportion of a disease in a population that is associated with (attributed to) a certain risk factor

results. We have discussed issues that help to determine whether associations are causal, as well as the role of intervention research in disease control. Such information serves as a foundation that will help readers address the more complex issues of chronic disease etiology and control. Some of the key epidemiologic concepts that the reader will encounter in other chapters are summarized in Table 2.4.

REFERENCES

1. Rothman KJ, Greenland S. *Modern Epidemiology,* 2nd ed. Philadelphia, Pa: Lippincott-Raven; 1998.
2. Kleinbaum DG, Kupper LL, Morgenstern H. *Epidemiologic Research: Principles and Quantitative Methods.* Belmont, Calif: Lifetime Learning Publications; 1982.
3. Schlesselman JJ. *Case-Control Studies: Design, Conduct, Analysis.* New York, NY: Oxford University Press Inc; 1982.
4. Fletcher RH, Fletcher SW, Wagner EH. *Clinical Epidemiology—The Essentials.* 2nd ed. Baltimore, Md: Williams & Wilkins; 1988.
5. Weiss NS. *Clinical Epidemiology. The Study of the Outcome of Illness,* 2nd ed. New York, NY: Oxford University Press Inc; 1996.
6. Hennekens CH, Buring JE. *Epidemiology in Medicine.* Boston, Mass: Little, Brown & Company; 1987.
7. Kelsey JL, Whittemore AS, Evans AS, Thompson WD. *Methods in Observational Epidemiology,* 2nd ed. New York, NY: Oxford University Press; 1996.
8. Lilienfeld DE, Stolley PD. *Foundations of Epidemiology.* New York, NY: Oxford University Press Inc; 1994.
9. Gordis L. *Epidemiology.* Philadelphia, Pa: WB Saunders Company; 1996.

10. Black WC, Welch HG. Advances in diagnostic imaging and overestimations of disease prevalence and the benefits of therapy. *N Engl J Med*. 1993;328:1237–1243.

11. McDowell I, Newell C. *Measuring Health: A Guide to Rating Scales and Questionnaires*. New York, NY: Oxford University Press Inc; 1996.

12. Fletcher SW, Black W, Harris R, Rimer BK, Shapiro S. Report on the International Workshop on Screening for Breast Cancer. *J Natl Cancer Inst*. 1993;85:1644–1656.

13. Wilson MC, Hayward RSA, Tunis SR, Bass EB, Guyatt G. User's guides to the medical literature: VIII. how to use clinical practice guidelines: B. What are the recommendations and will they help you in caring for your patients? *JAMA*. 1995;274:1630–1632.

14. Miller BA, Ries LAG, Hankey BF, Kosary CL, Harras A, Devesa SS, Edwards BK (eds). *SEER Cancer Statistics Review: 1973–1990*, Bethesda, Md: National Cancer Institute; 1993. NIH publication 93-2789.

15. Ries LAG, Miller BA, Hankey BF, Kosary CL, Harras A, Edwards BK (eds). *SEER Cancer Statistics Review, 1973-1991: Tables and Graphs,* Bethesda, Md: National Cancer Institute; 1994. NIH publication 94-2789.

16. Shapiro S, Venet W, Strax P, Venet L. *Periodic Screening for Breast Cancer: The Health Insurance Plan Project and Its Sequelae, 1963–1986*. Baltimore, Md: Johns Hopkins University Press; 1988.

17. Shore RE, Hildreth N, Woodward E, Dvoretsky P, Hempelmann L, Pasternack B. Breast cancer among women given x-ray therapy for acute postpartum mastitis. *J Natl Cancer Inst*. 1986;77:689–696.

18. Farquhar JW, Fortmann SP, Flora JA, et al. Effects of community-wide education on cardiovascular disease risk factors. The Stanford Five-City Project. *JAMA*. 1990;264:359–365.

19. Bracken MB. Methodologic issues in the epidemiologic investigation of drug-induced congenital malformations. In: Bracken MB, ed. *Perinatal Epidemiology*. New York, NY: Oxford University Press Inc; 1984:423–449.

20. Hill AB. The environment and disease: association or causation? *Proc R Soc Med*. 1965;58:295–300.

21. Saracci R. The interactions of tobacco smoking and other agents in cancer etiology. *Epidemiol Rev*. 1987;9:175–193.

22. Wolff M, Toniolo P, Lee E, Rivera M, Bubinn N. Blood levels of organo chlorine residues and risk of breast cancer. *J Natl Cancer Inst.* 1993;85:648–652.

23. Wynder EL. Workshop on guidelines to the epidemiology of weak associations. Introduction. *Prev Med.* 1987;16:139–141.

24. Morrison AS. *Screening in Chronic Disease,* 2nd ed. New York, NY: Oxford University Press Inc; 1992.

25. Glass GV. Primary, secondary and meta-analysis of research. *Educ Res.* 1976;5:3–8.

26. Petitti DB. Meta-analysis, decision analysis, and cost-effectiveness analysis: methods for quantitative synthesis in medicine. New York, NY: Oxford University Press Inc; 1994.

27. Greenland S. Quantitative methods in the review of epidemiologic literature. *Epidemiol Rev.* 1987;9:1–30.

28. Dickersin K, Berlin JA. Meta-analysis: State-of-the-science. *Epidemiol Rev.* 1992;14:154–176.

29. World Health Organization. *Assessment and Management of Environmental Health Hazards.* Geneva: 1989. Publication WHO/PEP/89.6.

30. Samet JM, Burke TA. Epidemiology and risk assessment. In: Brownson RC, Petitti DB, eds. *Applied Epidemiology: Theory to Practice.* New York, NY: Oxford University Press Inc; 1998:137–175.

31. Hertz-Picciotto I. Epidemiology and quantitative risk assessment: a bridge from science to policy. *Am J Public Health.* 1995;85:484–491.

32. National Research Council, Committee on the Institutional Means for Assessment of Risks to Public Health. *Risk Assessment in the Federal Government: Managing the Process.* Washington, DC; National Academy Press; 1983.

33. US Environmental Protection Agency. Guidelines for carcinogenic risk assessment. *Federal Register.* 1986;51:33992–34003.

34. Brownson RC. Epidemiology and health policy. In: Brownson RC, Petitti DB, eds. *Applied Epidemiology: Theory to Practice.* New York, NY: Oxford University Press Inc; 1998:349–387.

35. US Preventive Services Task Force. *Guide to Clinical Preventive Services.* 2nd ed. Baltimore, Md: Williams & Wilkins; 1996.

36. Pappaioanou M, Evans C. Developing a guide to community preventive services: a U.S. Public Health Service initiative. *J Public Health Manag Pract.* 1998 (in press).

37. Nelson NJ. The mammography consensus jury speaks out. *J Natl Cancer Inst.* 1997;89:344–347.

SUGGESTED READING

Brownson RC, Petitti DB, eds. *Applied Epidemiology: Theory to Practice*. New York, NY: Oxford University Press Inc; 1998.

Fletcher RH, Fletcher SW, Wagner EH. *Clinical Epidemiology—The Essentials*. 2nd ed. Baltimore, Md: Williams & Wilkins; 1988.

Hennekens CH, Buring JE. *Epidemiology in Medicine*. Boston, Mass: Little, Brown & Company; 1987.

Kelsey JL, Whittemore AS, Evans AS, WD Thompson. *Methods in Observational Epidemiology*, 2nd ed. New York, NY: Oxford University Press Inc; 1996.

Last JM, ed. *A Dictionary of Epidemiology*. 3rd ed. New York, NY: Oxford University Press Inc; 1995.

Morrison AS. *Screening in Chronic Disease*, 2nd ed. New York, NY: Oxford University Press Inc; 1992.

3

CHRONIC DISEASE SURVEILLANCE

S urveillance is the ongoing systematic collection, analysis, and interpretation of health data that are essential to the planning, implementation, and evaluation of public health practice. These activities must be closely integrated with the timely dissemination of these data to the appropriate audience. The final link in the surveillance chain is the application of surveillance findings to disease prevention and health promotion programs (Figure 3.1). A public health surveillance "system" includes a functional capacity for data collection, analysis, and dissemination linked to public health programs.[1]

Public health surveillance evolved during the 20th century as the health burden from chronic diseases increased. In the early 1900s, surveillance described the practice of monitoring people who had been in contact with patients with certain infectious diseases, such as plague, smallpox, or typhus (Table 3.1). In the 1950s, surveillance began to be used to describe the practice of monitoring populations for the occurrence of specific infectious diseases, such as polio, measles, or tetanus.[2] By the 1970s, surveillance techniques were being applied to a broader array of diseases, including cancer, childhood lead poisoning, and congenital malformations.[1]

Over the past 20 years, our understanding of the causes of chronic diseases has continued to increase. Studies have demonstrated that chronic diseases develop slowly over a lifetime and are the end result of years of exposure to behavioral and environmental risk factors. For example, dietary habits in early life lead to high blood cholesterol in adulthood and the subsequent development of coronary heart disease. In addition, numerous studies have demonstrated the consistent association between measures of socioeconomic status, such as education, poverty status, or social networks, and chronic diseases. This continuum—from health, to the exposure to risk factors, development of chronic disease conditions and

Patrick L. Remington, MD, MPH
Richard A. Goodman, MD, MPH

Table 3.1—Trends in the Application of Surveillance to Public Health, 1900 to Present

Period	Application	Examples
1900s	Individual contacts of infected patients	Surveillance of individuals who came in contact with a case of smallpox is conducted.
1950s	Communicable diseases	Cases of polio are reported to the public health agency as part of a communicable disease control program.
1970s	Selected chronic diseases	Cancer registries are established as part of the Surveillance, Epidemiology, and End Results (SEER) Program.
1990s	Behavioral, occupational, and environmental risk factors	Trends in the prevalence of cigarette smoking, determined through telephone surveys, are used to plan tobacco control programs.

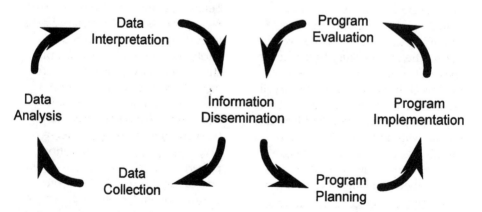

Figure 3.1—Organizational model for state-based chronic disease surveillance programs.

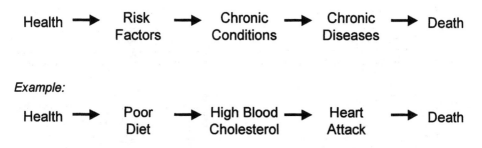

Example:

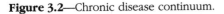

Figure 3.2—Chronic disease continuum.

diseases, and finally premature death—is shown in Figure 3.2.

In response to this greater understanding of the complex causes of chronic disease, surveillance systems have recently evolved to include monitoring trends behavioral, occupational, and environmental risk factors, as well as other health conditions, such as disabilities. This information is critical for the development and monitoring of prevention programs that focus on preventing risk factors, such as smoking and poor diet, or controlling chronic disease conditions, such as high blood cholesterol and hypertension.[3,4]

This chapter describes the three basic elements of a chronic disease surveillance system: (1) data sources, (2) analysis and interpretation, and (3) dissemination to public health programs and other important constituents. The chapter concludes by emphasizing the importance of linking these data to chronic disease prevention and control efforts.

DATA SOURCES

Seven types of information systems exist in the United States that routinely provide data for surveillance.[5] These data systems include notifiable diseases, vital statistics, sentinel surveillance, registries, health surveys, administrative data collection systems, and the US census (Table 3.2). Chronic disease surveillance may use data from one or more of these systems. For example, surveillance of the health effects of tobacco use relies on data from vital statistics, cancer registries, telephone surveys about tobacco use, and administrative records of tobacco sales tax.

Notifiable Disease Systems

Public health agencies classify diseases as "notifiable" if their occurrence requires prompt public health action. In each state, laws specify those conditions that physicians, other health care providers, and laboratories must report to the

Table 3.2—Selected Chronic Disease Data Sources and Surveillance Systems

Data System	Example	Strengths	Limitations
Notifiable diseases [a,b,c]	State-based lead poisoning reporting systems	• Data are available at the local level. • Usually coupled with a public health response (eg, lead paint removal). • Detailed information can be collected to aid in designing control programs. • Laboratory-based systems are inexpensive and effective.	• Requires participation by community-based clinicians. • Clinician-based systems have low reporting rates. • Active reporting systems are time-consuming and expensive.
Vital statistics [a,b,c]	Death certificates	• Data are widely available at the local, state, and national levels. • Population-based. • Can monitor trends in age-adjusted disease rates. • Can target areas with increased mortality rates.	• Cause of death information may be inaccurate (eg, lack of autopsy information). • No information about risk factors.
Sentinel Surveillance [b,c]	Sentinel Event Notification System for Occupational Risks (SENSOR)	• Low-cost system to monitor selected diseases. • Usually coupled with a public health response (eg, asbestos removal following report of mesothelioma). • Provides information on risk factors and disease severity.	• Requires motivated reporting providers. • May not be representative.

Method	Example	Advantages	Limitations
Disease registries[b,c]	Cancer registries	• Data are increasingly available throughout the United States. • Includes accurate tissue-based diagnoses. • Provides stage-of-diagnosis data.	• Systems are expensive. • Data are affected by patient out-migration from one geographic unit to another. • Risk factor information is seldom available.
Health Surveys[b,c]	Behavioral risk factor surveillance telephone surveys	• Monitors trends in risk factor prevalence. • Can be used for program design and evaluation	• Information is based on self-reports. • May be too expensive to conduct at the local level. • May not be representative due to non-response (eg, telephone surveys).
Administrative data collection systems[b,c]	Hospital discharge systems	• Reflects regional differences in disease hospitalization rates. • Can capture cost information. • Data are readily available. • One of few sources of morbidity data.	• Often lacks personal identifiers. • Rates may be affected by changing patterns of diagnosis based on reimbursement mechanisms. • Difficult to separate initial from recurrent hospitalizations.
US Census[a,b,c]	Poverty rates by county	• Required to calculate rates. • Important predictors of health status. • Available to all communities and readily available on-line.	• Collected infrequently (every 10 years). • May undercount certain populations (eg, the poor, homeless persons).

[a] Data are available from most local public health agencies.
[b] Data are available from most state departments of health.
[c] Data are available from many US federal health agencies (eg, Centers for Disease Control and Prevention, National Cancer Institute, Health Care Financing Administration, etc).

health department. These reports may trigger public health responses, such as immunizing or providing prophylaxis to contacts, reviewing food handling techniques, or closing a food establishment.

The Council of State and Territorial Epidemiologists, an organization consisting of the state epidemiologist from every state and territory in the United States, establishes the list of notifiable diseases. This list of reportable diseases and illnesses (numbering 56 in 1997) includes primarily infectious diseases, such as measles, salmonella, and AIDS. Some noncommunicable diseases, such as lead poisoning, have been included. Using reports from clinicians and laboratories, public health agencies follow up on people with high blood lead levels and provide appropriate control measures.

In 1996, the Council of State and Territorial Epidemiologists added the prevalence of cigarette-smoking to the list of conditions designated as reportable by states to the Centers for Disease Control and Prevention (CDC). This is the first time that a behavior, rather than a disease or illness, has been considered nationally reportable. The goals include monitoring the trends in tobacco use, guiding intervention resources, and evaluating public health interventions. The state-based Behavioral Risk Factor Surveillance System will be used as the source of data for trends in smoking.

Currently, the Council of State and Territorial Epidemiologists, in conjunction with the CDC, is developing an expanded list of reportable chronic diseases, conditions, and behaviors. As a result of this initiative, the list of nationally reportable diseases may be expanded to include chronic disease deaths, cancer incidence, and other youth and adult behavioral risk factors (in addition to cigarette smoking) and preventive health practices (Table 3.3). The addition of these indicators will serve as a critical step in the recognition of chronic diseases as a preventable public health problem.

Vital Statistics

Information collected at the time of birth and death constitute one of the cornerstones of surveillance in the United States.[5] Mortality records are the records most often used for chronic disease surveillance and constitute the oldest data systems used for disease surveillance. In 1850, the federal government began publishing US mortality statistics based on the decennial census of that year.[1] By the early part of the century, the death registration system had become an integral part of efforts to control tuberculosis, typhoid fever, and diphtheria. It was viewed as the foundation of all public health work.[6] Because chronic diseases are now the major cause of death in the United States, disease

Table 3.3—Proposed Priority Chronic Disease Surveillance Indicators

Category	Source	Indicator (subtype)
Mortality	Vital statistics	Cancer (lung, breast, cervical, colorectal, oral/pharyngeal, prostate, bladder, melanoma)
		Cardiovascular (total, ischemic heart disease, cerebrovascular, congestive heart disease)
		Diabetes (any listing on the death certificate)
		Chronic obstructive lung disease
		Asthma
		Cirrhosis
Morbidity	Registries	Cancer incidence by stage at diagnosis (total, lung, breast, cervical, colorectal, oral/pharyngeal, bladder, melanoma)
	Hospital discharge	Hip fractures, lower extremity amputations (diabetic)
Risk factors	BRFSS[a]	Adult cigarette smoking, obesity, physical inactivity, alcohol use, and smokeless tobacco use
	YBRS[b]	Youth cigarette smoking, physical inactivity, and smokeless tobacco use
Preventive Health Practices	BRFSS	Screening for breast, cervical, and colorectal cancer

[a]BRFSS, Behavioral Risk Factor Surveillance System.
[b]YRBS, Youth Risk Behavior Surveillance.

control programs will benefit similarly from the use of chronic disease mortality data for surveillance.

In the United States, mortality data are collected through the vital registration system. After a person dies, a physician or coroner completes the death certificate. He or she lists the immediate cause of death (eg, pneumonia), the sequence of events that led to the death (eg, lung cancer), and other contributing causes (eg, tobacco use). Subse-

quently, these listings are coded and a computerized algorithm is used to determine the "underlying cause of death" that is, the disease or condition that triggered the chain of events that eventually caused the death.[7] In the example cited above, lung cancer would be listed as the underlying cause of death and tobacco use and pneumonia would be listed as contributing causes.

One important limitation of using mortality data for surveillance is that death certificates are occasionally incomplete. The physician or coroner who is completing the certificate may not know the complete clinical history of the deceased person or may not take the time to properly complete the certificate. In addition, some conditions, such as diabetes, are often underreported as underlying or contributing causes.[8] Finally, even though some state death certificates provide a space to list risk factors such as tobacco use, some physicians may be reluctant to list this information as a contributing cause of death.

In most states, mortality data are readily accessible for chronic disease surveillance. State-specific data are collected and maintained by vital statistics departments in a standard format. The CDC has developed guidelines for the use of mortality data for chronic disease surveillance.[9] In addition, these mortality data are now easily accessible through the World Wide Web (http://www.wonder.cdc.gov).[10]

Sentinel Surveillance

The term *sentinel surveillance* encompasses a wide range of activities that focus on key health indicators in the population. A sentinel event is a preventable disease, disability, or untimely death whose occurrence serves as a warning that prevention may need to be improved. Sentinel surveillance

for chronic diseases most often focuses on occupational-related health conditions. The National Institute for Occupational Safety and Health (NIOSH) has developed the Sentinel Event Notification System for Occupational Risks (SENSOR), which depends on sentinel providers to report detailed information about people diagnosed with diseases such as silicosis, lead poisoning, or carpal tunnel syndrome.[11]

Chronic Disease Registries

Chronic disease registries are useful for monitoring trends in diseases that are not otherwise reported to public health agencies. In addition, more detailed information about each disease can be collected, such as personal characteristics, stage at diagnosis, or types of treatment provided. Although registries are extremely useful, they require considerable financial resources to implement and maintain.

Cancer registries are the most common type of disease registry used for chronic disease surveillance. Hospitals and clinics collect data on patients with cancer after they have been diagnosed with or treated for cancer. These data include demographic information and information about the cancer, such as primary site, histology, diagnostic confirmation, extent of disease, presence of other tumors, date of first diagnosis, place of first diagnosis, forms of definitive therapy, and date of definitive therapy.

Cancer registries vary according to the population surveyed and the extent of follow-up performed. Hospital-based registries collect information on patients diagnosed or treated at that facility. In contrast, population-based registries collect information on all people residing in a specific geographic area, such as a county or state. These registries are more useful because they can be related to a defined population at risk; thus, cancer incidence rates can be calculated over time and between geographic regions. However, patient migration out of the area for care often limits the accuracy of these systems.

Cancer registries were established to identify regional differences in cancer incidence rates and to better understand the reasons for these differences.[12] The first population-based cancer registry was established in Connecticut in 1936. The Surveillance, Epidemiology, and End Results (SEER) Program of the National Cancer Institute, established in 1972, is a population-based registry in 11 separate geographic areas in the United States. This system is used to determine national trends in both cancer incidence and mortality and to conduct epidemiologic studies of cancer.

In October 1992, Congress established the National Program of Cancer Registries (NPCR) by enacting The Cancer Registries Amendment Act (Public Law 102-515). As a result of this law, the Centers for Disease Control and Prevention (CDC) provides over $20 million annually to state and territorial health departments to establish and improve population-based cancer registries. As of September 1996, 42 states and the District of Columbia were receiving CDC support for cancer registries: 34 for enhancement of established registries and 9 for developing registries where none had been organized previously.

Health Surveys

Health surveys may be used to collect information about self-reported behaviors and health practices in the general population. In the United States, surveys such as the annual National Health Interview Survey (NHIS) are important sources of information for monitoring trends in the prevalence of health conditions and risk factors in the general population. These surveys, conducted annually since 1957, provide information on self-reported chronic conditions, health behaviors, and use of health services.

In order to obtain comparable information at the state or local level, CDC has developed an ongoing telephone surveillance system called the Behavioral Risk Factor Surveillance System. These data are collected using standardized methods and questionnaires, thus permitting comparison of the prevalence of behavioral risk factors, such as smoking and alcohol use, between states, over time, and for various sociodemographic groups.

In a typical state, about 150 adults are interviewed monthly throughout the year. The respondents are selected by random-digit dialing. Each interview takes about 15 minutes to complete and addresses a variety of risk factors, including tobacco use, alcohol consumption, exercise, diet, and the use of preventive health services. These data are usually entered directly into a computer and are summarized annually by CDC and state health departments. Data quality concerns include validity and reliability of the questions, sample bias, and reporting accuracy.[13]

Finally, the CDC supports the Youth Risk Behavior Surveillance.[14] Anonymous surveys are administered to a random sample of 9th to 12th grade students in each state and many cities throughout the United States. This surveillance system monitors six categories of priority chronic disease risk behaviors, including tobacco use, alcohol and other drug use, sexual behaviors, unhealthy dietary behaviors, and physical inactivity. Health and education officials are using these data to improve national, state, and local policies and programs designed to reduce risks associated with the leading causes of mortality and morbidity.

Administrative Data Collection Systems

Many data on chronic diseases are collected as part of the routine of health care administration. Hospital discharge data are the most widely available of these types of data. In particular, hospital discharge data may be used to characterize hospitalization patterns and reasons for hospitalization for chronic diseases.[15] Information is collected from the medical abstracts and billing records of each patient discharged from the hospital. Patient diagnoses and procedures are coded according to the *International Classification of Diseases, Ninth Revision, Clinical Modification* (ICD-9-CM).[16]

The usefulness of administrative databases is limited by incomplete records, unreliable or invalid coding, and missing important clinical variables. Measurement errors associated with hospital discharge data arise chiefly in the coding process, which requires coders to know clinical diagnoses and the organization of the ICD coding scheme. Although diagnoses are often listed on the face sheet of the medical record, the principal diagnoses may not be cited accurately when the hospital discharge form is completed. In addition, changing reimbursement systems, such as the use of diagnosis-related groups (DRGs), may influence the listing of diagnoses.

For example, an analysis of trends in hospitalization due to cerebrovascular disease (stroke) showed an increase in hospitalization rates from 1970 through 1984 and a decrease from 1985 to 1986.[17] The authors speculated that the increase resulted from increased detection and hospitalization of people with mild strokes and that the decrease probably resulted from fewer hospitalizations as a result of the implementation of DRGs in 1984.

Recently, the principles of surveillance have been used by state and national agencies to monitor the quality of health care.[18] For example, consumers and purchasers of health care use "HEDIS" (Health Plan Employer Data Information System) in order to have the information they need to reliably compare the performance of managed health care plans.[19] This system uses eight performance domains, including effectiveness of care, access/availability of care, satisfaction with the experience of care, cost of care, stability of the health plan, informed health care choices, use of services, and health plan descriptive information. As the percentage of the population enrolled in managed care continues to grow, these data may be useful to monitor the health of entire populations.

Census Data

Every 10 years, the US government conducts a census of the entire US population. In addition to counting the population, the census collects detailed information on individual and household characteristics, such as age, race, education, and income. These census data are essential for calculating rates in populations, in order to compare disease burden and trends between regions or over time.

Despite efforts to enumerate the entire population, however, the census misses some people in its count. In 1990, the census missed nearly 5 million people, who were disproportionately from minority racial and ethnic groups and concentrated in a small number of geographic areas. The potential for errors in the census must be taken into account when examining rates in these special populations.

In conclusion, chronic disease surveillance can be conducted using a wide variety of existing data sources. When using these data, public health practitioners must understand the advantages and limitations inherent in each system. Despite these limitations, a comprehensive surveillance system—using a wide variety of chronic disease data—can serve as a resource to improve the health of the entire population.[20]

Chronic disease surveillance systems must have the capacity to analyze data. Data analysis and interpretation require knowledge about chronic diseases and the relationship among risk factors, conditions, morbidity, and death. In addition, interpretation of analyses must include a thorough understanding of the data systems and statistical techniques used in all analyses. Because of the large number of cases involved, analysis has traditionally required the use of mainframe computers; however, with recent improvements in personal computers, subsets of the larger data sets are often downloaded to personal computers and analyzed using spreadsheet, statistical, or database software.

Chronic disease surveillance uses descriptive epidemiology and examines the distribution of diseases in the population by person, place, and time. Brief descriptions of these important analyses follow.

Person Analyses

Descriptive studies begin by examining how the distribution of a disease or condition varies in the population according to personal characteristics, such as age, race, or gender. For example, breast cancer mortality rates in the United States by age and race are shown in the following table (Table 3.4). Breast cancer mortality rates increase with increasing age, from only 1.3 deaths per hundred thousand women under the age of 35, to almost 200 deaths per hundred thousand women 85 years of age and older. In addition, Blacks have a higher mortality rate compared with Whites and persons of other races (Native Americans and Asian/Pacific Islanders). Recognizing and understanding the reasons for these differences is

Table 3.4—Female Breast Cancer Mortality Rates, per 100 000 women, United States, 1990-1994, by Race and Age

Age	White	Black	Other	All Races
<35	0.8	1.5	0.5	1.3
35 - 44	15.2	25.5	8.5	16.2
45 - 54	41.8	59.9	24.7	43.1
55 - 64	74.4	89.4	34.0	74.7
65 - 74	109.4	114.0	38.4	108.2
75 - 84	146.5	144.6	55.0	144.9
85+	200.2	200.6	74.7	198.8
All ages[a]	32.7	38.0	14.1	32.8

[a]Age adjusted to the 1990 US female population. Data obtained from CDC WONDER.

needed to design effective breast cancer prevention and control programs.

Place Analyses

A second type of analysis involves comparing the occurrence of a disease, condition, or risk factor between one geographic region and another. Typically, the rate in a city or county is compared with rates for the rest of the state or the nation. This information may be used to target a specific intervention in a region.[21] Figure 3.3 shows the differences in breast cancer mortality between states in the United States.

Regional analyses must account for differences in age structure between regions by using age-standardized rates. In addition, regional differences in disease rates may result from differences in diagnostic practices and/or disease definitions. Finally, these analyses are often limited because of the small number of cases typically occurring in small regions, such as cities, villages, or towns.

A specialized form of regional analysis involves the analysis of diseases that appear to "cluster" in a geographic area, such as a cluster of cancer cases that occur in a neighbor-hood. The investigation of these disease clusters poses a continuing challenge to state and local public health officials. Most often these

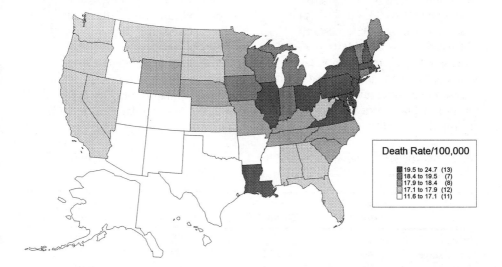

Death Rate/100,000

■ 19.5 to 24.7 (13)
▨ 18.4 to 19.5 (7)
▧ 17.9 to 18.4 (8)
▨ 17.1 to 17.9 (12)
□ 11.6 to 17.1 (11)

Figure 3.3—Female breast cancer mortality rates by state, age-adjusted to the 1990 US female population, 1990-1994.

disease clusters are reported by the public or by clinicians who are looking for explanations for the apparent increase in the incidence of a disease. For example, in response to a request from a legislator, the Wisconsin Division of Health analyzed breast cancer rates among women living in neighborhoods north of Milwaukee. This analysis found higher rates of breast cancer incidence and deaths in this community that might be attributable to differences in breast cancer risk factors in the community[22] (Table 3.5).

Public health agencies have developed systematic protocols to aid in the investigation of these apparent disease clusters.[23,24] These procedures involve defining the population at risk, ascertaining all cases, estimating rate ratios (ie, observed versus expected), and assessing exposure and biologic plausibility. Using this approach, few investigations identify specific environmental exposures responsible for the disease cluster. A major

difficulty in studying such clusters involves the small number of disease cases available for analysis. In fact, Rothman states that, with very few exceptions, there is little scientific or public health purpose in investigating individual disease clusters at all.[25]

Time Analyses

Finally, and perhaps most importantly, chronic disease surveillance systems must monitor the trends in chronic disease rates over time. The epidemic curve traditionally has been used to detect outbreaks, to better characterize transmission patterns, and to determine appropriate intervention strategies. Similarly, age-adjusted trends in smoking prevalence rates, per capita cigarette sales, and lung cancer mortality rates have been used to monitor the effects of tobacco use on health.[26–28]

Temporal trend analyses must consider changes in the age structure of the population over time, usually by using age standardization with a standard reference population. In

Table 3.5—Breast Cancer Mortality and Incidence in Milwaukee's North Shore Communities, 1989-1994

	Observed Number	Expected Number	Difference	p Value
Cases	394	336	+58	<0.01
Early stage	282	213	+69	<0.001
Late stage	94	104	-10	Not significant
Deaths	108	87	+21	<0.05

Note: From Remington and Park.[22]

addition, changes in diagnostic practices and disease definitions may cause apparent trends in disease incidence over time. Both temporal trend and regional analyses may be done for specific subgroups of the population. For example, although the rates of breast cancer appear to be declining among White women in the United States, they appear to be increasing among Black women (Figure 3.4). These findings have important implications in the development of programs to extend the progress seen among some groups, to the entire population.

DATA DISSEMINATION

The final step in chronic disease surveillance is to disseminate the information that has been collected. The increasing amount of surveillance data described above provides a wealth of information to public health agencies. However, too often these agencies simply analyze the data and report the results in agency reports or occasionally in state or national publications. These reports are often long and contain technical jargon. In addition, the information is seldom linked to program priorities, and the

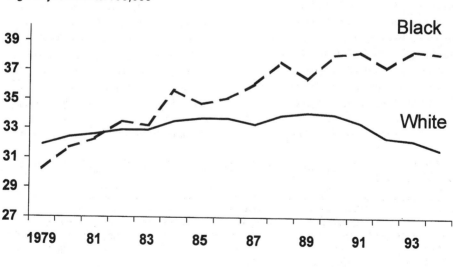

Figure 3.4—Trends in age-adjusted female breast cancer mortality rates in the United States, by race, 1979-1994.

reports are seldom used to promote public health practice or as a vehicle for setting priorities for action.

In the past, communicable disease surveillance systems typically produced surveillance reports and distributed them to health care providers. Today's chronic disease programs address a broader constituency, including policy makers, voluntary health organizations, professional organizations, and the general public. Thus, the information must be communicated through several channels using different strategies to assure that it reaches the appropriate target groups.

Epidemiologists working in public health agencies are frequently asked to disseminate the results of a surveillance report, often by publishing the information in a health department report. To increase application of surveillance findings to disease prevention and health promotion programs, a basic framework for communicating surveillance information can be used[29, 30] (Table 3.6).

Once the analysis has been completed, this framework has five additional steps:

Establish the Message

This is perhaps the most important step in disseminating health and surveillance information. Like businesses, public health agencies have a product (ie, information) that they need to sell (ie, communicate). An epidemiologist must convince the audience that it is worth their time to read, understand, and act on the information. An important adage in marketing the message is that "less is more."

Many reports produced by public health agencies are long, technical, and full of information. These reports might be mailed to the media, policy makers, or health care providers who, in turn, rarely take the time to read through the report to find the impor-

Table 3.6—Steps in Communicating Public Health Surveillance Information

Step	Question	Action
1	What do the data show?	Conduct the analysis
2	What should be said?	Establish the message
3	What is the communication objective?	Set an objective
4	To whom should the message be directed?	Define the audience
5	What communications medium should be used?	Select the channel
6	Was the communication objective achieved?	Evaluate the impact

Note: From Remington.[29]

tant information. In order to capture their attention, the main point of the report must be obvious and simple to understand. For example, the main message of the report describing the trends in breast cancer in the United States would be that these trends are different for Black and White women.

Set an Objective

Why is the information being reported? Public health agencies often report information without any specific goal, but simply "because it is there." Other times, the purpose is to educate the general public about a health issue. This is a worthy, but challenging goal, given the complexity of the message and the inability to shape the message for the intended audience.

Occasionally, surveillance findings point to a needed public health action. For example, the findings of increasing breast cancer mortality among Black women emphasize the need for effective breast cancer screening initiatives. Therefore, the intent of releasing this information might be to support a public health initiative, such the National Breast and Cervical Cancer Early Detection Program.

Define the Audience

Once the objective for communicating the information has been established, one can define the appropriate target audience. Local health departments and health care providers have been the long-standing audience of communicable disease surveillance information, since these professionals were responsible for implementing disease control strategies. In addition, physicians were the source of these reports, and reporting back to them showed the usefulness of the system and helped maintain their continued reporting.

The audience for public health surveillance information is much broader today and includes policy makers, voluntary health organizations, professional organizations, and the general public. A report that breast cancer death rates are increasing among Black women in a state could be communicated to the general public, or to women specifically. This would increase awareness of the importance of mammography and early detection. It might also be targeted to policy makers, such as legislators considering developing a breast cancer detection program focused on reducing breast cancer deaths among Black women. Finally, the report could be given to an advocacy organization, such as a statewide minority health council, to use in their efforts to advocate for minority health.

Select the Channel

A "channel" can be considered the medium through which messages must travel to reach the intended audience. Examples of channels include professional journals, direct mail, television, radio, or newspapers. Public health agencies traditionally report surveillance information in newsletters or statistical bulletins. These reports are routinely mailed to local public health agencies, physicians, health care institutions, the media, and other interested individuals in the community or the state. A press release is occasionally used to increase the media interest in the story.

Careful selection of a proper communication channel increases the likelihood that the information will reach the target audience. This requires a thorough understanding, based on market research, on how those individuals get their information. For example, children and teachers might best be reached through the school system newsletter. Policy makers might be reached through a direct mailing to their offices or via a constituent organization. Doctors might be reached through a state medical society journal.

In an effort to bring public health surveillance information to Wisconsin's doctors, the Wisconsin Division of Health established a "public health column" in the *Wisconsin Medical Journal*, the monthly journal of the state's medical society. Each month, one or more brief articles are published, present-

ing a wide variety of surveillance information. These articles are often cited in the media and are widely quoted by the journal's readership. This series represents one of the channels that a state division of health can use to bring information to the medical and health care community.

In addition, creative presentation of information can increase the media coverage of a health issue. An oft-cited example involves reporting the health impact from cigarette smoking in the United States. The government reports that over 400 000 persons die each year from smoking-related diseases. This health burden can be equated with the lives lost if two fully loaded 747s crashed every day for a year.

Evaluate the Impact

The final step in a communication plan is to evaluate how widely the information was disseminated and whether the information led to the intended outcome. The dissemination can be measured by determining the number of reports distributed, the readership of a journal, or by assessing the coverage in the media. Newspaper clipping services will search for all articles in a defined geographic area and provide copies of each article with the selected "key words." These articles can be reviewed by the program staff to assess the geographic distribution and extent of the media coverage. In addition, the content of the clippings can be reviewed to assess both the accuracy and appropriateness of the messages.

Determining the impact of the communication effort on public health action requires an evaluation of changes in outcomes, such as knowledge, behaviors, or disease rates. This type of evaluation often requires surveys of the target population before and after the surveillance information has been disseminated to detect these changes. These evaluations are often expensive, time-consuming, and difficult to interpret.

CONCLUSION

Data collection, analysis, and dissemination are important components of a chronic disease surveillance system. The final link in surveillance is the application of the data to prevention and control.[1] The long latency period of most chronic diseases often results in a perceived lack of urgency in developing and implementing control measures. For example, if the lung cancer epidemic that has evolved over the past three decades instead evolved over days or weeks, more public attention and resources would have been dedicated to prevention efforts. Therefore, the simple tabulation and reporting of increasing death rates

due to lung cancer over the past 30 years does not constitute a "public health surveillance system" unless these data are actively incorporated into a public health control program.

Recently, the importance of surveillance in chronic disease control has been acknowledged. The Institute of Medicine's report *The Future of Public Health* emphasizes that assessment is a key responsibility of public health, one that cannot be delegated to others.[31] State health departments are more frequently using chronic disease surveillance information to guide programs.[3,21] As more surveillance data are incorporated into chronic disease prevention and control programs, greater resources and public attention will be devoted to these important public health problems.

RERERENCES

1. Thacker SB, Berkelman RL. Public health surveillance in the United States. *Epidemiol Rev.* 1988;10:164–190.
2. Langmuir AD. The surveillance of communicable diseases of national importance. *N Engl J Med.* 1963;288:182–192.
3. Berkelman RL, Buehler JW. Public health surveillance of noninfectious chronic disease: the potential to detect rapid changes in disease burden. *Int J Epidemiol.* 1990;19:628–635.

4. Boss LP, Suarez L. Uses of data to plan cancer prevention and control programs. *Public Health Rep.* 1990;105:354–360.

5. Stroup NE, Zack MM, Wharton M. Sources of routinely collected data for surveillance. In: Teutsch SM, Churchill RE, eds. *Principles and Practice of Public Health Surveillance.* New York, NY: Oxford University Press, Inc; 1993.

6. Chapin CV. State health organization. *JAMA.* 1916;66:699–703.

7. Kirscher T, Anderson RE. Cause of death: proper completion of the death certificate. *JAMA.* 1987;258:349–352.

8. Centers for Disease Control. Sensitivity of death certificate data for monitoring diabetes mortality—Diabetic Eye Disease Follow-up Study, 1985–1990. *MMWR.* 1991;40:739–741.

9. Office of Surveillance and Analysis. *Using Chronic Disease Data: A Handbook for Public Health Practitioners.* Atlanta, Ga: National Center for Chronic Disease Prevention and Health Promotion, Centers for Disease Control; 1992.

10. Centers for Disease Control. Wide-ranging ONline Data for Epidemiologic Research (WONDER). USPHS, DHSS. June 1992.

11. *SENSOR: Sentinel Event Notification System for Occupational Risks.* Atlanta, Ga: US Department of Health and Human Services, Public Health Service, Centers for Disease Control, National Institute for Occupational Safety and Health; 1987.

12. Austin DF. Cancer registries: a tool in epidemiology. *Rev Cancer Epidemiol.* 1983;2:118–140.

13. Jackson C, Jatulis DE, Fortmann SP. The Behavioral Risk Factor Survey and the Stanford Five-City Project Survey: a comparison of cardiovascular risk behavior estimates. *Am J Public Health.* 1992;82:412–416.

14. Kann L, Warren CW, Harris WA, et al. Youth Risk Behavior Surveillance —United States, 1995. *MMWR* 1996;45(SS-4);1–83.

15. Centers for Disease Control. Lower extremity amputations among persons with diabetes–Washington; 1988. *MMWR.* 1991; 40:737–739.

16. *International Classification of Diseases, 9th Revision, Clinical Modification.* 2nd ed. Washington, DC: US Department of Health and Human Services; 1980. DHHS publication PHS 80-1260.

17. Centers for Disease Control. Cerebrovascular disease mortality and Medicare hospitalization—United States, 1980–1990. *MMWR.* 1992;41:477–480.

18. Chassin MR, Hannan EL, DeBuono BA. Benefits and hazards of reporting medical

outcomes publicly. *New Engl J Med.* 1996;334:394–398.

19. Iglehart JK. *The National Committee for Quality Assurance.* 1996;335:995–999.

20. Roos LL, Mustard CA, Nicol JP et al. Registries and administrative data: organization and accuracy. *Medical Care* 1993;31(3)201–212.

21. Brownson RC, Smith CA, Jorge NE, et al. The role of data-driven planning and coalition development in preventing cardiovascular disease. Public Health Rep. 1992;107:32–37.

22. Remington PL, Park S. Breast cancer incidence and mortality in Milwaukee's North Shore communities. *Wis Med J* 1997 March;96(3):46–47.

23. Fiore BJ, Hanrahan LP, Anderson HA. State health department response to disease cluster reports: a protocol for investigation. *Am J Epidemiol.* 1990;132(suppl 1):S14–S22.

24. Devier JR, Brownson RC, Bagby JR, Carlson GM, Crellin JR. A public health response to cancer clusters in Missouri. *Am J Epidemiol.* 1990;132(suppl 1):S23-S31.

25. Rothman KJ. A sobering start for the cluster buster's conference. *Am J Epidemiol.* 1990;132(suppl 1):S6–S13.

26. Remington PL, Fiore M. Trends in lung cancer mortality in Wisconsin. *Wis Med J.* 1989;88:34,36,38.

27. Peterson DE, Remington PL. Publicity, policy, and trends in cigarette smoking: Wisconsin 1950–1988. *Wis Med J.* 1989;88:40,42.

28. Remington PL, Anderson HA. Trends in cigarette smoking—Wisconsin, 1950–1988. *MMWR.* 1989;38:752–754.

29. Remington PL. Communicating epidemiologic information. In: Brownson RC, Petitti DB, eds. *Applied Epidemiology: Theory to Practice.* New York, NY: Oxford University Press, Inc; 1998:323–348.

30. Goodman R, Remington PL. Disseminating surveillance information. In: Teutsch SM, Churchill RE, eds. *Principles and Practice of Public Health Surveillance.* New York, NY: Oxford University Press, Inc; 1993.

31. Committee for the Study of the Future of Public Health. *The Future of Public Health.* Washington, DC: National Academy Press; 1988.

RESOURCES

Information on the availability of routinely collected chronic disease surveillance data are available from a variety of federal agencies:

- Centers for Disease Control and Prevention (CDC), including the National Center for Health Statistics, the National Center for

Chronic Disease Prevention and Health Promotion, and the Epidemiology Program Office (http://www.cdc.gov)

- National Institute of Health (NIH), including the National Cancer Institute (NCI), the National Heart, Lung, and Blood Institute (NHLBI), and the National Institute on Drug Abuse (NIDA) (http://www.nih.gov)

- Agency for Health Care Planning and Research (AHCPR)
- Health Care Financing Administration (HCFA)
- Bureau of the Census

In addition, mortality, disease registry, and behavioral risk factor surveillance information can be obtained from state health departments and many local public health agencies.

INTERVENTION METHODS FOR CHRONIC DISEASE CONTROL

This chapter provides an overview of chronic disease control intervention methods that can be used to address many of the risk factors discussed in Chapters 5 through 16. It includes a brief review of the basic psychological, sociological, and communication research supporting chronic disease control and distills a core set of principles for developing effective interventions. It identifies and characterizes basic intervention strategies and channels that are commonly used in chronic disease control. The latter sections of the chapter discuss practical issues such as coalition development, intervention planning, and program management. Examples are provided throughout the chapter to illustrate the principles and strategies that are discussed.

James R. Davis, PhD
Randy Schwartz, MSPH
Fran Wheeler, PhD
R. Brick Lancaster, MA, CHES

THE SCOPE OF CHRONIC DISEASE CONTROL

Chronic disease control interventions can focus at the individual level, at the system level, or at the community level, where both system-level and individual approaches are integrated into a comprehensive program. Interventions can address disease prevention, early detection, treatment, and/or management.

Many preventive interventions seek to change health risk behaviors by targeting messages directly at the individual. Primary risk factors for disease such as poor diet, tobacco use, alcohol consumption, physical inactivity, and noncompliance with work site safety precautions often are approached in this manner. Messages can be delivered through written materials, the mass media, health professionals, school teachers, and other individuals with direct access to high-risk populations.

Messages that are targeted at individuals also are used to encourage screening and compliance with treatment recommendations. These chronic disease control interventions are particularly important for identifying and treating cancer, diabetes, high blood pressure, and high blood cholesterol. Health care professionals usually play a major role in these interventions, but messages also can be delivered in written materials, by the mass media, and by other individuals in the community. Interactive computer systems also are becoming available for communicating health messages to patients and other consumers.

Managing the complications of disease and ensuring a continued quality of life are frequent goals of chronic disease control interventions. Examples include self-management of blood glucose by individuals with diabetes and regular exercise by heart disease patients. Health professionals are almost always involved in these interventions; however, written materials, family members, and self-help groups often play major support roles in maintaining long-term health behaviors.

Other chronic disease control interventions target specific system-level changes, including policies, economic factors, and professional behaviors. These interventions address issues such as mandatory nutrition labeling, insurance coverage for mammography, tobacco taxes, and the health care professional's recognition and treatment of tobacco use as an addictive behavior. They often include health advocacy communications that are directed at the broader community as well as at decision makers.

The most comprehensive interventions seek to change multiple aspects of the community environment that predispose people to develop chronic diseases. These interventions include a combination of activities that target changes in individual behavior as well as system-level change. These interventions often address the health inequities between high- and low-income populations. They seek to influence the social acceptability of harmful behaviors like drinking and driving, public smoking, and polluting the environment. Occasionally, these interventions will directly address the roots of chronic disease—that is, poverty and limited education. They also may attempt to provide widespread social support for positive health behaviors such as regular exercise, screening, and compliance with work site safety precautions. These interventions usually involve health advocacy and often require empowerment of individuals or communities to take action.[1-3]

THE SCIENTIFIC BASES OF CHRONIC DISEASE CONTROL INTERVENTIONS

Numerous studies have clearly demonstrated the major role of individual behavior change in chronic disease control.[4] Approximately one million deaths each year in the United States are attributable to four behavior-related disease precursors: tobacco use, high blood pressure, excess calorie and fat consumption, and alcohol consumption.[5]

Behavior change also is a factor in the success of chronic disease control interventions that target system-level changes. In order to reduce occupational hazards, corporate managers and direct supervisors will be required to change their behaviors. Changes in the economic and social conditions that cause chronic diseases will require changes in the behavior of policy makers, community leaders, and other decision makers.

Behavior change and maintenance strategies have been developed from basic psychology, sociology, and communications research. Research studies have demonstrated the difference between behavior change and preliminary increases in knowledge or changes in attitudes. The transtheoretical model of behavior change identifies several stages in the process of change.[6] Individuals move from a precontemplative stage through contemplative, action, and maintenance stages that lead to long-term health behavior change. A specific population segment may, on the whole, be at an earlier or later stage of change compared to another population segment. Different individuals within a population (eg, work site) also may be at different stages in the behavior change process.

Other research has identified the health beliefs that are most highly correlated with positive health behavior (ie, the health belief model). These beliefs include the person's perception of (1) personal susceptibility to the disease in question, (2) severity of the disease, (3) benefits of preventive actions or treatment, and (4) barriers to taking the recommended actions.[7, 8]

Numerous studies have examined the individual and identified characteristics that support or impede behavior change. Research on health locus of control has shown that health behaviors are motivated internally for some individuals and externally for others.[9, 10] For example, a self-help weight-loss intervention would be suitable for someone with an internal locus of control, whereas physician counseling or a work site program would be more effective for someone with an external locus of control.

Research by several investigators has examined behavioral intentions and found that they are related to two key factors: personal attitudes and perceived social norms.[11-14] Personal attitudes are a function of the belief that a specific outcome will result from a behavior as well as the value that is placed on the outcome. Perceived social norms are a function of what the individual perceives others believe should be done and of the individual's motivation to meet the expectations of others.

Other research has examined persuasive communication and has identified steps that individuals must pass through to change behavior.[15] These steps include exposure to, attention to, interest in, and understanding of a message; accepting and personalizing the message; remembering to incorporate the message in decision making; conducting the behavior; and receiving positive reinforcement for the behavior. Variables that determine the effectiveness of persuasive communications include the credibility of the message source, the content of the message, the delivery channel, the target audience, and the desired behavior.[16]

Social marketing studies have examined how to develop and disseminate health messages.[17] This research shows that the consumer should be the primary focus of all intervention strategies.[18] Program managers should fully understand the target audience and design messages or products that meet the needs of consumers, not the needs of the intervention program. Complete understanding of consumers requires information on community norms, peer influences, personal characteristics, and economic resources. Target audiences frequently must be segmented into homogeneous subgroups before program managers can develop messages that will result in behavior change.

The above findings have been expanded by social cognitive theory to include several concepts that provide guidance in developing interventions.[19] The concept of self-efficacy explores the individual's beliefs concerning his or her personal ability to make desired behavior changes.[20, 21] This includes the individual's assessment of personal knowledge and skills as well as the likely outcome of an effort to change behavior. The concept of modeling or observational behavior examines the direct influences of other individuals in the social environment and suggests opportunities for interventions, such as peer role models in school health education.[22] The concept of self-management explains a process of replacing external control of behavior with internal control of behavior. Strategies based on this concept establish internal cues that must come into play at specific times and places—for example, conscious avoidance of smoking after meals. Recent work has shown the importance of reinforcing self-management strategies with changes at the institutional and community level.[23] Concepts related to patient self-management have recently received increased attention in the literature and health policy discussions, associated with the growing emphasis on managed care and integrated health systems.

Social research has examined the health effects of individuals and population segments taking control of the interpersonal, economic, political, and social forces that affect their lives.[24–26] Empowerment of individuals and populations has led directly to individual health improvement and has influenced the broader determinants of health (eg, economic conditions, education). Empowered community leadership on specific health issues (eg, increased physical activity) also can enhance positive social norms that prompt and reinforce individual behavior change.

Research has also examined the impact of interventions that target system-level changes. The effects of economic incentives, changes in health policies, and promotion of professional norms have been demonstrated. Several studies have quantified the effects of economic factors on health-risk behaviors. These studies most often have focused on the impact of tobacco tax

increases on smoking rates.[27] Lewit and Coate found that increasing the federal excise tax on cigarettes in 1981 from $0.08 to $0.16 would result in a 4.8% decrease in smoking by the total US population.[28] Smoking among men aged 20 through 25 would decrease by as much as 16%. A more recent review article found that an increase of 10% in the price of cigarettes would cause a 3% to 5% decline in cigarette consumption.[29]

Other studies have documented the impact of policy changes on health-risk behaviors. Several investigators have examined the effects on smoking rates of restricting public smoking.[30] One study found a 17% decrease in the smoking rate among a work site population following the introduction of a no-smoking policy.[31] A second study found a 21% decrease in the smoking rate among soldiers after implementation of a no-smoking policy and an education program.[32]

Several investigators have examined peer group interactions that effect changes in professional behavior among health, education, and other professionals.[33] Interpersonal influences (eg, persuasion, role modeling) often are the most important factors in the adoption of new practices by professionals.

Other investigators have examined the effects of professional publications on professional behavior change. One study conducted by the

National Heart, Lung, and Blood Institute detected a substantial change in physicians' attitudes and practices regarding cholesterol levels following the release of results from the Lipid Research Clinics Coronary Primary Prevention Trial.[34] The percent of physicians who believed that interventions to reduce serum cholesterol levels would reduce the risk of coronary heart disease increased from 39% in 1983 to 64% in 1985.

Major community-based chronic disease control projects have demonstrated the success of interventions that address both individual behavior change and system-level change. The majority of the projects have focused on cardiovascular disease prevention (see Chapter 5). They include the North Karelia Project in Finland,[35,36] the Stanford Five-City Project,[37,38] the Pawtucket Heart Health Program,[39,40] the Minnesota Heart Health Program,[41] and others.[42] The ultimate goal of most of these interventions has been to modify the environment that influences health behaviors. The projects have included interventions delivered by the mass media, health professionals, education professionals, community leaders, coworkers, neighbors, friends, family members, and other individuals in the community.

During the past decade, there has been a significant growth in Healthy Cities / Healthy Communities initiatives in the United States. The Healthy Cities / Healthy Communities approach is based in the Canadian and European sociopolitical context of addressing the root causes of public health problems.[43,44] These interventions are based on the recognition that chronic disease problems must be addressed through an ecological model.[45,46] The ecological model "presents health as a product of the interdependence between the individual and subsystems of the ecosystem (family, community, culture, etc.). To promote health, this ecosystem must offer economic and social conditions conducive to health."[47] Healthy Communities uses citizen participation and "a collaborative problem-solving process that allows a broad spectrum of community stakeholders to create a vision of health and implement a plan to turn its vision into reality."[44] For example, a community wishing to address the contribution of tobacco to ill health will focus on such policy or environmental change strategies as creating smoke-free environments, restricting youth access to tobacco products, or restricting tobacco advertising.

THE BASIC PRINCIPLES OF CHRONIC DISEASE CONTROL INTERVENTIONS

The development of chronic disease control interventions has been guided by health promotion theory, research results, and direct experience from community-based interventions. Several basic principles can be distilled from theory, research results, and successful programs (Table 4.1).

1. Comprehensive approaches that address the economic, social, and political roots of health and sickness have proven to be more effective than traditional education approaches. New concepts of empowerment and community participation should be combined with direct efforts to modify lifestyles and specific health behaviors. Health advocates should remain aware of the lifestyle determinants of health and sickness but address these issues in the context of economic, social, and political forces. An important role of health advocates is to assure conditions in which people can be healthy by addressing issues of poverty, limited education, unemployment, discrimination, and poor access to information.[48]

2. Changes in underlying community norms are another key to *widespread and long-term improvements in health.*[3, 27, 42] To a large extent, individual health is determined by social expectations for personal health behavior. Affecting community norms concerning personal health behavior is an effective way to improve health. Interventions that facilitate frequent, value-laden communication among family members and peers concerning the basic determinants of health can influence community norms and can lead to widespread, long-term changes in health. Interventions that focus on changing community norms can mobilize the tremendous resources of neighborhoods, families, and other naturally occurring social groups.

3. Community-based approaches that target the whole population will contribute the most to reducing chronic disease mortality.[49] Several approaches are commonly used to reduce chronic disease mortality. The traditional medical approach focuses on individuals with disease and

Table 4.1—Key Concepts of Chronic Disease Control Interventions

Strategies focused on community norms
Community-based approach targeting the whole population
Active involvement of the priority population
Active involvement of community organizations
Clearly defined objectives
Strategies based on the needs of the priority population
Multiple intervention strategies
Ongoing evaluation

attempts to effectively address acute episodes—for example, providing emergency medical services for cardiovascular disease patients. The high-risk prevention approach seeks to identify at-risk individuals through screening and to provide intensive interventions that reduce the risk of disease—for example, screening for hypertension and using medications to reduce blood pressure. The community-based primary prevention approach attempts to reduce the risk of disease in the entire population— for example, by encouraging low-fat diets.[50] This third strategy generally has the greatest impact on total disease burden because it reaches a large number of individuals who are at relatively low risk of disease. The most effective interventions use high-risk prevention within the larger context of a community-based primary prevention approach.[51]

4. A chronic disease control program will be more effective if the at-risk population is actively involved in prioritizing, developing, and implementing all intervention activities.[39, 52–56] A full partnership between health professionals and local citizens can empower individuals and groups to be more effective in managing their own lives and influencing the broader economic, social, and political forces in the community. Initially, participation of local citizens provides a more accurate assessment of the commu-

nity, including its knowledge of and attitudes toward health issues, the priority health issues of the community, and the available resources within the community. Participation also facilitates community ownership of the intervention, which may provide better access to community leaders and ultimately influence changes in community norms affecting health issues. In addition, participation by local citizens shapes the intervention to fit the norms and values of the community and to ensure that the proposed intervention is culturally sensitive. Local citizens can play a key leadership role in intervention planning through community coalitions. They also can be involved in implementing the intervention by serving as paid health paraprofessionals, by coordinating local intervention activities (eg, activating a grassroots lobbying network), or by providing access to decision makers who influence the outcome of policy interventions.

5. A chronic disease control program will be more effective if community organizations (eg, schools, churches, social clubs) are actively involved in developing and implementing the intervention.[54] The participation of these mediating organizations will provide many of the same benefits as participation by at-risk population members. However, the participation of local organizations can strengthen these contributions (eg, by enhancing access to decision makers), provide extensive resources for implementing interventions, and facilitate long-term maintenance of the intervention. Representatives from community organizations should be involved in intervention planning as full partners. The entire community organization can be involved in implementing the intervention by providing access to organization members, adding local legitimacy to media communications, and coordinating local intervention activities.

6. *Chronic disease control interventions should build on traditional practices and cultural norms.* Communities and even segments within communities may have unique world views, priorities, social expectations, and cultural norms. Health advocates must understand these factors and help design interventions that fit the specific community. Local knowledge must be incorporated into new interventions. In some communities, new programs can be adapted to local conditions by linking them to existing programs. In other cases, expansion of an existing program may be the best way to accomplish new goals. Formative and process evaluation involving representatives from the community must be conducted to ensure that programs are meeting community needs and that interventions can be adapted if

programs are not accomplishing their goals.

7. *Clearly defined objectives are essential for planning and implementing effective interventions.*[16] An intervention objective should include a clear identification of the health issue or risk factor being addressed, the at-risk population that is being addressed, the current status of the health issue or risk factor in the at-risk population, and the desired outcome of the intervention. A clearly defined objective can guide both the development of intervention content and the selection of appropriate communication channels. It also facilitates the development of quantitative evaluation measures that can be used to monitor the success of the intervention and to identify opportunities for improvement. Most important, a clearly defined objective will improve the coordination of activities among the various organizations participating in the intervention.

8. *Intervention strategies should be selected based on the needs of the specific at-risk population.*[16, 17] A complete understanding of the at-risk population is necessary to identify appropriate interventions that are compatible with the population's knowledge, attitudes, perceptions, and economic circumstances. System-level interventions that focus on policies, economic incentives, or organizational change will affect

different populations in different ways. Communication messages that do not meet the needs of the specific population will be ignored. Understanding the specific population is also essential for identifying appropriate communication channels (eg, the media, the health care system, the work site). Different social, cultural, and economic circumstances require different channels for the successful delivery of messages.

9. *Multiple intervention strategies will increase the effectiveness of health programs.*[57] Multiple intervention strategies are essential for establishing and maintaining community norms that enable system-level changes and changes in individual health behaviors. In general, single strategies are more likely to be overwhelmed by the broader community conditions and norms that determine health.

10. *Effective interventions require ongoing evaluation and the appropriate adjustment of strategies.*[16] Incomplete knowledge of at-risk populations, social conditions, communication channels, and future events precludes the planning of a fully effective intervention. As new information is encountered or problems arise in implementing intervention components, program managers must evaluate the impact on achievement of the intervention objectives. By initially linking evaluation methods to quantifiable objectives and well-defined process measures, program managers can easily assess the situation and make rapid changes in strategies.

INTERVENTION STRATEGIES

This section describes several different types of interventions that have been used in comprehensive community-based intervention programs. In practice, these types of interventions are integrated in a mutually reinforcing way that provides multiple strategies with multiple messages.

Modify Community Conditions and Norms

Programs that directly address health-related community conditions and norms can have a substantial impact on health. These interventions generally seek to empower individuals or groups in the community, work site, or family to affect changes in community conditions or norms that directly affect them or their families. Interventions often include components to increase knowledge, to frame an issue as a legitimate social issue, and to facilitate dialogue about the issue.

Community conditions and norms can be changed, to some degree, through all of the channels discussed in the following section, but media advocacy and mobilization of community organizations are among the most effective strategies. Media advocacy can create awareness of a social issue, initiate controversy concerning the issue, and prompt local advocacy for change. The involvement of a community organization can provide access to community leaders who can frame the issue as a legitimate community issue and can encourage members of the organization to become involved in local advocacy efforts.

The most important role of health advocates in this type of intervention is to empower individuals or groups in the community to take action.[58] Health advocates can assist in defining health problems, accessing information for developing solutions, supporting local leadership, strengthening local mediating organizations by increasing citizen participation, increasing local problem solving skills, and linking communities with problems to communities that have solved the problems.[59, 60] The successful health advocate must often place a higher priority on local empowerment than on accomplishing specific health objectives that were set by external agencies or organizations. This can be accomplished by creating an atmosphere and program structure where local citizens can take control of the program and intervention activities.

A familiar example of the change that can result from this type of intervention is the tremendous shift that has occurred in the social acceptability of public smoking.[27] Ten years ago, secondhand tobacco smoke was perceived as an acceptable component of indoor air, and very few people even considered speaking out against it. Aggressive media advocacy for nonsmokers' rights and the involvement of community leaders in efforts to pass clean indoor air legislation have empowered individuals to speak out. The designation of secondhand tobacco smoke as a major cancer causing agent is likely to further accelerate this trend.[61]

Establish and Enforce Health Policies

Health policies can be effective in changing health behaviors and initiating system-level changes that promote health.[27, 58] An extremely wide array of policies can affect health. Health policies can be established at the federal, state, and community levels (eg, laws and local ordinances) and at the organizational level (eg, association accreditation standards, mandatory work site policies, and voluntary community organization policies). Examples include requirements for food labeling; requirements for certification of breast cancer screening facilities and cytology laboratories; restrictions on public smoking, the sale of tobacco to minors, tobacco vending machines, and tobacco advertising; requirements for workplace safety; and environmental protection laws.

Health policies can be promoted through several channels. In addition to directly focusing on legislators to pass laws and local ordinances, policy advocates often must garner media support and mobilize community organizations to form a grassroots network. Establishing meaningful public policies usually requires changes in the community norms that influence policy decision makers. An effective comprehensive strategy is needed to combine direct public policy advocacy with interventions focused on community norms. Other important health policies can be pursued through work sites, health institutions, health professional associations, school systems, and community organizations.

Adoption of work site smoking policies has expanded dramatically over the past decade. Work site policies severely restricting or banning smoking protect employees and visitors from the detrimental effects of involuntary exposure to secondhand tobacco smoke. Research also has shown that work site smoking policies contribute to reducing smoking among employees. A smoke-free policy in the Duke University Medical Center resulted in a significantly increased smoking cessation rate of 22.5% compared to adjacent buildings on the campus.[62] A study in California found that work

site smoking policies encourage changes in smoking behavior and that individuals who leave a work site with a strong policy may increase their cigarette consumption if they obtain employment in a work site that allows smoking in work areas.[63] Another study found that work site smoking restrictions altered daytime smoking patterns and reduced cotinine levels (a chemical biomarker of smoking behavior).[64]

The enforcement of a health policy is as important as the initial development of the policy. Policy enforcement probably will be the responsibility of a different individual or agency. Specific intervention efforts also need to be directed at this individual or agency to ensure that a policy is fully enforced. Unfortunately, responsibility for policy enforcement is often ambiguous. In such cases, community norms must be promoted that motivate and empower local citizens to request enforcement by local agencies.

Establish Economic Incentives

The purposes of economic incentives are to directly change individual health behaviors and to reinforce system-level changes that affect health. Incentives that focus on health behavior include tobacco taxes, weight loss contests, and reduced insurance rates for safe drivers. Incentives that influence system-level changes include fines for industries that violate worker safety regulations, Medicare reimbursement for mammography screening, reduced insurance rates for work sites that offer health promotion programs, and insurance reimbursement to physicians for nicotine replacement therapy.

Economic incentives can be promoted through several channels, including work sites and public policy makers. As is true with other types of policies, community norms often need to be modified to support changes in economic incentives. Thus, media advocacy and mobilization of community organizations also may be important for successful economic interventions.

Enhance Knowledge and Skills

Traditional health education programs seek to enhance individual knowledge and skills to support changes in health behavior. Major examples include diabetes self-management, comprehensive school health education, and weight loss programs. Although knowledge and skills do not necessarily result in behavior change, they usually are required before other broader social forces can influence behavior change.

Health education can be provided through all of the channels discussed in the next section. The mass media, health care professionals, and school personnel are most commonly involved in these types of interventions. All of the planning steps described in the Intervention Planning Steps section (p. 69) apply directly to knowledge and skills enhancement.

Provide Screening and Follow-Up Services

The purposes of screening and follow-up services are to detect and treat disease at an early, curable stage. Examples include screening for hypertension, cholesterol, diabetes, and cancer. Although these interventions appear to be straightforward, they are complex and require careful attention to several issues. In addition to providing the screening service, program managers also need to motivate the public to participate in screening, establish rigorous screening quality standards, train health professionals in proper screening and follow-up procedures, track all clients with detected disease, ensure treatment for all clients with detected disease, and motivate clients to fully participate in the recommended treatment.

Screening and follow-up services are almost always provided by health professionals. However, the cost and labor associated with these services can be moderated through collaboration with other organizations. Screening services are often provided through work sites and community organizations.

Several intervention channels provide opportunities for reaching individuals with health messages or making system-level changes to support healthy communities. The initiators and planners of chronic disease control programs can personally implement interventions through these channels; they can collaborate closely with several individuals or institutions in the channel (eg, school teachers) to implement interventions; or they can develop strategies to encourage the implementation of interventions by all individuals or institutions in the channel.

Health Care System

The health care system is a very effective channel for implementing chronic disease control interventions.[4, 27, 65–69] The United States is undergoing a rapid and extensive change in how health care systems are organized and what services they provide. Managed care organizations and integrated health systems have an increased presence and mission to interact with public health, work sites, and other community settings to prevent disease in the communities where they provide services. Many states and major employers who are the primary purchasers of health care services have begun to designate required prevention

services in contracts, clinical guidelines, and community benefit accountability standards. This provides new opportunities for chronic disease surveillance, prevention, and disease self-management.

The types of clinical health care settings that are appropriate for interventions include public health agencies, federally funded community health clinics, family planning clinics, private physician and dental practices, and hospitals. Physicians, dentists, nurses, health educators, dental hygienists, occupational therapists, nutritionists, dietitians, support staff, and volunteers can all contribute to interventions that are implemented in these clinical health care settings.

The health care system is most effective for providing screening and follow-up services. Model screening and follow-up interventions include the National High Blood Pressure Control Program, funded by the National Institutes of Health,[70] and the Breast and Cervical Cancer Control Project, funded by the national Centers for Disease Control and Prevention.[71]

The health care system can enhance the knowledge and skills of patients through direct health education.[72, 73] Effective health education by those in the health care system should include long-term counseling of patients, should use existing intervention materials that have been developed for the health care setting (eg, the National Cancer Institute's guide for physician counseling of patients who smoke),[27] and should be integrated with other health education resources in the community (eg, referral to a community nutrition program). When possible, family members and other caretakers should be recruited to support patients' behavior changes (eg, asthma management in children).[74]

In addition to conducting these activities, managed care organizations, integrated health systems, and individual hospitals or clinics also can reinforce community norms that support health by promoting policies in their institutions, such as eliminating public smoking and the sale of tobacco products on site.[67] Managed care organizations and individual health professionals also can contribute substantially to system-level changes, especially the adoption of local ordinances and organizational (eg, worksite) policies that promote health.[27] They also can participate in media advocacy[75] and mobilization of community organizations to help establish community conditions and norms that support health.[27]

Train-the-trainer programs are an effective strategy for increasing the skills of health professionals and promoting their involvement in chronic disease control.[72] The National Cancer Institute and American Cancer Society have developed a train-the-trainer program to recruit and train physicians, who can then train other health professionals on how to conduct tobacco cessation counseling.[27]

Schools

The Youth Risk Behavior Surveillance System (YRBSS) developed by the Centers for Disease Control and Prevention gathers national and local data on youth health behaviors (ie, tobacco use, diet, injuries, physical activity, alcohol use, and other activities). Recent data from the YRBSS indicate that a substantial proportion of high school students exhibit poor health behaviors.[76] For example, in 1993, 70% of high school students reported having tried cigarettes and 34% reported not having participated in any vigorous physical activity during the past week.[77]

Schools can be an effective channel for implementing chronic disease control interventions for youth.[78, 79] More than 48 million youth attend school each day in the United States.[4] Schools provide a structured opportunity to reach youth with chronic disease control interventions that modify health-related norms, establish school health policies, and enhance knowledge and skills that support positive health behaviors. Early learning and behavior choices also can influence adult behaviors and provide the groundwork for the development of adult values.

Comprehensive school health education is a very important approach for influencing health-related knowledge, behaviors, skills, and norms.[80, 81] The Institute of Medicine, Committee on Comprehensive School Health Programs has adopted a provisional definition of comprehensive school health.[82] "A comprehensive school health program is an integrated set of planned, sequential, school-affiliated strategies, activities, and services designed to promote the optimal physical, emotional, social, and educational development of students. The program involves and is supportive of families and is determined by the local community, based on community needs, resources, standards, and requirements. It is coordinated by a multidisciplinary team and accountable to the community for program quality and effectiveness."

Chronic disease control interventions occurring within broad comprehensive school health education programs commonly address such topics as tobacco, alcohol, drugs, nutrition, physical fitness, and injury prevention. Comprehensive school health programs can increase student understanding of the biological and social aspects of these health issues; establish health-related values, including personal responsibility for one's health; enhance self-esteem and decision-making skills; and

strengthen peer-resistance skills. Individual health issues, such as diet and physical activity, can be addressed in a larger program that enables skill building and behavioral change as well as understanding.

Occasionally, chronic disease control topics will be integrated into other school subjects such as physical education, social studies, science, and history. In some schools, separate programs address individual risk factors, such as physical fitness, tobacco use prevention, and other drug use prevention programs.

Many "packaged" school health education programs are available for use.[80, 83] These programs target specific age groups and usually have several core components, including curriculum guides, teaching activities, student activities, materials, and evaluation guidelines. Many of these programs have been extensively tested in controlled settings or in practice.

The National Cancer Institute has summarized the results of extensive research on the effectiveness of programs to prevent tobacco use.[84] The review revealed five major findings: (1) many programs are effective in delaying the onset of tobacco use, but success appears to be limited to low-risk groups; (2) programs should address social influences on tobacco use, especially from peers, family, and the media; (3) programs should focus on grades

6 to 9; (4) involving peers and parents enhances the effectiveness of programs; and (5) comprehensive training of teachers is essential for success.

Schools also provide an ideal opportunity for establishing health policies that will influence behaviors and norms. For example, bans on all tobacco use on school grounds directly limit student tobacco use and send a clear message to students that tobacco use is also socially unacceptable for adults.[27] Banning tobacco also clearly communicates the tobacco control message to teachers, staff, parents, and other members of the community who are not allowed to use tobacco on school property. Other school-based policies can affect the availability of healthy choices, such as nutritious food selections in school cafeterias and vending machines. One study in Minnesota demonstrated that nutrition policies designed to reduce cancer risks were feasible and resulted in a healthier diet for students.[85]

The Centers for Disease Control and Prevention has recently implemented a School Policies and Programs Study (SHPPS).[86] The study was designed to measure policies and programs at the state, district, school, and classroom levels. Data from the study will provide national policy makers with the information needed to effectively promote comprehensive school health programs in the United States.

Work Sites

Work sites provide an opportunity to reach a captive adult audience with interventions that influence social norms, establish health policies, provide incentives for positive health behavior, enhance health knowledge and skills, facilitate screening and follow-up activities, and reduce occupational hazards.[87] Work site programs are especially important for delivering interventions to high-risk populations such as blue-collar workers.

A comprehensive 1992 survey of work sites in the United States with 50 or more employees found that nearly two-thirds sponsored one or more health promotion activities.[88] The most common chronic disease control services were focused on exercise and fitness (41%), smoking cessation (40%), stress management (37%), back problem prevention and care (32%), nutrition (31%), high blood pressure control (29%), and cholesterol control (27%).

Social norms can be strongly influenced through work site programs, because most employees spend at least a third of their waking hours at work. Interpersonal advocacy concerning issues like secondhand tobacco smoke, dietary fat consumption, exercise, and other risk factors can play a major role in behavior change. Health policies in the work site can influence health behaviors directly as well as through changes in social norms. Effective health promotion policies can address secondhand tobacco smoke, dietary options in cafeterias and vending machines, and worker safety, among many others. Economic incentives, such as bonuses for employees who participate in health promotion activities, insurance reductions for nonsmokers, and contests that promote physical fitness can be very effective in motivating behavior change. Health knowledge and skills can be enhanced through structured programs or distribution of self-help materials.

Employers also can facilitate disease screening and follow-up activities by establishing relationships with local health care providers. This strategy is especially important for cancer and heart disease screenings.[89] In addition, employers can play a unique role in reducing occupational exposures to organic chemicals, radiation, metals, dusts, fibers, and other substances that cause chronic diseases.

Work site interventions also can reach beyond employees to address family members and the broader community. Many large employers establish support relationships with local schools to promote programs that benefit students. Employers also can participate as active members in community interventions and provide local support for changes in community policies.

Extensive research has been conducted to identify the best ways to design, promote, implement, and evaluate work site interventions.[90, 91] The success of work site interventions depends in part on support by corporate and union leaders, support by employees, the cost-effectiveness of interventions, the amount of employee time consumed by health promotion activities, and maintenance of employee confidentiality.[91, 92] Work site programs also have been evaluated for their impact on employee health and corporate cost-benefits.[93] Examples include the Live for Life Program at Johnson & Johnson[94, 95] and the Staywell Program at Control Data Corporation.[96]

Community Organizations

Community organizations can contribute substantially to chronic disease control interventions.[27, 87] Community organizations include religious groups, unions, clubs, professional associations, community action groups, sports groups, voluntary health agencies, social service groups, and others. Community organizations are especially important for reaching underserved groups such as undereducated, economically disadvantaged, rural, or minority populations.

Community organizations can provide access to organization members and their families to enhance their health knowledge and skills and to coordinate the delivery of screening and follow-up services. The access they provide for education and screening is similar to that discussed above for work sites. These types of interventions are commonly implemented through faith communities.[97-99] Involving churches and other community organizations in interventions also provides access to decision makers and to extensive resources, and it may ensure long-term maintenance of the intervention.

More important, community organizations can play leadership roles in changing health-related community conditions and norms, promoting health policies, and creating economic incentives for positive health behavior. Addressing the underlying causes of chronic diseases, such as poverty and lack of education, requires resources and influence beyond that available within a single health agency or even a coalition comprised of several health agencies. The participation of community organizations is essential to empower the community to achieve changes in these areas.

Community organizations can contribute to changing a community norm by increasing the public's knowledge of an issue, framing the issue as a legitimate social concern, and stimulating public discussion about the issue. Organization leaders and other opinion leaders within the organization can speak out in group meetings, public forums, or to the media. Organization members also can work behind the scenes to influence the attitudes of other leaders in the community. This type of intervention has proven successful, for example, in curtailing the marketing of tobacco products to minorities, young people, and women.[27]

The development of health policies and economic incentives for healthy behavior benefit tremendously from the participation and support of community organizations. Voluntary health, youth, and women's organizations have provided substantial support for policies restricting the sale of tobacco to minors and efforts to raise tobacco taxes.

Media

Media include television and radio stations, daily and weekly newspapers, and an array of smaller outlets such as cable television stations, magazines, billboards, newsletters, and local computer networks. Media can be divided into news, features, entertainment, editorials, and advertisements. Different media channels and categories are appropriate for communicating different types of messages and accessing different populations. Given this variability, the planning process described in the Intervention Planning Steps section (p. 69) is particularly important for designing and implementing media interventions.

Flora and Cassady[100] identified four roles for the media in interventions targeting the health behavior of individuals: (1) primary change agent, (2) complement to other interventions, (3) means of recruiting and promoting services and programs, and (4) provider of support for lifestyle changes. Media interventions targeted at system-level change include two additional roles: (1) means of reframing an issue from one of personal health behavior to one of public policy and (2) agent for stimulating and empowering organizations and individuals to participate in the process of generating policy.[101]

Several major interventions that have effectively used the media to enhance health knowledge and skills and to promote participation in screening and follow-up include the North Karelia Project in Finland,[35, 36] the Stanford Five-City Project,[37, 38] the Pawtucket Heart Health Program,[39, 40] and the Minnesota Heart Health Program.[41] These large community-based projects have found that using the media, in combination with other community-based interventions, is an effective way to influence health behaviors.

Flynn and colleagues[102] have conducted a well-controlled research trial to document the effect of television and radio spots, in conjunction with school-based interventions, on the smoking behavior of youth. The media component of the intervention reduced smoking by more than a third among study participants. The success of the project was attributed to several characteristics of the media intervention: sufficient duration; use of multiple channels and messages; population segmenting; placement at appropriate times and places for reaching each population segment; use of surveys and focus groups to identify appeals to each population segment; appropriate peer role modeling; and direct attention to behavioral skills, alternatives, and reinforcement.

Media have a key role to play in efforts to modify health-related community conditions, norms, and policies and to establish economic incentives for healthy behavior.[101, 103] Media interventions that target these issues are often referred to as media advocacy. Media advocacy is defined as the use of media to promote a social or policy initiative.[101, 104] The goal of media advocacy is to change the way that an issue is understood by the public and by policy makers and to empower groups or individuals to take action.

Although media advocacy rarely determines health-related attitudes or behaviors, it often increases a community's knowledge about a public health issue, frames the issue, and stimulates public discussion about it.[101] The creative use of epidemiology is very important in media advocacy. Accurate and well-known statistics can be packaged creatively so that they are interesting to the public and highlight the importance of the issue being addressed. Creative presentation of epidemiologic results also enhances the interest of media professionals and provides an opportunity to communicate to the public and policy makers through editorials and news reports (see Chapter 3).

Interventions that target public smoking and the associated hazards of secondhand tobacco smoke have benefited substantially from media advocacy.[27] Creative epidemiology has presented information on the health hazards of secondhand tobacco smoke in a way that is understandable to the public—for example, by comparing secondhand tobacco smoke to other health hazards. Focusing on the health effects of secondhand tobacco smoke for special populations— young people, pregnant women, and people with asthma—has defined public smoking as a health issue for nonsmokers rather than a personal rights issue for smokers. Focusing on the lobbying tactics of the tobacco industry has stimulated public

discussion of secondhand tobacco smoke and empowered health advocates to take action in the policy arena.

Public Policy Makers

Changing public health policies is a cost-effective way to modify individual health behavior as well as to induce system-level change. Policy promotion usually focuses on the legislative branch of government. Access to health care, insurance coverage, nutrition labeling, tobacco advertising restrictions, quality assurance for cancer screening, and worker right-to-know laws are several of the policy issues related to chronic disease that have been addressed recently at the national level. Public smoking limitations, restricted tobacco sales to minors, tobacco taxes, radon monitoring, and mandatory insurance coverage for mammography are several issues that have been addressed at the state and local levels.

Clear and concise communication with legislators is essential for effective policy promotion. Health policy advocates should employ strong media advocacy and grassroots lobbying through existing community organizations.[27] Obtaining the services of a professional lobbyist also may be necessary, depending on the lobbying strength of the organizations that are opposing the health policy.

A coalition of organizations can provide an opportunity for implementing an intervention that includes all of these components. Special attention should be paid to recruiting coalition member organizations that can provide accurate and timely epidemiologic data, directly communicate with policy makers, access the media, mobilize grassroots support, and hire a lobbyist. Frequently, some coalition member organizations, such as public health agencies, will be precluded from direct involvement in lobbying or media advocacy.

There almost always will be substantial opposition to changing or initiating a health policy. Achieving a health policy objective usually requires several years of commitment. A policy intervention must be approached with the same rigor and thoroughness as are other chronic disease control interventions. Specific policy objectives should be identified, and a process for modifying these objectives (eg, accepting amendments) should be established at the beginning of the program. An implementation plan should be developed, and the roles of all intervention participants should be clearly defined. Lobbyists and grassroots supporters should be thoroughly trained. A rapid communication system should be established and tested on a regular basis. Strong media relationships should be established before the intervention is

initiated and should be reinforced regularly. The selection of communication messages and channels should be based on a detailed understanding of the target audiences and their needs (especially legislators), and all communications should be pretested.

COALITION DEVELOPMENT AND MAINTENANCE

A coalition is an alliance of organizations working together to achieve a common purpose. A chronic disease control program usually is strengthened when several organizations are involved in planning, implementing, and evaluating interventions. A coalition can provide direct access to intervention channels within a community, such as the health care system, schools, and work sites. It also can provide an opportunity to involve local community organizations and representatives from at-risk populations. A coalition can mobilize the human resources that are needed to plan and implement a culturally sensitive community-based intervention.

Several key issues in the development and maintenance of a coalition have been identified through experience in numerous community-based projects (Table 4.2). Although circumstances vary from one community to the next, these issues must be addressed to assure that the

Table 4.2—Issues in Coalition Development and Maintenance

Committed lead agency
Effective core planning group
Planned recruitment of coalition members
Functional coalition structure
Clearly defined staff roles
Formally accepted mission and goals
Respected leadership
In-depth education of coalition members
Ownership and commitment by coalition members
Successful implementation of a pilot project
Recognition of coalition members

---

coalition will include the necessary partners, address pertinent health issues, and implement one or more successful interventions.[54, 56, 105, 106]

A coalition *lead organization* should be selected, and its members should be fully educated about health issues and coalition support expectations. This lead organization is often, but not always, a public health agency in the geographic area covered by the coalition. Voluntary health organizations, major work sites, or community-based organizations also can act as the lead organization in a coalition. A lead organization is necessary to provide a stable source of staffing and operating resources for the coalition. It also can act as the financial manager for the coalition and supply the primary spokesperson for communicating with the media and policy makers.

The coalition lead organization should identify a *core planning group* to provide leadership and guidance for the coalition. This group should include three to six individuals who represent organizations in the community and the at risk population. The core planning group should initially focus on expanding the coalition to include additional member organizations, each carefully selected for a specific reason. Additional member organizations should have a workable relationship with the lead organization and other members of the core planning group. Member organizations also should provide access to community leaders and policy makers that have influence over the determinants of health affecting the at-risk populations. Other potential coalition members should be approached because they can provide access to planning and intervention resources, including staff support.

The coalition structure must be defined very early in the development process. Clear guidelines or bylaws should be developed, fully discussed, and formally accepted by the entire coalition. A complete understanding of committee structure, leadership roles, leadership transition, and rules of order will allow the coalition to address pertinent health issues without continually discussing and redefining structural issues. Special attention should be paid to empowering representatives from at-risk populations to be major contributors and decision makers in the coalition.

The roles of program staff should also be clarified very early in the development process. Some coalitions are able to function without dedicated staffing, but this often limits the scope of the coalition's activity and demands a higher level of commitment from coalition members. In general, dedicated coalition staffing must be maintained throughout the project to assure effective planning and coordination of interventions. In either situation, coalition membership should have realistic expectations for staff support.

The coalition also should quickly define its mission and goals. This will productively limit the scope of the coalition's activities and will enable new members to determine their level of commitment to coalition projects. A clear definition of the coalition's mission and goals also may assist in identifying additional

organizations that may participate in the coalition.

After the structure, roles, and mission are clarified, coalition leadership must be identified. Individuals selected for leadership roles should have the time to participate fully in all of the coalition's planning and intervention activities. However, it is most important that coalition leadership should reflect informal leadership in the community and give voice to at-risk populations. Coalition members should select individuals for leadership roles.

As indicated previously, coalition member organizations may be selected for a variety of reasons. A successful coalition should reach out to the broader community and involve organizations that are not traditional partners in health programs, such as minority or youth organizations. In-depth education of coalition members will be necessary to ensure that nonhealth organizations are knowledgeable on health issues and are able to participate in leadership roles within the coalition. Educational presentations or dissemination of concise educational materials also provide an opportunity for program initiators to create awareness of health data and effective intervention strategies.

Development of ownership and commitment by coalition members is critical for the successful implementation of the coalition's projects. The plans developed by coalition members should reflect the needs and potential solutions expressed by coalition members. Program initiators usually need to set the broad parameters for the coalition's activities and provide in-depth education on relevant issues; however, at a very early stage in the planning process, leadership must shift to the coalition members. If full ownership and commitment is not achieved, coalition members may lose interest or expect external agencies to implement projects, thus undermining the primary benefits of a community-based coalition.

Most coalitions require early implementation of a successful project to establish an atmosphere of accomplishment and to maintain their members' commitment to the coalition's mission and goals. Although community assessment and detailed planning are essential for long-term success, these initial activities should be supplemented with at least one project that is visible to the community and that legitimizes commitment of resources to the coalition. The project selected for implementation should be acceptable to all coalition members and highly likely to succeed. However, it should require only a limited commitment of time so that it does not detract from important planning activities.

Of critical importance is the need to provide frequent and public recognition of coalition members' contributions. This recognition should not be limited to verbal praise during coalition meetings. Special efforts should be made to communicate the contributions of member organizations to the broader community. Participating in coalition media events and including organization logos on published materials will provide a minimal level of recognition. Whenever possible, the contributions of individual members of the coalition should be communicated to the organizations they represent. This can often be accomplished by providing brief newsletter articles that explain the coalition and the special role of the representative.

INTERVENTION PLANNING STEPS

An effective chronic disease control intervention requires a conscious focus on the process used to plan, implement, and evaluate the intervention.[16, 56] Several key steps should be taken during intervention planning (Table 4.3). Limited resources may restrict the staff's capacity to fully accomplish all of these activities, but all should be addressed at some level.

First, program staff and coalition members must review available health data for the defined geographic area of the program and

Table 4.3—Key Intervention Planning Steps

Review health data
Assess demographic, economic, social, political, and environmental conditions
Review intervention literature
Assess current community intervention activities and resources
Precisely define health issue and priority population
Segment the priority population
Identify potential intervention channels
Select intervention channels and strategies
Pretest existing procedures, messages, and materials
Develop and pretest new procedures, messages, and materials
Pilot test intervention
Expand program implementation plan
Provide evaluation feedback

determine the health issues and at-risk populations that will be addressed. This step is necessary to focus efforts on a specific, achievable goal and to reinforce the importance of data in decision making. (For a list of chronic disease data sources, see Chapter 3.) Other factors such as staff expertise and available resources also may be important in determining the health issues and at-risk populations selected. Frequently, health issues and at-risk populations will be determined by the funding agency. However, coalition members and staff often are responsible for further refining these basic guidelines to develop a focused, achievable program.

Program staff should also assess demographic, economic, social, political, and environmental conditions that affect the health issues and

at-risk populations in the defined geographic area. Information collection at this level often is called community diagnosis or needs assessment.[107] It combines quantitative information from existing databases (eg, census data) with qualitative information from interviews with members of the community. Community diagnosis provides an opportunity for coalition members and others from the community to participate in developing interventions. The information collected at this stage should be used to identify opportunities for addressing the health issues in the defined geographic area. Again, many of these variables may be directly determined by the funding agency, and coalition members will be requested to adapt strategies to the local geographic area.

Using the information collected in the previous steps, program staff now should review available intervention literature to identify intervention strategies that have been used under similar conditions. Access to the literature can be provided through the many projects described in this book and the references at the end of each chapter. General descriptions of interventions are usually all that is available from published reports. Detailed information often can be obtained by calling the program managers and asking for examples of intervention materials or implementation plans. Information concerning ongoing projects can be obtained by calling funding agencies that are sponsoring projects on similar topics.

The program staff should assess current intervention activities and resources in the defined geographic area.[107] Most information on existing activities and programs can be obtained from informal interviews with coalition members or others in the community. Identification of existing programs provides an opportunity for collaboration and avoids competition or conflict. Expanding existing programs is often the most cost-effective and culturally sensitive way of implementing an intervention. This strategy also may provide access to community leaders and other decision makers who are already involved with the at-risk populations or health issues. Understanding existing programs will also

help intervention planners to identify additional interventions that may be needed in the community.

After all of this preliminary information is collected and analyzed, coalition members and staff are in a position to precisely define health issues and at-risk populations for the program. These selections should be quantified in the form of specific outcome objectives. The objectives should include baseline measures that indicate the current health status of people in the defined geographic area. Information collected on the depth of the problem, the availability of resources, and the success of comparable interventions should be considered in setting realistic objectives. Each objective should be accompanied by a detailed description of how the baseline and the outcome will be assessed—that is, the source of existing data or data collection instrument and methods. The objectives should be consulted frequently to guide all future intervention development and evaluation.

After specific objectives are determined, the staff should collect additional information to characterize and segment each at-risk population into subpopulations that may respond differently to specific interventions; subpopulations may be characterized, for example, by demographics, economic and social status, health care access, health knowledge and attitudes, readiness to change behavior, potential environmental exposures, or media use patterns. This information can be collected through key informant interviews, focus groups, surveys, or secondary data sources (eg, existing surveys of media habits).[16, 108]

Another necessary step is to identify potential intervention channels for affecting changes in the selected at-risk subpopulations. (Major intervention channels are discussed previously in this chapter.) Information should be collected to determine the appropriateness of each intervention channel for achieving program objectives, including access to and ability to influence members of the at-risk subpopulations, current level of health activity, potential support for change, and barriers to change. Individual interviews and telephone surveys with members of the community are often the best methods for collecting this type of information.[16]

After the community, subpopulations, and channels are understood, intervention planners can select specific intervention channels and strategies for the program. As discussed above, it is important to intervene through multiple channels to reach at-risk subpopulations with multiple strategies addressing system-level changes as well as individual health behavior changes.

The next steps are to review and pretest existing intervention procedures, messages, and materials that may be appropriate for the specific at-risk subpopulations and channels. The best way to assess these items is to conduct focus groups or individual interviews with members of the subpopulations and representatives from the channel (eg, a physician).[16] Specific intervention procedures, messages, and materials should be identified for use with each specific combination of subpopulation and channel.

In many cases, an appropriate procedure, message, or material may not be available for a specific combination of subpopulation and channel. At this point, a decision must be made to exclude a particular subpopulation from the intervention or to develop and pretest a new procedure, message, or material that is appropriate. Using an inappropriate procedure, message, or material will not contribute to achieving program objectives; however, developing a new item may be costly and time consuming. The final decision should be based on a careful analysis of what will contribute the most to achieving program objectives.

If possible, staff should pilot test the total intervention in a small portion of the defined geographic area. The intervention should be implemented within the normal routine of the selected channels and should target a representative sample of the at-risk subpopulations. Rigorous outcome and process evaluation should be conducted on this smaller sample. Preliminary activities for the overall intervention—for example, program promotion with the media and other channels—can be initiated while this pilot test is being conducted.

Intervention planning does not end with the implementation of the intervention. The program design should provide evaluation feedback that allows continual modification of the intervention. Modifications should be based on progress toward desired outcomes as well as the acceptability of intervention activities to representatives of both the subpopulations and channels. The flexibility to increase activities in some areas and cease activities in other areas must be maintained. Coalition members and representatives from the subpopulations and channels should be active participants in this evaluation process.

KEY ISSUES IN INTERVENTION PROGRAM MANAGEMENT

Several issues are important for effective organizational management of a large community-based intervention program. Probably the most important is upper-level management support. Community-based interven-

tion programs are collaborative efforts between organizations in the community, including the organization initiating the program. Upper-level managers need to fully understand the program and provide the consistent administrative, financial, and public support that is necessary to maintain a coalition effort. Without this stability and public support, program staff may not be able to maintain the support of coalition organizations in the face of competing priorities and resistance from the community (eg, tobacco industry resistance to efforts to modify community norms concerning tobacco use). Staff need to actively seek out such support by providing regular program briefings to upper-level managers and selectively involving them in the program's implementation.

Adequate staffing is essential for planning and implementing a community-based intervention. It is important not to underestimate the staff time needed to conduct a meaningful community analysis, recruit and educate coalition members, staff coalition planning meetings, and coordinate the implementation of projects. Inadequate staffing can undermine coalition member participation and limit the effective implementation of interventions. Program leaders need to accurately assess the availability of staff resources and limit the scope of the community-based program to maximize the effectiveness of available staff.

The development of a detailed program implementation plan is essential for identifying and coordinating implementation of all program activities. A formal plan is necessary for staying focused on the most important program activities and managing human resources efficiently. The plan should list all activities in chronological order and highlight the dates of major events or documents (eg, annual action plans). The plan should be developed by program staff in consultation with coalition leadership, and it should be used at all staff meetings to guide discussion of upcoming events and preliminary activities for future events.

A detailed implementation plan will help to clarify staff roles. Defining lines of authority and communication is crucial for a community-based program in which numerous activities may occur simultaneously. Decision-making authority for specific components of the program needs to be clarified (eg, final content of a newsletter). Clear guidelines need to identify which staff members can communicate with coalition members about specific topics or issues. In particular, the guidelines must clearly identify who is authorized to speak to the media or to policy makers about the

program. The primary responsibilities of each staff person should be documented and fully discussed before program implementation. Where possible, specific responsibilities should be indicated in the program implementation plan.

In addition, adequate staff training is essential for smooth functioning of the program and effective implementation of interventions. Formal training should be provided for staff members who have limited backgrounds in specific program areas such as health issues, health behavior change, media communications, and coalition building. Special attention also should be given to basic skills such as planning, budgeting, personnel management, written and verbal communication, and cultural sensitivity. Too often, these basic skills are taken for granted until a serious problem develops in the program.

CONCLUSIONS

The science of chronic disease control has advanced to the stage at which clear guidance is available for developing, implementing, and evaluating interventions. Epidemiologic research has identified many of the causes of chronic diseases. Although uncertainties remain, health promotion theory, the scientific literature, and in-depth experience from numerous community-based projects have demonstrated the value of chronic disease control interventions.

Public health agencies and other organizations can adapt the basic empowerment and intervention strategies discussed in this book for implementation in their unique settings. The capacity of individual organizations can be enhanced through community-based coalitions that provide access to multiple channels for implementing proven intervention strategies. The key steps for effective coalition building, intervention planning, and program management have been defined. Public health is now in a position to seriously address the burden of chronic diseases.

REFERENCES

1. Ashton J, Grey P, Barnard K. Healthy cities: WHO's new public health initiative. *Health Promotion*. 1986;1:319–324.
2. Minkler M. Building supportive ties and sense of community among the inner city elderly: the Tenderloin senior outreach project. *Health Educ Q*. 1985;12:303–314.
3. Minkler M. Health education, health promotion, and the open society: an historical perspective. *Health Educ Q*. 1989;16:17–30.
4. Tolsma DD, Koplan JP. Health behaviors and health promotion. In: Last JM, Wallace RB, eds. *Maxcy-Rosenau-Last Textbook of Public Health and Preventive Medicine*. 13th ed. Norwalk, Conn: Appleton & Lange; 1992:701–714.
5. Amler RW, Eddins DL. Cross-sectional analysis: precursors of premature death in the United States. In: Ambler RW, Dull HD, eds. *Closing the Gap: The Burden of Unnecessary Illness*. *Am J Prev Med*. 1987;3:181–187.
6. Prochaska JO, DiClemente CC. Stages and processes of self-change of smoking: toward an integrative model of change. *J Consult Clin Psych*. 1983;51:983–990.
7. Maiman LA, Becker MH. The health belief model: origins and correlates in psychological theory. *Health Educ Monogr*. 1974;2:336–353.
8. Strecher VJ, Rosenstock IM. The health belief model. In: Glanz K, Lewis FM, Rimer BK, eds. *Health Behavior and Health Education: Theory, Research, and Practice*. 2nd ed. San Francisco, Calif: Jossey-Bass; 1997:41–59.
9. Rotter JB. Generalized expectancies for internal versus external control of reinforcement. *Psychol Monogr*. 1966;80:1–28.
10. Lewis FM, Morisky DE, Flynn BS. A test of the construct validity of Health Locus of Control: effects on self-reported compliance for

hypertensive patients. *Health Educ Monogr.* 1978;6:138–148.

11. Fishbein M, Ajzen I. *Beliefs, Attitudes, Intention, and Behavior: An Introduction to Theory and Research.* Reading, Mass: Addison-Wesley; 1975.

12. Ajzen I, Fishbein M. *Understanding Attitudes and Predicting Social Behavior.* Englewood Cliffs, NJ: Prentice Hall; 1980.

13. Ajzen I. From intentions to actions: a theory of planned behavior. In: Kuhl J, Beckman J, eds. *Action Control: From Cognition to Behavior.* New York, NY: Springer-Verlag; 1985:11–39.

14. Monta'o DE, Kasprzyk D, Taplin SH. The theory of reasoned action and the theory of planned behavior. In: Glanz K, Lewis FM, Rimer BK, eds. *Health Behavior and Health Education: Theory, Research, and Practice.* 2nd ed. San Francisco, Calif: Jossey-Bass; 1997:85–112.

15. McGuire W. Theoretical foundations of campaigns. In: Rice RE, Paisley WJ, eds. *Public Communication Campaigns.* Newbury Park, Calif: Sage Publications; 1981:41–70.

16. National Institutes of Health, US Dept of Health and Human Services. *Making Health Communication Programs Work: A Planners Guide.* Bethesda, Md: National Cancer Institute; 1989. NIH publication 89-1493.

17. Lefebvre RC, Rochlin L. Social marketing. In: Glanz K, Lewis FM, Rimer BK, eds. *Health Behavior and Health Education: Theory, Research, and Practice.* 2nd ed. San Francisco, Calif: Jossey-Bass; 1997:384–402.

18. Kotler P, Andreason AR. *Strategic Marketing for Nonprofit Organizations.* 3rd ed. Englewood Cliffs, NJ: Prentice-Hall; 1987.

19. Baranowski T, Perry CL, Parcel GS. How individuals, environments, and health behavior interact: social cognitive theory. In: Glanz K, Lewis FM, Rimer BK, eds. *Health Behavior and Health Education: Theory, Research, and Practice.* 2nd ed. San Francisco, Calif: Jossey-Bass; 1997:153–178.

20. Bandura A. *Social Learning Theory.* Englewood Cliffs, NJ: Prentice-Hall; 1977.

21. Rodin J. Personal control through the life course. In: Heise R, ed. *Implications of the Lifespan Perspective for Social Psychology.* Hillsdale, NJ: Erlbaum; 1987:103–119.

22. Bandura A. *Social Foundations of Thought and Action.* Englewood Cliffs, NJ: Prentice-Hall; 1986.

23. Group Health Cooperative of Puget Sound. *An Index Bibliography on Self-Management for People with Chronic Disease,* 1st ed. Washington, DC: The Center

for the Advancement of Health
and The Center for Health
Studies; 1996.

24. Freudenberg N, Eng E, Flay B,
Paarcel G, Rogers T, Wallerstein
N. Strengthening individual and
community capacity to prevent
disease and promote health: In
search of relevant theories and
principles. *Health Educ Q.*
1995;22(3):290–306.

25. Wallerstein NB, Sanchez-Merki V.
Freirian praxis in health education: Research results from an
adolescent prevention program.
Health Educ Res 1994;9:105—118.

26. Israel B, Checkoway B, Schulz A,
Zimmerman M. Health education
and community empowerment:
conceptualizing and measuring
perceptions of individual,
organizational, and community
control. *Health Educ Q.* 1994;21:
149–170.

27. US Dept of Health and Human
Services. *Strategies to Control
Tobacco Use in the United States:
A Blueprint for Public Health
Action in the 1990's. Smoking
and Tobacco Control Mono-
graphs 1.* Bethesda, Md: National
Cancer Institute; 1991. NIH
publication 92-3316.

28. Lewit E, Coate D. The potential
for using excise taxes to reduce
smoking. *J Health Econ.* 1982;1:
121–145.

29. Coalition on Smoking OR
Health. *Saving Lives and Raising
Revenues.* Washington, DC:
Coalition on Smoking OR
Health; 1993.

30. Rigotti NA. Trends in the adoption of smoking restrictions in
public places and worksites. *NY
State J Med.* 1989;89:19–26.

31. Mackay JM, Barnes GT. Effects of
strong government measures
against tobacco in Hong Kong.
Br Med J. 1986;292:1435–1437.

32. Hagey A. Implementation of a
smoking policy in the United
States Army. *NY State J Med.*
1989;89:42–44.

33. Rogers EM. *Diffusion of Innovations.* New York, NY: Free Press;
1983.

34. Schucker B, Wittes JT, Cutler JA,
et al. Change in physician
perspective on cholesterol and
heart disease: results from two
national surveys. *JAMA.* 1987;
258:3521–3526.

35. McAlister A, Puska P, Salonen JT,
Tuomilehto J, Koskela K. Theory
and action for health promotion:
illustrations from the North
Karelia Project. *Am J Public
Health.* 1982;72:43–50.

36. Puska P. Community based
prevention of cardiovascular
disease: the North Karelia
Project. In: Matarazzo JD, Weiss
SM, Herd JA, Miller NE, Weiss
SM, eds. *Behavioral Health: A
Handbook of Health Enhance-
ment and Disease Prevention.*
New York, NY: Wiley-Inter-

science Publication; 1984:1140–1147.

37. Farquhar JW, Fortmann SP, Maccoby N, et al. The Stanford Five-City Project: design and methods. *Am J Epidemiol.* 1985;122:323–334.

38. Farquhar JW, Fortmann SP, Flora JA, Maccoby N. Methods of communication to influence behavior. In: Holland WW, Detels R, Knox G, eds. *Oxford Textbook of Public Health.* 2nd ed. New York, NY: Oxford University Press; 1991;2:__-__.

39. Lasater T, Abrams D, Artz L, et al. Lay volunteer delivery of a community-based cardiovascular risk factor change program: the Pawtucket experiment. In: Matarazzo JD, Weiss SH, Herd JA, Miller NE, Weiss SW, eds. *Behavioral Health: A Handbook of Health Enhancement and Disease Prevention.* New York, NY: Wiley-Interscience Publication; 1984:1166–1170.

40. Elder JP, McGraw SA, Abrams DA. Organizational and community approaches to community-wide prevention of heart disease: the first two years of the Pawtucket Heart Health Program. *Prev Med.* 1986;15:107–115.

41. Blackburn H, Luepker RV, Kline FG, et al. The Minnesota Heart Health Program: a research and demonstration project in cardio-vascular disease prevention. In: Matarazzo JD, Weiss SM, Herd JA, Miller NE, Weiss SM, eds. *Behavioral Health: A Handbook of Health Enhancement and Disease Prevention.* New York, NY: Wiley-Interscience Publication; 1984:1171–1178.

42. Thompson B, Kinne S. Social change theory: applications to community health. In: Bracht N, ed. *Health Promotion at the Community Level.* Newbury Park, Calif: Sage Publications; 1990.

43. Flynn B. Healthy Cities: a model of community change. *Family Commun Health* 1992;15(1):13–23.

44. Norris T. *The Healthy Communities Handbook.* Denver, CO: The National Civic League; 1993.

45. McLeary KR, Bibeau D, Steckler A, Chang K. An ecological perspective on health promotion programs. *Healthy Educ Q.* 1988;15:351–378.

46. Stokols AJ, Ballingham RL. The social ecology of health promotion: Implications for research and practice. *Am J Health Promotion.* 1996;10(4):247–251.

47. Green LW, Richard L, Potvin L. Ecological foundations of health promotion. *Am J Health Promotion.* 1996;10(4):270–281.

48. Institute of Medicine, Committee for the Study of the Future of Public Health. *The Future of*

Public Health. Washington, DC: National Academy Press; 1988.

49. Shea S, Basch CE. A review of five major community-based cardiovascular prevention programs. Part I: rationale, design, and theoretical framework. *Am J Health Promotion.* 1990;4:203–213.

50. Safer MA. A comparison of screening for disease detection and screening for risk factors. *Health Educ Res.* 1986;1:131–138.

51. Kottke TE, Puska P, Salonen JT, Tuomilehto J, Nissinen A. Projected effects of high-risk versus population prevention strategies in coronary heart disease. *Am J Epidemiol.* 1985; 121:697–704.

52. Rothman J. Three models of community organization practice. In: Cox FM, Erlich JL, Rothman J, Tropman JE, eds. *Strategies of Community Organization.* Itasca, Ill: Peacock Press; 1970.

53. Levine S, Sorenson JR. Social and cultural factors in health promotion. In: Matarazzo JD, Weiss SM, Herd JA, Miller NE, Weiss SM, eds. *Behavioral Health: A Handbook of Health Enhancement and Disease Prevention.* New York, NY: Wiley-Interscience Publication; 1984:222–229.

54. Bracht N, Gleason J. Strategies and structures for citizen partnerships. In: Bracht N, ed. *Health Promotion at the Community*

Level. Newbury Park, Calif: Sage Publications; 1990:109–124.

55. Bracht N, Kingsbury L. Community organization principles in health promotion: a five stage model. In: Bracht N, ed. *Health Promotion at the Community Level.* Newbury Park, Calif: Sage Publications; 1990:66–88.

56. *J Health Educ.* 1992;23(3). Entire issue dedicated to descriptions and accounts of PATCH program.

57. Thompson B, Hunkeler EF, Biener L, Orleans CT, Perez-Stable EJ. Interdependence and synergy among smoking control activities. In: National Cancer Institute. *Strategies to Control Tobacco Use in the United States: A Blueprint for Public Health Action in the 1990s.* Bethesda, Md: National Institutes of Health, US Dept of Health and Human Services; 1991. NIH publication 92-3316.

58. Steckler A, Allegrante JP, Altman D, Brown R, Burdine JN, Goodman RM, Jorgensen C. Health education intervention strategies: recommendations for future research. *Health Educ Q.* 1995;22(3):307–329.

59. Steckler A, Dawson L, Israel B, Eng E. Community health development: an overview of the works of Guy W. Steuart. *Health Educ Q.* 1993;1(suppl):S3–S20.

60. Cottrell LS. The competent community. In: Lyon WR, ed.

New Perspectives on the American Community. Homewood, Ill: Dorsey Press; 1983.

61. US Environmental Protection Agency. *Respiratory Health Effects of Passive Smoking: Lung Cancer and Other Disorders.* Washington DC: US Environmental Protection Agency, Office of Research and Development; 1993. EPA publication EPA/600/6-90/006F.

62. Stowe GM, Jackson GW. Effect of a total worksite smoking ban on employee smoking and attitudes. *J Occup Med.* 1991; U33(8):884–890.

63. Patten CA, Gilpin E, Cavin SW, Pierce JP. Workplace smoking policy and changes in smoking behavior in California. *Tobacco Control.* 1995;4:36–41.

64. Brigham J, Gross J, Slitzer ML, Felch LJ. Effectos of a restricted work site smoking policy on employees who smoke. *Am J Public Health.* 1994;84:773–778.

65. Lindeman C. Nursing and health education. In: Matarazzo JD, Weiss SM, Herd JA, Miller NE, Weiss SM, eds. *Behavioral Health: A Handbook of Health Enhancement and Disease Prevention.* New York, NY: Wiley-Interscience Publication; 1984:1214–1217.

66. US Preventive Services Task Force. *Guide to Clinical Preventive Services.* 2nd ed. Baltimore, Md: Williams & Wilkins; 1996.

67. Luepker RV, Rastam L. Involving community health professionals and systems. In: Bracht N, ed. *Health Promotion at the Community Level.* Newbury Park, Calif: Sage Publications; 1990:185–198.

68. Roter DL, Hall JA. Patient-provider communication. In: Glanz K, Lewis FM, Rimer BK, eds. *Health Behavior and Health Education: Theory, Research, and Practice.* 2nd ed. San Francisco, Calif: Jossey-Bass; 1997: 206–226.

69. Centers for Disease Control and Prevention. Prevention and managed care: opportunities for managed care organizations, purchasers of health care, and public health agencies. *MMWR Morb Mort Wkly Rep.* 1995; 44(RR-14)

70. National High Blood Pressure Education Program. *Working group report on primary prevention of hypertension.* National Heart, Lung, and Blood Institute, NIH. *Arch Intern Med.* 1993;153: 186–208.

71. Henson RM, Wyatt SW, Lee NC. The National Breast and Cervical Cancer Early Detection Program: A comprehensive public health response to two major health issues for women. *J Public Health Manag Pract.* 1996;2:36–47.

72. Kottke TE, Battista RN, Defriese GH, Brekke ML. Attributes of successful smoking cessation

interventions in medical practice. A meta-analysis of 39 controlled trials. *JAMA*. 1988;259:2883–2889.

73. Glynn TJ, Manley MW, Pechacek TF. Physician initiated smoking cessation program: the National Cancer Institute trials. *Prog Clin Biol Res*. 1990;339:11–25.

74. Clark NM, Feldman CH, Evans D. The effectiveness of education for family management of asthma in children: a preliminary report. *Health Educ Q*. 1981;8:166–174.

75. Doctors ought to care. Counter promotion—tennis elbows tobacco company sponsorship at sports. *DOC News Views*. 1989; summer:4-5.

76. *School Health Programs: an investment in our future. At-A-Glance*. Atlanta, Ga: Centers for Disease Control and Prevention, National Center for Chronic Disease Prevention and Health Promotion;1996.

77. Kann L, Warren CW, Harris WA, Collins JL, Douglas KA. Youth risk behavior surveillance— United States, 1993. *MMWR Morb Mort Wkly Rep*.1995;44(SS-1):1–56.

78. Connell DB, Turner RR, Mason EF. Summary of findings of the school health education evaluation. *J School Health*. 1985;55: 316–320.

79. *J School Health*. 1989;59(5). Entire issue dedicated to cancer education and prevention in the schools.

80. Kolbe LJ, Iverson DC. Comprehensive school health education programs. In: Matarazzo JD, Weiss SM, Herd JA, Miller NE, Weiss SM, eds. *Behavioral Health: A Handbook of Health Enhancement and Disease Prevention*. New York, NY: Wiley-Interscience Publication; 1984:1094–1116.

81. Murray DM, Richards PS, Luepker RV, Johnson CA. The prevention of cigarette smoking in children: two- and three-year follow-up comparisons of four prevention strategies. *J Behav Med*. 1987;10:595–611.

82. Allensworth D, Wyche J, Lawson E, Nicholson L. eds. *Defining A Comprehensive School Health Program: An Interim Statement*. Washington, DC: National Academy Press; 1995:2.

83. National Center for Health Education. *A Compendium of Health Education Programs Available for Use by Schools*. Atlanta, Ga: US Center for Health Promotion and Education; 1982.

84. Glynn TJ. Essential elements of school-based smoking prevention programs. *J School Health*. 1989;59:181–188.

85. Bishop DB, Slater JS, Taylor GL, Brand W. St. Cloud area cancer prevention project: a public health model for community-based health promotion. Paper presented at the meeting of the

Society of Behavioral Medicine; March 1992; New York, NY.

86. Kann L, Collins JL, Pateman BC, Small ML, Ross JG, Kolbe LJ. The School Health Policies and Programs Study (SHPPS): rationale for a Nationwide Status Report on School Health Programs. *J School Health* 1995;65(8).

87. Sorensen G, Glasgow RE, Corbett K. Involving worksites and other organizations. In: Bracht N, ed. *Health Promotion at the Community Level.* Newbury Park, Calif: Sage Publications; 1990:158–179.

88. US Public Health Service. 1992 *National Survey of Worksite Health Promotion Activities.* Summary Report. Washington, DC: Office of Disease Prevention and Health Promotion; 1993.

89. Eriksen MP. Cancer prevention in the workplace. *Cancer Bull.* 1987; 39(3):176–178.

90. Fielding JE. Health promotion and disease prevention at the workplace. *Ann Rev Public Health.* 1984;5:237–265.

91. Sloan RP, Gruman JC, Allegrante JP. *Investigating Employee Health: A Guide to Effective Health Promotion in the Workplace.* San Francisco, Calif: Jossey-Bass; 1987.

92. O'Donnell MP, Ainsworth T. *Health Promotion in the Workplace.* New York, NY: John Wiley; 1984.

93. Johnson K, LaRosa JH, Scheirer CJ, Wolle JM. *Methodological Issues in Worksite Research. Proceedings of a Workshop April 10–12, 1988.* Washington, DC: National Heart Lung and Blood Institute, US Dept of Health and Human Services; 1989.

94. Nathan PE. Johnson & Johnson's Live for Life: a comprehensive positive lifestyle change program. In: Matarazzo JD, Weiss SM, Herd JA, Miller NE, Weiss SM, eds. *Behavioral Health: A Handbook of Health Enhancement and Disease Prevention.* New York, NY: Wiley-Interscience Publication; 1984:1064–1070.

95. Bly JL, Jones RC, Richardson JE. Impact of worksite health promotion on health care costs and utilization. *JAMA.* 1986;256: 3235–3240.

96. Naditch MP. The Staywell Program. In: Matarazzo JD, Weiss SM, Herd JA, Miller NE, Weiss SM, eds. *Behavioral Health: A Handbook of Health Enhancement and Disease Prevention.* New York, NY: Wiley-Interscience Publication; 1984: 1071–1078.

97. Hatch HW, Lovelace K. Involving the southern rural church and students of the health professions in health education. *Public Health Rep.* 1980;95:23–25.

98. Lasater T, Wells BL, Carleton RA, Elder JP. The role of churches in

disease prevention studies. *Public Health Rep.* 1986;101:125–131.

99. Levine JS. The role of the black church in community medicine. *J Nat Med Assoc.* 1984;76:477–483.

100. Flora JA, Cassady D. Roles of media in community-based health promotion. In: Bracht N, ed. *Health Promotion at the Community Level.* Newbury Park, Calif: Sage Publications; 1990:143–157.

101. Wallack L. Media advocacy: promoting health through mass communication. In: Glanz K, Lewis FM, Rimer BK, eds. *Health Behavior and Health Education: Theory, Research, and Practice.* San Francisco, Calif: Jossey-Bass; 1990:370–386.

102. Flynn BS, Worden JK, Secker-Walker RH, Badger GJ, Geller BM, Costanza MC. Prevention of cigarette smoking through mass media intervention and school programs. *Am J Public Health.* 1992;82:827–834.

103. Erickson AC, McKenna JW, Ramano RM. Past lessons and new uses of the mass media in reducing tobacco consumption. *Public Health Rep.* 1990;105:239–244.

104. Advocacy Institute. *Smoking Control Media Advocacy Guidelines.* Bethesda, Md: National Cancer Institute, National Institutes of Health; 1989.

105. Minkler M, Wallerstein N. Improving health through community organization and community building. In: Glanz K, Lewis FM, Rimer BK, eds. *Health Behavior and Health Education: Theory, Research, and Practice.* 2nd ed. San Francisco, Calif: Jossey-Bass; 1997:241–269.

106. Butterfoss FD, Goodman RM, Wandersman A. Community coalitions for prevention and health promotion. *Health Educ Res.* 1993. In press.

107. Haglund B, Weisbrod RR, Bracht N. Assessing the community: its services, needs, leadership, and readiness. In: Bracht N, ed. *Health Promotion at the Community Level.* Newbury Park, Calif: Sage Publications; 1990:91–108.

108. Stewart DW, Shamdasani PN. *Focus Groups: Theory and Practice.* Newbury Park, Calif: Sage Publications; 1990.

SUGGESTED READING

Bracht N, ed. *Health Promotion at the Community Level.* Newbury Park, Calif: Sage Publications; 1990.

Glanz K, Lewis FM, Rimer BK, eds. *Health Behavior and Health Education: Theory, Research, and Practice,* 2nd ed. San Francisco, Calif: Jossey-Bass; 1997.

Hanauer P, Barr G, Glantz S. *Legislative Approaches to a Smokefree Society.* Berkeley, Calif: American Non-Smoker's Rights Foundation; 1986.

Health Education Research. 1993;8(3). Entire issue dedicated to community coalitions for health promotion.

Health Education Quarterly 1995;22(4). Entire issued dedicated to policy advocacy interventions for health promotion and education.

Matarazzo JD, Weiss SM, Herd JA, Miller NE, Weiss SM, eds. Behavioral Health: *A Handbook of Health Enhancement and Disease Prevention.* New York, NY: Wiley-Interscience Publication; 1984.

National Cancer Institute. *Making Health Communication Programs Work: A Planners Guide.* Bethesda, Md: US Dept of Health and Human Services; 1989. NIH publication 89-1493.

Pertschuk M. *Smoke Signals.* Atlanta, Ga: American Cancer Society; 1987.

Tolsma DD, Koplan JP. Health behaviors and health promotion. In: Last JM, Wallace RB, eds. *Maxcy-Rosenau-Last Textbook of* *Public Health and Preventive Medicine.* Norwalk, Conn: Appleton & Lange; 1992:701–714.

US Dept of Health and Human Services. *Strategies to Control Tobacco Use in the United States: A Blueprint for Public Health Action in the 1990's. Smoking and Tobacco Control Monographs 1.* Bethesda, Md: National Cancer Institute, 1991. NIH publication 92-3316.

RESOURCES

Planned Approach to Community Health (PATCH)
Division of Chronic Disease Control and Community Intervention
Centers for Disease Control and Prevention
4770 Buford Highway, MS K-46
Atlanta, GA 30341
(770) 488-5426
Community Health Promotion Kit: Mobilizing Your Community to Promote Health
Center for Health Promotion
Minnesota Department of Health
717 SE Delaware Street
P.O. Box 9441
Minneapolis, MN 55440-9441
(612) 623-5479

TOBACCO USE

ICD-9 405.1

Tobacco use is a behavior with complex biochemical, social, political, and behavioral interrelationships. This chapter will deal with tobacco use and its consequences as a disease entity. Mental and behavioral disorders due to use of tobacco have been assigned a code (F17.2) in the *International Statistical Classification of Diseases and Related Health Conditions, Tenth Revision.*[1] Some researchers have urged regular coding on death certificates in the assignment of contributory causes of death.[2] In 1996, the Council of State and Territorial Epidemiologists added prevalence of cigarette smoking to the list of conditions designated as reportable by states to the Centers for Disease Control and Prevention (CDC).[3]

The 1988 Report of the Surgeon General on nicotine addiction[4] concluded that nicotine met the primary criteria for "drug dependency." The conclusions in this Report were that (1) cigarettes and other forms of tobacco are addicting; (2) nicotine is the drug in tobacco that causes addiction; and (3) the pharmacologic and behavioral processes that determine tobacco addiction are similar to those that determine addiction to drugs such as heroin and cocaine. Smokeless tobacco (snuff and chewing tobacco) also contains high levels of nicotine, and using these products provides more nicotine per dose and greater persistence of blood nicotine levels than smoking. Smokeless tobacco use may lead to nicotine addiction and later longterm cigarette use as a substitute source for nicotine.[5]

In August 1995, the Food and Drug Administration (FDA) asserted jurisdiction over cigarettes and smokeless tobacco under the Federal Food, Drug, and Cosmetic Act. Under this act, the FDA determined that nicotine "is intended to affect the structure or any function of the body" through its pharmacologic and addictive effects and is thus under its jurisdiction.[6]

In addition, tobacco industry documents were cited by the FDA to

Thomas E. Novotny, MD, MPH
Gary A. Giovino, PhD

show that nicotine's drug effects are the primary reason people use these products. The industry has known of the pharmacological role of nicotine in tobacco use, including its ability to affect brain function and behavior and to produce dependence.[7] Currently, FDA jurisdiction is being challenged in the US court system.

SIGNIFICANCE

Cigarette smoking caused more than 400 000 deaths each year in the United States in 1990 to 1994.[8] This is approximately 20% of total US annual mortality. Of these annual deaths, approximately 181 000 resulted from cardiovascular diseases, 155 000 resulted from cancers, 91 000 resulted from respiratory diseases, 3 000 from environmental tobacco smoke (ETS)-induced lung cancer, 1 600 resulted from diseases among infants, and 1100 resulted from cigarette-caused fires. It has also been estimated that between 35 000 and 62 000 ischemic heart disease deaths in the United States are caused by ETS.[9] In addition, cigarette smoking caused over 1.1 million years-of-potential-life lost (YPLL) before the age of 65 and over 5.7 million YPLL to life expectancy (excluding ETS-related or burn deaths).[8]

The relative risk of premature deaths among male smokers compared with men who have never smoked is 2.34, and the relative risk of premature deaths among female smokers compared with women who have never smoked is 1.90.[10] Smoking causes coronary heart disease, atherosclerotic peripheral vascular disease, cerebrovascular disease, a variety of cancers (lung, larynx, mouth, esophagus, bladder), chronic obstructive pulmonary disease, intrauterine growth retardation, and low-birthweight babies. It is a probable cause of unsuccessful pregnancies, increased infant mortality, and peptic ulcer disease, and it is a contributing factor for cancers of the pancreas, kidney, and cervix.[10,11] Recent studies indicate that ETS is a cause of lung cancer in nonsmokers and increases the risk of ischemic heart disease.[12,13] Meta-analysis of pediatric studies indicate that ETS exposure in the home is associated with lower respiratory tract illness causing death, up to 2.2 million yearly episodes of otitis media, and over 3 million physician visits for asthma, bronchitis, and pneumonia among children.[14] Smoking interacts with certain occupational and environmental exposures and some medications to produce and multiply their adverse effects.[10] The relative risks for death due to diseases caused by or associated with smoking and the smoking-attributable mortality for each of the diseases listed above based on 1990 to 1994 data are shown in Tables 5.1 and 5.2.

Smokeless tobacco use is a cause of oral cancers and oral leukoplakia. It also increases risk of tooth attrition, tooth abrasion, and gingival recession. Other effects may include adverse outcomes of pregnancy, coronary artery disease, hypertension, and upper digestive tract cancers.[5,15]

Cigar and pipe smoking can cause oral, esophageal, laryngeal, and lung cancers.[10,16] Regular cigar smoking, especially when the smoke is inhaled and several cigars are smoked each day, increases the risk for coronary heart disease and chronic obstructive pulmonary disease.[16]

In 1993, the CDC estimated total direct costs for smoking-related medical care at $50 billion.[17] Further research using data from the 1987 National Medical Expenditures Survey applied to the Medicaid system found that 14.4% (range 8.6% in Washington DC to 19.2% in Nevada) of total state Medicaid expenses was attributable to cigarette-caused illnesses. In 1993, a total of $12.9 billion was spent on smoking-attributable illnesses by the Medicaid system.[18] Currently, more than 40 states have sued the tobacco industry to recover these damages.[19]

In addition to the direct costs of medical care, other losses caused by cigarette smoking may be considered. For 1993, indirect losses due to morbidity were estimated at $2.9 billion per year (Leonard Miller, personal communication, January 1998). Indirect mortality losses may reach another $50 billion.[20] Additional burdens of smoking are the pain, suffering, and other social and emotional losses incurred when friends and family members die prematurely from tobacco-related diseases. However, these burdens are not usually taken into account in research that emphasizes compensatory increases in societal costs due to increased longevity among nonsmokers.[21]

PATHOPHYSIOLOGY

Cardiovascular Disease

Cigarette smoking is one of the major independent coronary heart disease (CHD) risk factors that is amenable to public health intervention. Smoking acts in combination with the other major risk factors (eg, hypertension, elevated blood cholesterol) to greatly increase a person's risk for CHD.[22] Atherosclerosis (the buildup of fat and cholesterol in the arteries) is the underlying condition leading to the increased risk of death due to cardiovascular disease, and cigarette smoking is one of the most important risk factors for atherosclerosis. The effects of nicotine and carbon monoxide on blood vessel walls and the decreased oxygen-carrying capacity of the blood of smokers contribute to the overall effect of cigarette smoking on cardiovascular disease.

Table 5.1—Relative Risks[a] (RR) for Smoking-Attributable Mortality and Average Annual Number of Smoking-Attributable Mortalities (SAM[b]) among Current and Former Smokers, by Sex and Disease, United States, 1990-1994

	Men			Women			Total SAM
	Current Smokers RR	Former Smokers RR	SAM	Current Smokers RR	Former Smokers RR	SAM	
Cancers							
Lip, oral cavity, pharynx	27.5	8.8	4 864	5.6	2.9	1 447	6 311
Esophagus	7.6	5.8	6 007	10.3	3.2	1 668	7 675
Pancreas	2.1	1.1	2 21	2.3	1.8	3 660	6 381
Larynx	10.5	5.2	2 476	17.8	11.9	683	3 159
Trachea, lung, bronchus	22.4	9.4	81 710	11.9	4.7	38 656	120 365
Cervix uteri	NA	NA	NA	2.1	1.9	1 303	1 303
Urinary bladder	2.9	1.9	3 171	2.6	1.9	1 026	4 197
Kidney or other part of urinary tract	3.0	2.0	2 981	1.4	1.2	385	3 366
Total			103 931			48 827	152 757
Cardiovascular diseases							
Hypertension	1.9	1.3	3 535	1.7	1.2	2 345	5 880
Ischemic heart disease							
Persons aged 35-64 years	2.8	1.8	25 097	3.0	1.4	7,546	32,643
Persons aged >65 years	1.6	1.3	38 751	1.6	1.3	26,619	65,370
Other heart diseases	1.9	1.3	24 078	1.7	1.2	12 872	36 949
Cerebrovascular disease							
Persons aged 35-64 years	3.7	1.4	4 571	4.8	1.4	4 086	8 657
Persons aged >65 years	1.9	1.3	10 668	1.5	1.0	4 304	14 972
Artherosclerosis	4.1	2.3	3 561	3.0	1.3	2 617	6 179
Aortic aneurysm	4.1	2.3	5 767	3.0	1.3	1 460	7 227
Other arterial disease	4.1	2.3	2 197	3.0	1.3	1 254	3 450
Total			118 224			63 103	181 327

Respiratory diseases							
Pneumonia, influenza	2.0	1.6	11 267	2.2	1.4	8 060	19 327
Bronchitis, emphysema	9.7	8.8	9 642	10.5	7.0	6 475	16 116
Chronic airway obstruction	9.7	8.8	32 132	10.5	7.0	21 893	54 025
Other respiratory diseases	2.0	1.6	776	2.2	1.4	721	1 497
Total			53 817			37 148	90 965
Other diseases/conditions							
Environmental tobacco smoke lung cancer deaths			1 110			1 890	3 000
Burn deaths			691			409	1 100

[a] Relative to people who have never smoked.
[b] SAM is the estimated number of annual US deaths due to smoking.

121

Table 5.2—Relative Risks (RR) for Smoking-Attributable Mortality and Average Annual Number of Smoking-Attributable Mortalities among Infants of Current Smokers, by Sex and Contributor to Death, United States, 1990-1994

	Male Children		Female Children		Total
	RR	SAM	RR	SAM	SAM
Contributors to Death					
Short gestation, low birth weight	1.8	299	1.8	245	544
Respiratory distress syndrome	1.8	171	1.8	112	283
Other respiratory conditions affecting newborns	1.8	187	1.8	138	325
Sudden infant death syndrome	1.5	269	1.5	171	439
Total		926		666	1592

ETS increases the risk of cardiovascular disease among exposed nonsmokers through reduced myocardial oxygen uptake, increased platelet adhesiveness, influences on established atherosclerosis, and increased damage after preexisting infarction. These effects are mediated by several components of passively inhaled cigarette smoke, including carbon monoxide, nicotine, and polycyclic aromatic hydrocarbons.[23]

Cancer

Mainstream (MS) cigarette smoke contains nearly 5 000 chemicals.[24] This mixture contains 43 chemicals that have met the criteria of a known human or animal carcinogen established by the International Agency for Research on Cancer.[25] These carcinogens include polycyclic aromatic hydrocarbons, nitrosamines, and aldehydes. Large-scale epidemiologic studies have provided convincing evidence that confirms the findings of toxicologic studies in animals and clinical observations of the relationship between tobacco use and cancer (epidemiologic criteria used to infer that tobacco use causes cancer are discussed in Chapter 2).

Recent studies have addressed unresolved issues concerning the relationship between smoking and lung cancer,[26] including the possible role of genetic predisposition, sex, and race/ethnicity. However, twin studies do not show that genetic factors predict lung cancer risk in male smokers older than 50, the age group in which most such cancers occur.[27]

Smokeless tobacco contains tobacco-specific nitrosamines and other carcinogens, often at levels hundreds of times higher than what foods and beverages may legally contain. Smokeless tobacco use and oropharyngeal cancer are causally related. Snuff contains other carcinogenic agents, including polonium-210, uranium-235, nickel, and formaldehyde.[5]

According to a 1992 report by the Environmental Protection Agency, ETS is a Group A (known human) carcinogen, to which there is no safe level of exposure.[28] Exposure to ETS is causally associated with lung cancer in adults, and ETS is qualitatively similar in composition to MS smoke. In fact, many of the carcinogens found in MS appear in greater concentration in ETS. ETS is a major cause of indoor air contamination and thus may have a significant impact on population health.

Chronic Lung and Other Respiratory Diseases

Cigarette smoking causes almost 90% of chronic obstructive pulmonary disease and emphysema mortality. No other single risk factor is significant in the causation of these diseases, and the effects of most other lung disease risk factors (such as asbestos exposure) are greatly exacerbated by smoking. Cigarette smoke paralyzes respiratory ciliary action, increases mucus production and small airway plugging, and causes an inflammatory response in respiratory syncitial cells. These processes facilitate the breakdown of alveolar membranes to cause emphysema.

Airflow obstruction due to these changes leads to poor exchange of oxygen and carbon dioxide and ultimately air starvation (hypoxemia) for the victim. Hypoxemia is further exacerbated by carbon monoxide produced by smoking cigarettes.[26]

ETS exposure among adults can contribute to chronic respiratory impairment and the occurrence of a variety of lower respiratory symptoms.[9,29] Of arguably greater concern are reports on the effects of ETS exposure among young (less than 5 years old) children, 50% to 60% of whom may be exposed in the home. In fact, the EPA reported that some structural and functional properties of the lung are altered by prenatal exposure through maternal smoking. ETS causes bronchial hyperresponsiveness in children that may lead to asthma. Lower respiratory tract infections are more common among children of smokers, and these infections may have long-term effects on lung growth and development. Children of smokers experience increased middle ear effusion leading to reduced patency of the euschacian tube. Reduced mucociliary function, well documented in smokers, may also predispose children exposed to ETS to acute and chronic otitis media, one of the most common reasons for seeking medical attention.[9,28]

High-Risk Groups

In order to use national and state data on smoking to examine secular trends and identify high-risk groups, public health professionals must understand the uniform definitions used for various levels of smoking because these definitions permit useful comparisons between and within surveys. *Ever smokers* are defined as persons who report that they have smoked at least 100 cigarettes in their entire life. *Current smokers* are ever smokers who report smoking every day or some days at the time of the interview (the question is "Do you now smoke cigarettes every day, some days, or not at all?"). *Former smokers* are ever smokers who do not smoke currently.[30] The *quit ratio* is the proportion of ever smokers who are former smokers.[10]

The National Health Interview Surveys (NHIS) provide data on US adults, aged 18 years and older, from household interviews of large sample populations (eg,17 213 in 1995) over the last 33 years. Despite significant changes in the prevalence of smoking since 1965 (among men, decreasing from 50.2% in 1965 to 27.0% in 1995; among women, decreasing from 31.9% in 1965 to 22.6% in 1995), more than 47 million Americans continue to smoke (Table 5.3).[31]

Overall, 20.1% were every-day smokers, and 4.6% were some-day smokers (total current smokers, 24.7% in 1995).

In 1995, the patterns of smoking reflect previous findings in the United States. By race/ethnicity, the highest prevalence of smoking was reported among American Indians/Alaskan Natives (36.2%), and the lowest prevalence among Asians/Pacific Islanders (16.6%). The prevalence of smoking according to level of education was highest among persons with 9 to 11 years of education (37.5%) and lowest among those with ≥16 years of education (14.0%). Those living below the poverty level had approximately 36% higher prevalence of smoking than did those below the poverty level. In contrast to past analyses, non-Hispanic Blacks and Whites differed only slightly in prevalence (25.8% versus 25.6%). Prevalence among Southeast Asian males ranged from 36% to 48% in several population-based studies conducted in the 1990s.[32]

The highest risk groups in terms of initiation of tobacco use are children and adolescents. Currently, there are three national surveys that assess tobacco use among youth on a regular basis: the Monitoring the Future Survey (MTFS) and the Youth Risk Behavior Survey (YRBS) are school-based, and the National Household Survey on Drug Abuse

Table 5.3—Percentage of Adults Who Smoke Cigarettes, by Sex, Age, Race, Hispanic Origin, and Level of Education, United States, 1995

	Men		Women		Total	
	%	(95% CI[a])	%	(95% CI)	%	(95% CI)
Age (y)						
18-24	27.8	(23.9–31.7)	21.8	(18.8–24.8)	**24.8**	**(22.4–27.2)**
25-44	30.5	(28.7–32.3)	26.8	(25.2–28.4)	**28.6**	**(27.4–29.8)**
45-64	27.1	(25.0–29.2)	24.0	(22.0–26.0)	**25.5**	**(24.0–27.0)**
≥65	14.3	(12.2–16.4)	11.5	(10.0–13.0)	**13.0**	**(11.7–14.3)**
Race/Ethnicity						
White, non-Hispanic	27.1	(25.6–28.6)	24.1	(22.8–25.4)	**25.6**	**(24.6–26.6)**
Black, non-Hispanic	28.8	(25.1–32.5)	23.5	(20.4–26.6)	**25.8**	**(23.2–28.4)**
Hispanic	21.7	(18.8–24.6)	14.9	(12.8–17.0)	**18.3**	**(16.5–20.1)**
Asian/Pacific Islander	29.4	(20.8–38.0)	4.3	(1.2–7.4)	**16.6**	**(12.0–21.2)**
American Indian/ Alaska Native	37.3	(20.1–54.5)	35.4	(21.5–49.3)	**36.2**	**(25.6–46.8)**
Education						
<8 years	28.4	(24.2–32.6)	17.8	(15.0–20.6)	**22.6**	**(20.1–25.1)**
9-11 years	41.9	(37.5–46.3)	33.7	(30.2–37.2)	**37.5**	**(34.6–40.4)**
12 years	33.7	(31.4–36.0)	26.2	(24.4–28.0)	**29.5**	**(28.1–30.9)**
13-15 years	25.0	(22.4–27.6)	22.5	(20.3–24.7)	**23.6**	**(22.0–25.2)**
≥16 years	14.3	(12.5–16.1)	13.7	(11.9–15.5)	**14.0**	**(12.6-15.4)**
Poverty Status						
At or Above	25.9	(24.6–27.2)	21.8	(20.7–22.9)	**23.8**	**(22.9–24.7)**
Below	36.9	(32.6–41.2)	29.3	(26.4–32.2)	**32.5**	**(30.0–35.0)**
Unknown	26.9	(21.2–32.6)	21.0	(17.5–24.5)	**23.5**	**(20.3–26.7)**
Total	**27.0**	**(25.8–28.2)**	**22.6**	**(21.5–23.7)**	**24.7**	**(23.9–25.5)**

[a]95% confidence interval.

Note: National Health Interview Survey 1995.[31]

(NHSDA) is household-based. In addition, the Teenage Attitudes and Practices Survey (TAPS) is a telephone-based household survey of young people conducted in 1989 and 1993. In 1994, the Report of the Surgeon General, *Preventing Tobacco Use Among Young People* summarized data from these surveys, and emphasized that almost all first use (more than 80%) occurs before age 18 and that initiation is occurring at younger ages among more recent birth cohorts of girls.[33] Each day, approximately 3000 young people begin smoking in the United States.[34]

In 1997, 65.4% of high school seniors reported ever trying cigarettes, while 36.5% reported using any cigarettes in the last 30 days, and 24.6% reported daily use of cigarettes.[35] Prevalence of use within the last 30 days among White seniors is significantly higher than among Blacks (40.7% versus 14.3%), and among males and females, prevalence is now approximately equal (37.3% and 35.2% respectively).[35]

Between 1970 and 1986, among males aged 17 to 19 years, the prevalence of snuff use increased fifteenfold, and use of chewing tobacco increased more than fourfold.[10] In 1987 and 1991 combined, 6.2% of adults used smokeless tobacco (SLT), with highest rates among American Indian/Alaska Native men (7.8%) and White men (6.8%). Only 0.6% of women used SLT.[30,36] Initiation of this product appears to begin in childhood and early adolescence. In 1997, 25.3% of high school seniors had ever tried SLT, and 9.7% report use within the last 30 days.[35] Among high school seniors who had ever tried SLT, 73% did so by the ninth grade.[33] In studying the incidence of regular SLT use among children and adolescents, males showed higher use than females (10.4% versus 0.3%) and Whites showed higher use than Hispanics or Blacks (10.4%, 4.1% and 0.8%, respectively).[37]

Geographic distribution

The CDC's Behavioral Risk Factor Surveillance System (BRFSS) reports state-specific tobacco use data. The BRFSS now collects yearly data for smoking and other behavioral risk factors on persons aged 18 and older in 50 states and the District of Columbia. Regional variation in state smoking patterns is shown, with higher smoking prevalence in the East and South and higher quit rates in the West. In 1994 to 1995, daily smoking among adults ranged from 15.0% in the District of Columbia to 29.1% in Nevada.[38] This represents approximately a twofold difference. Similarly, the smoking-related death rate is highest in Nevada (469 deaths per 100 000 population).[39] Among youth in grades 9 to 12, prevalence of current cigarette use ranged from 16.4% in Utah to 47.0% in Kentucky.[40]

Smokeless tobacco use varies even more. In 1992 to 1993, the prevalence among male adults age ≥18 years ranged from 0.1% in Connecticut to 15.6% in West Virginia.[39] In 1997, the prevalence of use among male students in grades 9 to 12 ranged from 6.4% in Hawaii to 34.7% in Wyoming.[40]

Time Trends

The most important phenomenon revealed by analyses of trends in adult cigarette smoking is the flattening of the previously noted downward trend among all groups since 1990. Although previous analyses[41] provided optimistic forecasts for reaching the Year 2000 Objective for the Nation for current smoking prevalence of 15%, it is now clear that with these recent trends, the Year 2000 Objective for the Nation will not be met (Figure 5.1).[30,31]

An earlier NHIS analysis of trends over time by educational status showed diverging trends for those with higher education compared with those with lower educational status.[42] These absolute differences persist, although the rate of change for all educational groups appears also to be level.[30,31]

Using combined NHIS data sets to analyze health care professionals, researchers found that between 1974 and 1991, cigarette smoking declined most rapidly among physicians (18.8% to 3.3%), intermediately

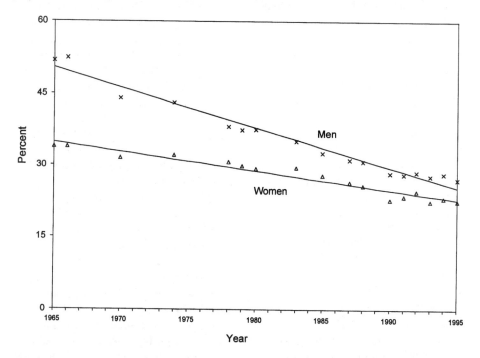

Figure 5.1—Prevalence of current smokers among adults (aged 18 years and older), United States, 1965-1995.[30,31]

among registered nurses (31.7% to 18.3%), and slowest among Licensed practical nurses (37.1% to 27.2%).[43] Using 1983 to 1993 NHIS data, researchers have found that persons below the poverty level are consistently more likely than persons above the poverty level to be current smokers and to have a lower quit ratio. This phenomenon persists even when the sociodemographic variables of education, age, employment status, marital status, sex, and race are controlled.[44]

The prevalence of smoking among Blacks had been higher than that among Whites in every year since 1965. However, the rate of change in current smoking prevalence among Blacks was not significantly different from that among Whites from 1974 to 1985, and since 1992, the prevalence of smoking among Blacks has been similar to that among Whites.[30–32]

Of particular concern relative to illness among children is the prevalence of smoking among women of reproductive age (18 to 44 years on the NHIS). This declined only modestly from 1987 to 1992 (29.6% to 26.9%).[45]

Because most smokers begin to smoke during the teenage years, the trends in smoking among youth deserve particular attention. Among high school seniors, the prevalence of daily smoking declined from almost 30% in 1978 to about 19% in 1990. Since 1991, prevalence has increased among all teens regardless of age, gender, or race.[35] Rates among females were higher than rates among males in every year from 1976 to 1989 (Figure 5.2).[35] Of increasing interest is the wide disparity between white and black youth smoking prevalence. Data from several different surveys show a similar pattern, with significantly lower smoking prevalence among non-Hispanic Blacks compared with non-Hispanic Whites (eg, among high school students in 1997, 40% of non-Hispanic White versus 17% of non-Hispanic Black females and 40% of non-Hispanic White versus 28% non-Hispanic Black males were current smokers.[35,46,47]

Recently reported data from the 1997 Youth Risk Behavior Survey[47] indicated that the prevalence of cigarette smoking among US high school students increased by 32%, from 27.5% in 1991 to 36.4% in 1997. Among White students, current cigarette smoking increased 28%, from 30.9% in 1991 to 39.7% in 1997. Among Black students, current smoking increased by 80%, from 12.6% to 22.7% in 1997. Among Hispanic students, current smoking increased by 34%, from 25.3% in 1991 to 34.0% in 1997. All of these increases were statistically significant ($p < 0.001$). In 1997, 9.3% of high school students (including 15.8% of males and 1.5% of females) reported

Percent

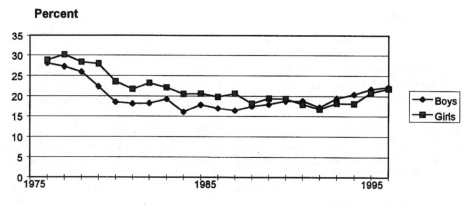

Figure 5.2—Prevalence of daily smokers among high school seniors, United States, 1976-1997.[35]

current smokeless tobacco use. Additionally, 22.0% of high school students (including 31.2% of males and 10.8% of females) reported current cigar use. Overall, 42.7% of high school students (including 48.2% of males and 36.0% of females) used cigarettes, smokeless tobacco, or cigars during the 30 days preceding the 1997 survey.

RISK FACTORS

Magnitude of Risk Factors

No single factor causes a young person to begin using tobacco, and no single intervention modality will be effective in preventing or treating tobacco use among adults or adolescents. Unlike risk factors for disease, relative risk estimates for tobacco use are difficult to precisely quantify because of the complexity of their interactions. In addition to sociodemographic factors, other important factors that encourage people to start using tobacco or discourage them from quitting include the effects of nicotine, public attitudes about smoking, tobacco advertising, parental and peer influences, and weight gain that often follows smoking cessation (Table 5.4).

Biochemical Determinants of Tobacco Use. When tobacco smoke is inhaled, nicotine is rapidly absorbed through the lung's alveolar membranes and small airways. Peak nicotine blood concentrations of approximately 16 ng/mL are reached within 15 minutes. The half-life of nicotine is approximately 2 hours. Studies of blood nicotine levels in regular cigarette smokers show peaks and troughs following each

129

Table 5.4—Modifiable Risk Factors for Tobacco Use, United States[a]

- Nicotine addiction and withdrawal symptoms
- Psychosocial support for smoking, including social norms
- Advertising and promotion of tobacco products
- Weight gain after cessation
- Psychoactive effects of nicotine (stimulation, relaxation, ability to concentrate, stress reduction)
- Low self-esteem or self-image
- Affordability of tobacco
- Lack of services/skills to support smoking cessation
- Parental smoking
- Lack of parental support and involvement
- Peer and best-friend smoking
- Low academic support and school involvement
- Perceptions among adolescents that smoking is normative
- Legislation and policies that allow smoking in public places
- Ease of access to tobacco products (eg, un-enforced minors' access laws)
- Lack of knowledge of health risks of smoking and smokeless tobacco use
- Positive imagery in media and sports

[a]Not in order of importance.

cigarette smoked. Nicotine accumulates over 6 to 8 hours of regular smoking and persists at significant levels for 6 to 8 hours after cessation. Smokers thus dose themselves throughout the day, maintaining blood levels sufficient to avoid withdrawal symptoms.[4] Smokeless tobacco users also maintain sustained levels of blood nicotine through slower absorption but more prolonged blood nicotine elevation.[5]

Although some US smokers only smoke occasionally or only a few cigarettes per day, most (70%) report smoking 15 or more cigarettes per day.[30] Withdrawal symptoms linked to the physical dependence on nicotine begin within 24 hours of abrupt cessation and appear to peak within a few days. Symptoms may persist for 10 days or more, and cravings for cigarettes may be sustained for years. Withdrawal symptoms include (1) a craving for nicotine; (2) irritability, frustration, or anger; (3) anxiety; (4) difficulty concentrating; (5) restlessness; (6) decreased heart rate; (7) increased appetite; and (8) weight gain.[4]

Nicotine is a psychoactive, or mood-altering, drug. Its pleasurable effects contribute to the initiation of smoking, or at least encourage people to switch from experimental to regular use of tobacco. Once the smoker establishes a level of nicotine tolerance, however, the primary physiologic effect of smoking is psychopharmacologic.[4,48] Thus, the addictive properties of nicotine are strong risk factors for continued tobacco use.[33]

Smoking and nicotine do not improve cognitive tasks for non-smokers, but smokers perform better on some tasks if they are not deprived of nicotine. Smokers also use cigarettes to reduce stress, and this function has been identified as a risk factor for smoking initiation. Importantly, nicotine and body weight are related. Smokers weigh, on average, 7 pounds less than nonsmokers. The 1990 Report of the Surgeon General emphasizes, however, that the benefits of smoking cessation far exceed any risks from weight gain or any adverse psychological effects that may follow quitting.[11]

Psychosocial Determinants of Tobacco Use. Children and adolescents have been studied extensively for psychosocial determinants of tobacco use. Despite widespread school health education and public information on the health consequences of smoking and smokeless tobacco use, several misconceptions about smoking may persist, especially among economically disadvantaged youth. At-risk youths may have a poor awareness of the long- and short-term health consequences and the addictive potential of smoking. They may be strongly influenced by peer and family norms and youth-oriented advertisements that positively portray smokers and smoking. Using cohort analyses from the 1989 and 1993 TAPS, the factor found most strongly associated with progression to established smoking from experimentation was exposure to other smokers (family and best friends, odds ratio 2.46, 95% confidence interval 1.73, 3.51), while cognitive susceptibility is the strongest predictor of experimentation (odds ratio 3.15, 95% confidence interval 2.37, 4.17).[49]

Adolescents who are extroverted and who demonstrate problem behaviors are more likely to begin smoking.[33] Interestingly, increased rates of children's behavior problems were found to be associated with exposure to maternal cigarette smoking during and after pregnancy. Thus, smoking may be related both to parental behavioral modeling and to actual behavior problems among children of mothers who smoke. Smoking may be used as a coping mechanism for dealing with boredom and frustration, seen as enjoyable and as a way to have fun; used as a strategy to reduce stress, seen as a transition to adulthood, seen as a way of gaining admission to a peer group, or used as a way to remain energetic.[33,48] Young persons at high risk for SLT use initiation include those who have the following characteristics: reside in the South, live with someone else who uses in the home, have peers who use SLT, are current smokers, participate in organized sports, display other risk behaviors, had a steady girlfriend, and perceive indifference or approval of SLT use from best friends.[37]

Environmental stimuli also play an important role in initiating and reinforcing cigarette use. These stimuli may include social interactions, conditioned responses to other behaviors such as eating, and supportive media imagery. Returning to smoking after cessation, or relapse, is in part determined by these external stimuli. Studies of cessation show that most smokers (65%) relapse within 3 months after quitting. Those who have maintained abstinence for at least 6 months are much less likely to relapse. However, about one-third of all former cigarette smokers who have maintained abstinence for at least 1 year eventually relapse.[45]

Economic Determinants of Tobacco Use. Economic determinants of tobacco use are commonly defined within the rubric of "negative price elasticity of demand," meaning that as price increases, demand decreases. This is particularly true for tobacco use by youth, who tend to have a lower spending capability than adults. It is estimated that a 10% increase in price would decrease the number of teenagers who smoke by 7%.[50]

Cigarette taxes and therefore prices affect consumption in a variety of ways. Conscious decisions were made in Canada to increase taxes as a *health policy*, whereas in most US states cigarette taxes are applied to *generate revenue*. In California, Massachusetts, Arizona, and Michigan, earmarked cigarette taxes also support strong tobacco control programs. In addition to the negative price elasticity of demand, these tax-supported programs have measurable effects on per capita cigarette consumption attributed to program content.[51,52]

In a study of state excise tax changes on per capita consumption, an average annual decrease of 3.0 in packs per capita consumed was observed in states with *any* tax increase.[53] The magnitude of the decrease in consumption was directly associated with the size of the tax increase. With time (approximately 3 years), the effects of a tax may become attenuated. That is, the rate of decline in per capita cigarette consumption levels off.[51] In addition, several small increases in the tax levy over time tend to be much less effective than large increases applied at longer intervals.

Legislative and Policy Determinants of Tobacco Use. Unenforced minors' access laws, laws that permit smoking in public places, and tobacco product advertising and promotion may facilitate initiation of smoking among youths or inhibit smoking cessation by supporting the social acceptability of smoking.

Employers who prohibit smoking may observe favorable changes in employees' attitudes, decreases in the number of cigarettes consumed daily by smokers, and improvements in ambient air quality.[54] Conversely, legislation permitting smoking in workplaces increases costs of building maintenance and ventilation and may send a mixed message about social norms to workers who smoke. In addition, evidence suggests that a total ban on smoking in the workplace may be the only way to protect the health of nonsmokers.[55] Data from several national surveys show that approximately 80% of employees support smoking restrictions in the workplace. The primary reasons for adopting workplace smoking policies are management concern for employees' health (71%), complaints from employees (54%), state or local laws (39%), executive order (17%), insurance cost concerns (10%), absenteeism concerns (10%), and productivity concerns (8%).[56] In an industry-wide study (hospitals, where the Joint Commission and Accreditation of Healthcare Organizations mandated smokefree buildings in 1993), quitting among employees after implementation of a smoking ban was significantly greater than among employees in matched communities

who did not have a worksite smoking ban.[57]

Restrictive legislation has increased in states and local jurisdictions throughout the United States. The presence of such legislation usually indicates and reinforces widespread psychosocial changes in populations supporting it. Preemption clauses, which restrict local communities from enacting more restrictive clean indoor air legislation, usually indicate successful efforts by tobacco lobbyists to limit the effect of state laws. Since 1990, several preemption clauses have appeared in state legislation.[58]

Of particular interest is the recent Environmental Protection Agency finding that ETS is a Group A Carcinogen to which there is no safe level of exposure.[28] This designation amplifies the health risks of cigarette smoke to nonsmokers and may result in increased regulation by agencies such as the Occupational Safety and Health Administration. Regulatory and licensing agencies now effectively use their authority to stimulate restrictive smoking policies.[57]

Cigarettes are the most heavily advertised consumer product. National restrictions on electronic media advertising of tobacco products have been circumvented, in part, by the use of outdoor advertising and cigarette logos that appear on televised events. This widespread marketing is a strong risk factor for tobacco use. Of interest are recent studies on the recognition of a cartoon character ("Old Joe") used by Camel cigarettes indicating that this logo was particularly effective among children and adolescents.[59] Further, advertising appeared to influence market share for specific brands primarily through its effect on children.[60] In a recent California study, one third of all cigarette experimentation among youth could be attributed to tobacco promotional activities.[61] Marketing tactics may affect cigarette consumption in four ways[10]:

• Encouraging children or young adults to experiment with tobacco and to start using it regularly.

• Prompting smokers to light up by creating attitudes and images that reinforce the desirability of smoking and that remind smokers of enjoyable occasions associated with smoking.

• Reducing smokers' motivation to quit through attractive imagery and implicit alleviation of fears about the health consequences of smoking.

• Using images to remind former smokers of the reasons and situations in which they smoked, to encourage them to relapse.

The evidence culled from published studies is sufficient to conclude that tobacco marketing has a causal relationship to smoking initiation among youth.[62]

Population-Attributable Risk

Estimates of the proportion of tobacco use in the population related to various modifiable risk factors cannot be made. These estimates are not possible because (1) precise relative risk estimates for these factors are not available and (2) no data are available on the proportion of the population exposed to many of these risk factors or exposure is ubiquitous (eg, tobacco product advertising).

PREVENTION AND CONTROL MEASURES

Prevention

School-based education alone will not prevent tobacco use among youths, yet anti-tobacco education in schools is an essential component of tobacco control.[63] Such education appears to work most effectively when combined with other community-based components such as mass media anti-smoking messages. The following interventions should also contribute to reducing tobacco use among youth and other high-risk groups:

• Enforcing state legislation to control sales of tobacco to minors. Merchant education and criminal or civil penalties are not sufficient to deter sales unless licensing and license revocation are used to ensure merchant compliance.

• Prohibiting free distribution of tobacco products and logo items.

- Eliminating sales of candy cigarettes and loose single cigarettes.
- Restricting advertising from outdoor and print media.
- Decreasing television and movie imagery supporting tobacco use.
- Eliminating tobacco company promotion of sports and cultural events.
- Developing media activities that effectively discourage tobacco use.
- Prohibiting smoking in all enclosed public places and workplaces, especially those where youths are likely to congregate.

In 1992, national legislation took effect that linked enforcement of state-based laws against sales of tobacco products to youth to federal funding for alcohol and drug abuse prevention block grants. As a result of this legislation, the sale of tobacco products to minors is illegal in all states and the District of Columbia.[58]

Results of the 1993 TAPS show that 61.9% of children smokers aged 12 to 17 usually bought their own cigarettes, indicating the ease with which minors can purchase tobacco products over the counter and from vending machines despite existing legislation.[64] In 1996, the Substance Abuse and Mental Health Services Administration issued final regulations to implement enforcement of state laws on purchase of tobacco products by minors. These regulations require states to develop a strategy to achieve noncompliance rates of $\leq 20\%$.[65] The proposed FDA regulatory action will be based on a youth-centered strategy that is intended to reduce the risk that future generations of Americans will become dependent on nicotine without prohibiting access to these products by adults. The FDA recognizes the need for cigarettes and smokeless tobacco products to remain available to adults, because millions of American adults use and are addicted to these products. The potential disruption to society resulting from the elimination of tobacco products would be great, and therefore FDA does not intend to remove them from the market.[59,62] A comprehensive and effective regulatory approach should be designed to reduce the many avenues of easy access to tobacco products available to children and teenagers, and to make it harder for young people to buy these products. The Agency should also act to reduce the powerful and alluring imagery used in tobacco advertising and promotion that tends to encourage impressionable young people to initiate tobacco use, and should attempt to enhance the positive image of a smoke-free generation. Further, such actions should seek to educate people about the specific and relevant health risks associated with tobacco use and to disseminate information about quitting.

Media dependence on cigarette advertising revenues is substantial, and acceptance of smoking and health messages have been shown to be negatively associated with acceptance of cigarette advertising by magazines.[10] Sports, cultural, and minority organizations have become financially dependent on contributions from tobacco companies and thus may be less likely to speak out against tobacco and risk withdrawal of this funding. Although more research establishing the causal nature of tobacco advertising and use of tobacco products by youth may be important, recent studies show evidence of the association between advertising expenditures and youth brand preference, tobacco marketing exposure and initiation, and favorable beliefs toward smoking in response to marketing exposure[33,61,66-68]

Screening and Early Detection

Although traditional screening and early detection tests (eg, those used in cholesterol screening) do not apply to tobacco use, several screening-related issues in evaluation and cessation warrant discussion. One of the most important screening strategies for health care professionals is to ask about a patient's smoking history. Information on a patient's smoking status should be included as part of any medical record and should be ascertained on every visit, similar to blood pressure and weight measurements.[69]

In addition, numerous biochemical measures are available to assess whether a person is a smoker. For example, cotinine (the major metabolite of nicotine) can be measured in various body fluids to identify smokers or nonsmokers passively exposed to environmental tobacco smoke.[70] Cotinine can be measured in plasma, urine, saliva, and even cervical secretions.

Treatment, Rehabilitation, and Recovery

Treatment for tobacco use, commonly called smoking cessation, will be briefly discussed in this section. Among smokers, 68.2% wanted to quit smoking completely in 1995[28]; yet, many health care finance systems do still not provide coverage for smoking cessation, including 45 of the 51 state Medicaid programs.

The success of formal smoking cessation programs varies according to clientele, methods used, and the definition of "success." In general, follow-up evaluation studies show about 20% to 40% success at 1 year of follow-up, with most recidivism within the first 6 weeks of quitting.[71] Approximately 90% of successful quitters have used a self-help quitting strategy (without formal assistance), most by quitting abruptly. Wide dissemination of self-help materials, may assist a substantial number of smokers as a very cost-effective public health intervention.[72]

Clinicians have excellent opportunities for improving cessation. An expert panel of the Agency for Health Care Policy and Research (AHCPR) concluded that effective smoking cessation treatments are available and should be offered to every patient who smokes.[73] These include nicotine replacement therapy (NRT), social support, and skills training/problem solving. NRT is now available over the counter in both nicotine gum and transdermal patch form. The gum and the patch are used as adjuncts to appropriate brief counseling or referral to more comprehensive programs. The AHCPR-supported guideline recommends that clinicians:
• Ask every patient at every visit if he or she smokes.
• Write a patient's smoking status in the medical chart under vital signs.
• Ask patients about their desire to quit, and reinforce their intentions.
• Motivate patients who are reluctant to quit.
• Help motivated smokers set a quit date.
• Recommend or prescribe nicotine replacement therapy.
• Help patients resolve problems that result from quitting.
• Refer for counseling, which may be helpful to some patients to increase the likelihood of successful quitting.
• Encourage relapsed smokers to try quitting again.

Cessation of smoking among youth is an untapped intervention modality. The 1993 TAPS provided information on youth advice from health care providers regarding cessation. Only approximately half of those who were current tobacco users received any communication about the use of tobacco from providers.[74]

Economic incentives to quit smoking offer great potential as cessation interventions and are generally underused. These include the following:
• Health insurance programs that pay for cessation services.
• Differential health insurance rates for smokers and nonsmokers.
• Employers' electing not to hire smokers.
• Employers' offering workplace-based cessation programs.
• Employers' offering bonuses or other incentives to workers who make healthy lifestyle choices.
• Periodic and substantial increases in cigarette excise taxes.

Interventions against smokeless tobacco use may begin with dental health providers, who treat 62% of the US population in any given year. Screening for leukoplakia, a hallmark lesion of smokeless tobacco use, by all providers will help prevent oropharyngeal cancer and begin a dialogue of education by the health professional.[5] Other specific efforts to control smokeless tobacco use include banning distribution of smokeless tobacco free samples, enforcing laws against purchase of any tobacco product by minors, banning advertising using logos in sporting events, banning smokeless tobacco use in schools, improving health education messages against smokeless tobacco use in schools, and separating major league baseball, a source of role models for youth and for outright production promotion, from tobacco use.[5]

EXAMPLES OF PUBLIC HEALTH INTERVENTIONS

Because no single educational or policy action will eliminate tobacco use, several essential elements of a comprehensive tobacco control program must be put into place[75]:
• Surveillance (monitor adult and adolescent tobacco use, per capita cigarette consumption, high-risk behavior, determinants of use, ETS exposure, and public opinion regarding tobacco use and tobacco control).
• Problem assessment (measure the attributable disease and economic impact of tobacco use, and assess the status of community prevention and control measures).

• Technical information collection and dissemination.
• Public information campaigns.
• Legislation and policies.
• Health agency and community-based programs (coalition-building, school-based education, self-help interventions, and advice from health care providers to quit).
• Cessation programs (including pharmacologic interventions).

State and local health departments are the central forces in public health. Tobacco use must be strongly addressed by these agencies to reduce smoking rates. Currently, state health departments display a wide variation in the scope and nature of their tobacco prevention and control measures.

The National Cancer Institute, in collaboration with the American Cancer Society, has recently evaluated the American Stop Smoking Intervention Study for cancer prevention (ASSIST). ASSIST implemented comprehensive tobacco control programs in 17 states in 1993, with approximately $114 million. The overall goal of ASSIST is to reduce current smoking prevalence to less than 15%. High-risk groups (ie, children and adolescents, women, Blacks and Hispanics, blue-collar workers, people of low-income status, and undereducated persons) are targeted. Specific interventions include (1) legislative and policy initiatives (eg, restricting tobacco sales to minors), (2) media interventions, (3) programs to increase counseling for tobacco prevention and cessation by health care providers, and (4) school- and workplace-based prevention and cessation classes. By 1996, intervention states consumed about 7% fewer cigarettes per capita than nonintervention sites, even after accounting for differences in price among states.[76] ASSIST states had developed 220 tobacco control coalitions with more than 6200 organizational and individual members.

State programs are augmented by funding from the Robert Wood Johnson Foundation (the SmokeLess States Program), supporting increased state tobacco excise taxes, promotion of tobacco free workplaces and public places, policy actions to inhibit access to tobacco products among children and youth, and changes in Medicaid health insurance coverage to include tobacco cessation services. In addition, the goals of the CDC's Initiatives to Mobilize for the Prevention and Control of Tobacco Use (IMPACT) Program are to build tobacco control capacity and to establish a comprehensive and coordinated national effort. This is accomplished through tobacco control plans in each state, statewide tobacco-control coalitions, resource development and training, funding of communities, media campaigns,

surveillance, and evaluation. Key strategies include (1) provision of smokefree indoor air, (2) economic incentives, (3) reducing minors' access to tobacco products, (4) countermarketing strategies, (5) tobacco product regulation, and (6) prevention and cessation activities.

State tobacco control programs supported by earmarked tobacco taxes have provided some of the most innovative actions against tobacco use in the 1990s. For example, in California, the tax itself and the state's paid advertising campaign against tobacco use appear to have contributed to a significant decline in cigarette smoking.[77,78] However, because of intense opposition of the tobacco industry, these programs have suffered setbacks and obstructions. An important lesson from the review of California programs is that continued vigilance and political involvement of the constituency groups supporting them is needed so that the intent of these programs is not willfully or neglectfully diverted by actions of the tobacco industry and their political allies.[79] Evidence from both California and Massachusetts suggests that a tobacco tax increase combined with a media-based campaign can be more effective than a tax increase alone.[52]

Perhaps the most important action to date by the states is the lawsuits brought by Attorneys General against the tobacco industry to recover damages incurred by years of state payments for medical care attributable to cigarette smoking.[80] At this writing, numerous pieces of legislation have been introduced in Congress to permit a financial settlement between the states and the tobacco industry, some of which involve providing immunity to the industry from future legal actions. Liability suits and other legal actions, combined with widespread disclosure of heretofore secret industry documents on tactics, intentions, and risk obfuscation arguably have caused more progress in controlling the actions of the industry than any previous intervention.[19,81]

AREAS OF FUTURE RESEARCH AND DEMONSTRATION

Research on the effect of various public health actions against tobacco use will be important in shaping interventions for the future. Key issues will include the following:
• Evaluating the effects of strictly enforced laws that restrict minors' access to tobacco.
• Evaluating the effects of tobacco advertising and promotion, product placement in movies and other mass media, and bans on tobacco advertising and promotion.
• Evaluating the effect of workplace policies on smoking (eg, hiring practices, smoking restrictions,

economic incentives, and cessation programs), on the health, and on the productivity of workers.
• Evaluating the long-term effects of school health education to prevent tobacco use.
• Understanding relapse prevention among smokers who quit.
• Evaluating alternatives for tobacco farmers and retailers dependent on tobacco sales.
• Evaluating the effects of national and state-based programs on tobacco use, mortality, and morbidity.
• Developing and evaluating the effect of widely disseminated self-help program materials and pharmacologic therapies to assist individual smoking cessation.
• Evaluating the effects of the shrinking domestic cigarette market on international tobacco markets, disease impact, and political strategies of the tobacco industry.
• Understanding the determinants of the recent increase in youth smoking, the lack of change in adult smoking prevalence, and the racial disparities in cigarette smoking among youth.
• Evaluating smoking cessation programs for youth.

Tobacco control actions have erupted dramatically in the past several years. With strengthened FDA regulatory approaches, Presidential leadership, industry document disclosures, litigation, AHCPR guidelines, OSHA rules on ETS exposure, and state programs, one could expect equally dramatic results in reducing tobacco use.[82] However, the power and money of the tobacco industry, the lack of political will to control the industry, and the lack of attention to the global effects of tobacco are liabilities that prevent progress against tobacco use. Research efforts, particularly those that are policy based, should be strengthened, with collaborative approaches among multinational organizations such as the World Bank, the World Health Organization, and UNICEF; national and state public health agencies; academic institutions; and communities. A research agenda needs to be coordinated at the federal level to identify the most pressing problems, allocate resources, convene expert panels to determine priorities, and find ways to translate research findings into action.[83]

REFERENCES

1. World Health Organization. *International Statistical Classification of Diseases and Related Health Problems,* Vol 3. Geneva: World Health Organization; 1994.
2. Pollin W, Ravenholt RT. Tobacco addiction and tobacco mortality. implication for death certification. *JAMA.* 1984;252:2849–2854.
3. Centers for Disease Control and Prevention. Addition of preva-lence of cigarette smoking as a nationally notifiable condition—June 1996. *MMWR.* 1996;45:537.
4. US Dept of Health and Human Services. *The Health Consequences of Smoking—Nicotine Addiction: A Report of the Surgeon General.* Rockville, Md: US Dept of Health and Human Services, Public Health Service, Centers for Disease Control, Center for Health Promotion and Disease Prevention, Office on Smoking and Health; 1988. DHHS publication (CDC)88-8406.
5. US Dept of Health and Human Services. National Cancer Institute. *Smokeless Tobacco or Health: An International Perspective. Smoking and Tobacco COntrol Monographs, no. 2.* Washington, DC: US Govt Printing Office; 1992.
6. Kessler DA, Barnett PS, Witt A, et al. Legal and scientific basis for FDA's assertion of Jurisdiction over cigarettes and smokeless tobacco. *JAMA.* 1997;277:405–409.
7. US Food and Drug Administration. Nicotine in cigarettes and smokeless tobacco products is a drug and these products are nicotine delivery devices under the The Federal Food, Drug, and Cosmetic Act. *Federal Register.* 1995;60:41583–41620.
8. Malarcher AM, Chrismon JC, Giovino GA, Eriksen MP. 1997

editorial note in: Smoking-attributable mortality and years of potential life lost—United States, 1984. *MMWR.* 1997;46: 444-451.

9. California Environmental Protection Agency. *Health Effects of Exposure to Environmental Tobacco Smoke.* Final Report. Sacramento, CA: California Environmental Protection Agency, Office of Environmental Health Hazard Assessment; September 1997.

10. US Dept of Health and Human Services. *Reducing the Health Consequences of Smoking—25 Years of Progress: A Report of the Surgeon General.* Rockville, Md: US Dept of Health and Human Services, Public Health Service, Centers for Disease Control, Center for Chronic Disease Prevention and Health Promotion, Office on Smoking and Health; 1989. DHHS publication (CDC)89-8411.

11. US Dept of Health and Human Services. *The Health Benefits of Smoking Cessation: A Report of the Surgeon General.* Rockville, Md: Office on Smoking and Health; 1990. DHHS publication (CDC) 90-8416.

12. Law MR, Morris JK, Wald NJ. Environmental tobacco smoke exposure and ischaemic heart disease: an evaluation of the evidence. *Br Med J.* 1997; 314:973-980.

13. Hackshaw AK, Law MR, Wald NJ. The accumulated evidence on lung cancer and environmental tobacco smoke. *BMJ.* 1997;315:980-988.

14. DiFranza JR Lew RA. Morbidity and mortality in children associated with the use of tobacco products by other people. *Pediatrics.* 1996;97:560-568.

15. Robertson PB, Walsh, MM, Greene JC. Oral effects of smokeless tobacco use by professional baseball players. *Adv Dent Res* 1997;11:307-312.

16. US Dept of Health and Human Services. National Cancer Institute. *Cigars: Health Effects and Trands. Smoking and Tobacco Control Monographs, no. 9.* Washington, DC: US Govt Printing Office; 1998.

17. Centers for Disease Control and Prevention. Medical-care expenditures attributable to cigarette smoking—United States, 1993. *MMWR.* 1994;43:469-472.

18. Miller LS, Zhang X, Novotny T, Rice DP, Max W. State estimates of Medicaid expenditures attributable to cigarette smoking, Fiscal Year 1993. *Public Health Rep.* 1998;113:140-151.

19. Glantz SA, Fox BF, Lightwood JM. Tobacco litigation: issues for public health and public policy. *JAMA.* 1997;277:751-752.

20. Herdman R, Hewitt M, Laschover M. Smoking-related deaths and

financial costs: Office of Technology Assessment Estimates for 1990—OTA testimony before the Senate Special Committee on Aging. Washington, DC: US Congress, Office of Technology Assessment Testimony; May 6, 1993.

21. Brendregt JJ, Bonneux L, van der Mass PJ. The health care costs of smoking. *N Engl J Med.* 1997;337:1052–1057.

22. US Dept of Health and Human Services. *The Health Consequences of Smoking—Cardiovascular Disease: A Report of the Surgeon General.* Rockville, Md: US Dept of Health and Human Services, Public Health Service, Office on Smoking and Health; 1983. DHHS publication (PHS)84-50204.

23. Glantz SA, Parmley WW. Passive smoking and heart disease: mechanisms and risk. *JAMA.* 1995;273:1047–1053.

24. Repace JL. Tobacco smoke pollution. In: Orleans CT, Slade J, eds. *Nicotine Addiction; Principles and Management.* New York, NY: Oxford University Press Inc; 1993:129–142.

25. International Agency for Research on Cancer. *Environmental Carcinogens: Methods of Analysis and Exposure Measurement.* Vol 9. *Passive Smoking.* O'Neill IK, Brunnemann KD, Dodet B, Hoffmann D, eds.

Lyon, France: International Agency for Research on Cancer; 1987.

26. Wynder EL, Hoffmann D. Smoking and lung cancer: scientific challenges and opportunities. *Cancer Res.* 1994;54: 5284–5295.

27. Braun MM, Caporaso NE, Page WF, Hoover RN. Genetic component of lung cancer: cohort study of twins. *Lancet.* 1994;344:440–443.

28. US Environmental Protection Agency. *Respiratory Effects of Passive Smoking: Lung Cancer and Other Disorders.* Washington, DC: Office of Health and Environmental Assessment, Office of Research and Development, US Environmental Protection Agency; 1992. EPA/600/6-90/006F.

29. US Dept of Health and Human Services. *The Health Consequences of Smoking—Chronic Obstructive Lung Disease: A Report of the Surgeon General.* Rockville, Md: US Dept of Health and Human Services, Public Health Service, Office on Smoking and Health; 1984. DHHS publication (PHS)84-50205.

30. Giovino GA, Henningfield JE, Tomar SL et al. Epidemiology of tobacco use and dependence. *Epidemiol Rev.* 1995;17:48–65.

31. Centers for Disease Control and Prevention. Cigarette smoking

among adults—United States, 1995. *MMWR.* 1997;46:1218–1220.

32. US Dept of Health and Human Services. *Tobacco Use Among U.S. Racial/Ethnic Minority Groups—African Americans, American Indians and Alaska Natives, Asian Americans and Pacific Islanders, and Hispanics: A Report of the Surgeon General.* Atlanta, Georgia: US Dept of Health and Human Services, Centers for Disease Control and Prevention, National Center for Chronic Disease Prevention and Health Promotion, Office on Smoking and Health; 1998.

33. US Department of Health and Human Services. *Preventing Tobacco Use Among Young People: A Report of the Surgeon General.* Atlanta, Ga: US Department of Health and Human Services, Public Health Service, Centers for Disease Control and Prevention, National Center for Chronic Disease Prevention and Health Promotion, Office on Smoking and Health; 1994.

34. Centers for Disease Control and Prevention. Incidence of cigarette smoking—United States, 1965–1996. *MMWR* 1998;47:837–840.

35. Monitoring the Future Project Home Page. Available at: http://www.isr.umich.edu/src/mtf/. Accessed August 22, 1998.

36. Giovino GA, Schooley MW, Zhu BP, et al. Surveillance for se-lected tobacco-use behaviors—United States, 1900–1993. *MMWR Surveill Summ.* 1994;43(SS-3).

37. Tomar SL, Giovino GA. Incidence and predictors of smoke-less tobacco use among US youth. *Am J Public Health.* 1998;88:20–26.

38. Centers for Disease Control. State- and sex-specific prevalence of selected characteristics—Behavioral Risk Factor Surveillance System, 1994 and 1995. *MMWR Surveill Summ.* 1997;46(SS-3).

39. Centers for Disease Control and Prevention. State and National Tobacco Control Highlights Home Page. Available at: http://www.cdc.gov/nccdphp/osh/statehi/statehi.htm. Accessed September 30, 1998.

40. Kann L, Kinchen SA, Williams, BI, et al. Youth risk behavior surveillance—United States, 1997. *MMWR.* 1998;47(SS-3).

41. Pierce JP, Fiore MC, Novotny TE, Hatziandreu EJ, Davis RM. Trends in cigarette smoking in the United States—projections to the year 2000. *JAMA.* 1989;261: 61–65.

42. Pierce JP, Fiore MC, Novotny TE, Hatziandreu EJ, Davis RM. Trends in cigarette smoking in the United States—educational differences are increasing. *JAMA.* 1989;261:56–60.

43. Nelson DE, Giovino GA, Emont SL, Brackbill R, Cameron LL,

Peddicord JP, Mowery PD. Trends in Cigarette Smoking Among Physicians and Nurses in the United States. *JAMA* 1994; 271:273–275.

44. Flint AJ, Novotny TE.Poverty status and cigarette smoking prevalence and cessation in the United States, 1983–1993: the independent risk of being poor. *Tobacco Control*. 1997;6:14–16.

45. Centers for Disease Control and Prevention. Cigarette smoking among women of reproductive age—United States, 1987–1992. *MMWR*. 1994;43:789–797.

46. Novotny TE. Smoking among black and white youth: differences that matter. *Ann Epidemiol*. 1996;6:474–475.

47. Centers for Disease Control and Prevention. Tobacco use among high school students—United States, 1997. *MMWR*. 1998;47: 1229–233.

48. Centers for Disease Control and Prevention. Reasons for tobacco use and symptoms of nicotine withdrawal among adolescent and young adult tobacco users—United States, 1993. *MMWR*. 1994;43:745–750.

49. Pierce JP, Choi WS, Gilpin EA, Farkas AJ, Merritt RF. Validation of susceptibility as a predictor of which adolescents take up smoking in the United States. *Health Psych*. 1996:355–361.

50. Grossman M, Chaloupka FJ. Cigarette taxes. The straw to break the camel's back. *Public Health Rep*. 1997;112:290–297.

51. Hu T, Sung H, Keeler TE. Reducing cigarette consumption in California: tobacco taxes vs an anti-smoking media campaign. *Am J Public Health*. 1995;85: 1218–1222.

52. Centers for Disease Control and Prevention. Cigarette Smoking Before and After an Excise Tax Increase and an anti-smoking campaign—Massachusetts, 1990–1996. *MMWR*. 1996;45:966–970.

53. Peterson DE, Zeger SL, Remington PL, Anderson HA. The effect of state cigarette tax increases on cigarette sales, 1955 to 1988. *Am J Public Health*. 1992;82:94–96.

54. Brownson RC, Eriksen MP, Davis RM, Warner KE. Environmental tobacco smoke: health effects and policies to reduce exposure. *Annu Rev Public Health*. 1997;18:163–185.

55. Borland R, Pierce JP, Burns DM, Gilpin E, Johnson M, Bal D. Protection from environmental tobacco smoke in California. The case for a smoke-free workplace. *JAMA*. 1992;268:749–752.

56. Fielding JE. Smoking control at the workplace. *Annu Rev Public Health*. 1991;12:209–234.

57. Longo DR, Brownson RC, Johnson JC, et al. Hospital

smoking bans and employee smoking behavior—results of a national survey. *JAMA.* 1996;275:1252–1257.

58. Shelton DM, Alciati MH, Chang MM, et al. State laws on tobacco control—United States, 1995. *MMWR.* 1995;44(SS-6).

59. DiFranza JR, Richards JW, Paulman PM, et al. RJR Nabisco's cartoon camel promotes Camel cigarettes to children. *JAMA.* 1991;266:3149–3153.

60. Pierce JP, Gilpin E, Burns DM, et al. Does tobacco advertising target young people to start smoking?—Evidence from California. *JAMA.* 1991;266:3154–3158.

61. Pierce JP, Choi WS, Gilpin EA, Farkas AJ, Berry CC. Tobacco industry promotion of cigarettes and adolescent smoking. *JAMA.* 1998;279:511–515.

62. US Food and Drug Administration. Regulations Restricting the Sale and Distribution of Cigarettes and Smokeless Tobacco to Children and Adolescents; Final Rule. *Federal Register* 1996;61:44395–44618.

63. Centers for Disease Control and Prevention. Guidelines for school health programs to prevent tobacco use and addiction. *MMWR.* 1994;43 (RR-2).

64. Centers for Disease Control and Prevention. Accessibility of tobacco products to youths aged 12–17 years—United States, 1989 and 1993. *MMWR.* 1996;45:125–130.

65. US Department of Health and Human Services, Substance Abuse and Mental Health Services Administration. Tobacco regulations for substance abuse prevention and treatment block grants. *Federal Register.* 1996; 12:1492–1509.

66. Pollay R, Siddarth S, Siegel M, et al. The last straw? Cigarette advertising and realized market shares among youths and adults, 1979–1993. *J. Market.* 1996;60:1–16.

67. Pierce JP,Lee, and Gilpin. Smoking initiation by adolescent girls, 1944–1988. An association with targeted advertising. *JAMA.* 1994;271:608–611.

68. Pechman C, RatneshawR. The effects of antismoking and cigarette advertising on young adolescents' perceptions of peers who smoke. *J. Consumer Res.* 1994;21:236–251.

69. Glynn T, Manley M. *How to Help Your Patients Stop Smoking: A National Cancer Institute Manual for Physicians.* Bethesda, Md; US Department of Health and Human Services; 1989. NIH publication 89-3064.

70. Etzel RA. A review of the use of saliva cotinine as a marker of tobacco smoke exposure. *Prev Med.* 1990;19:190–197.

71. Schwartz JL. *Review and Evaluation of Smoking Cessation Methods: The United States and Canada. 1978-1985.* Bethesda, Md: National Cancer Institute; 1987. NIH publication (DHHS)87-2940.

72. Centers for Disease Control. Public health focus: effectiveness of smoking-control strategies—United States. *MMWR.* 1992;41:645–653.

73. Agency for Health Care Policy and Research. *Smoking Cessation: Clinical Practice Guideline No. 18.* Washington, DC: US Government Printing Office; 1996. GPO publication 017-026-00159-0)

74. Centers for Disease Control and Prevention. Health care provider advice on tobacco use to persons aged 10-22 years—United States, 1993. *MMWR.* 1995;44:826–830.

75. Novotny TE, Romano RA, Davis RM, Mills SL. The public health practice of tobacco control: lessons learned and directions for the states in the 1990s. *Annu Rev Public Health.* 1992;13:287–318.

76. Manley MW, Pierce JP, Gilpin EA, et al. The impact of the American Stop Smoking Intervention Study (ASSIST) on cigarette consumption. *Tobacco Control* 1997;6(suppl 2):12–16.

77. Breslow L, Johnson M. California's Proposition 99 on tobacco, and its impact. *Annu Rev Public Health.* 1993;14:585–604.

78. Glantz SA. Changes in cigarette consumption, prices, and tobacco industry revenues associated with California's Proposition 99. *Tobacco Control* 1993;2:311–314.

79. Novotny TE, Siegel MB. California's tobacco control saga. *Health Affairs.* 1996;15:58–72.

80. Skolnick AA. Spate of lawsuits may finally find chink in tobacco industry's 'impenetrable armor.' *JAMA.* 1995;273:1080–1081.

81. Glantz SA, Slade J, Bero LA, et al. *The Cigarette Papers.* Berkeley, Calif: University of California Press; 1995.

82. Davis RM. The ledger of tobacco control—is the cup half empty or half full? *JAMA.* 1996;275:1281–1284.

83. Bauman KE. On the future of applied smoking research: is it up in smoke? *Am J Public Health.* 1992;82:14–16.

SUGGESTED READING

Agency for Health Care Policy and Research. *Smoking Cessation: Clinical Practice Guideline No. 18.* Washington, DC: US Government Printing Office; 1996. GPO publication 017-026-00159-0.

Orleans CT, Slade J, eds. *Nicotine Addiction; Principles and*

Management. New York: Oxford University Press Inc; 1993

US Dept of Health and Human Services. *The Health Consequences of Smoking—Nicotine Addiction: A Report of the Surgeon General.* Rockville, Md: Office on Smoking and Health; 1988.

US Dept of Health and Human Services. *Reducing the Health Consequences of Smoking—25 Years of Progress: A Report of the Surgeon General.* Rockville, Md: Office on Smoking and Health; 1989.

US Dept of Health and Human Services. National Cancer Institute. *Strategies To Control Tobacco Use in the United States: A Blueprint for Public Health Action in the 1990s. Smoking and Tobacco Control Monographs, no. 1.* Washington, DC: US Govt Printing Office; 1991.

US Dept of Health and Human Services. *Preventing Tobacco Use Among Young People: A Report of the Surgeon General.* Atlanta, Ga: US Department of Health and Human Services, Public Health Service, Centers for Disease Prevention and Control, National Center for Chronic Disease Prevention and Health Promotion, Office on Smoking and Health, 1994.

US Environmental Protection Agency. *Respiratory Effects of Passive Smoking: Lung Cancer and Other Disorders.* Washington, DC: Office of Health and Environmental Assessment, Office of Research and Development, US Environmental Protection Agency; 1992. EPA/600/6-90/006F.

RESOURCES

Office on Smoking and Health
Centers for Disease Control and Prevention
4770 Buford Highway, NE (Mailstop K-50)
Atlanta, GA 30341
(770) 488-5705; 1-800-CDC-1311
http://www.cdc.gov/tobacco

National Cancer Institute
Cancer Information Service
Building 31, Room 10A-18
9000 Rockville Pike
Bethesda, Md 20892
1-800-4-CANCER

American Cancer Society
46 5th Street, NE
Atlanta, GA 30308
1-800-ACS-2345

American Heart Association
7272 Greenville Avenue
Dallas, TX 75231-4596
(214) 373-6300

American Lung Association
1740 Broadway
New York, NY 10019
(212) 315-8700

6

ALCOHOL USE

Consumption of alcoholic beverages has been a part of many societies since the dawn of prehistory. Ancient texts from Persia, Egypt, Babylon, and China as well as Biblical writers have documented that people have been aware of alcohol's beneficial and harmful effects for nearly as long as people have been drinking.[1] Like tobacco use, alcohol use has complex physiological, behavioral, social, and political interrelationships. Unlike tobacco use, however, alcohol use per se is clearly not considered to be a disease entity. Rather, alcohol consumption should be viewed on a continuum from use to abuse, dependence, and other consequences.

SIGNIFICANCE

Alcohol consumption clearly is also a part of contemporary American life. As a result, although most people drink moderately and without ill-effect, alcohol abuse and alcohol

Mary C. Dufour, MD, MPH

dependence are major health problems in the United States. In 1992, nearly 14 million Americans age 18 and older met the criteria of the American Psychiatric Association's *Diagnostic and Statistical Manual of Mental Disorders,* 4th ed. (DSM-IV)[2] for alcohol abuse and dependence.[3] In human terms, the alcohol-related costs to the nation have been estimated to include over 100 000 deaths[4] accounting for approximately 5% of the total deaths each year and making alcohol the fourth leading cause of death after heart disease, cancer, and stroke.[5] Mortality from all causes is markedly elevated in alcoholics.[6]

In economic terms, alcohol-related costs approach $100 billion annually.[7] Of these costs, more than 70% are in the form of productivity losses due to premature mortality and excess morbidity attributed to alcohol, while less than 10% are for medical treatment of alcoholism and alcohol abuse.[7] Alcohol dependence contributes to other health problems and thereby increases the use of health care services. Between 15%

and 30% of patients in short-stay general hospitals have alcohol problems, regardless of their admitting diagnosis. Unfortunately, only a fraction of these alcohol diagnoses are reflected in discharge diagnoses.[8] In addition, the families of alcoholics consume more health care services than do those of nonalcoholics.[9] Beyond its impact on health and economic productivity, alcohol misuse exacts an enormous toll in terms of human suffering. Failed marriages, anguished families, stalled careers, criminal records, and the pain of having loved ones killed or disabled in alcohol-related traffic crashes attest to its destructive power.

Although moderate alcohol use has been sanctioned in the United States for a long time, its objective benefits have begun to be quantified only recently. For example, a substantial body of literature now exists describing the protective effects of low-level alcohol consumption against coronary heart disease, as evidenced primarily by the reduced risk of death from acute heart attacks.[10]

The public has also become aware of alcohol's general risks and benefits: News of grisly, alcohol-related, post-prom car crashes shares the media spotlight with reports on the cardioprotective effects of low-level alcohol consumption. Traffic statistics and news reports, however,

do not delineate the health risks and benefits of alcohol consumption for a given individual.

Hence, alcohol use may be beneficial or nonproblematic, or it may have negative consequences, some of which directly affect physical or mental health. Other consequences, such as divorce or loss of a job, are not health related, although they may negatively affect health indirectly through loss of income and concomitant access to health care.

Negative health consequences are of three broad types: the acute consequences of ingesting large doses of alcohol in a short period of time, such as alcohol-related motor vehicle crash injuries and alcohol poisoning; chronic disease consequences, such as alcoholic liver disease and alcoholic cardiomyopathy; and the primary chronic disease of alcoholism, or becoming dependent on alcohol. Individuals who suffer from alcoholism often sustain the acute and chronic health effects as well.

It is vitally important for public health practitioners to keep in mind, however, that an individual need not be alcoholic in order to suffer these other negative health consequences of alcohol consumption. For example, a teenager may die in an alcohol-related crash following his or her first drinking episode. It is also quite possible to drink enough to damage one's liver without becoming dependent on alcohol.

In the introductory portion of this chapter, numerous terms appeared, *including alcohol abuse, alcohol dependence, alcoholism, alcohol-related, alcohol problems*, and *heavy alcohol consumption*. All of these terms have multiple interpretations. The lack of one standard, universally agreed on set of definitions has made it difficult for epidemiologic research in the alcohol field to keep pace with that of other chronic diseases. The issue of the diagnosis of alcohol use disorders is closely linked to the problems of nomenclature and classification. Efforts to develop reliable and effective classification systems and well-founded diagnostic procedures have led to many modifications of the terms used to describe these disorders. *The Diagnostic and Statistical Manual of Mental Disorders,* 4th ed. (DSM-IV) of the American Psychiatric Association[2] and the *International Classification of Diseases, 10th Revision* (ICD-10) of the World Health Organization[11] have emphasized the concept of "alcohol dependence" introduced by Edwards and Gross in 1976.[12] Despite this diagnostic use of the term *alcohol dependence*, the term *alcoholism* continues to be widely used both among health professionals and the general public. The National Council on Alcoholism and Drug Dependency

and the American Society of Addiction Medicine recently formulated the following definition: "Alcoholism is a primary chronic disease with genetic, psychosocial, and environmental factors influencing its development and manifestations. The disease is often progressive and fatal. It is characterized by impaired control over drinking, preoccupation with the drug alcohol, use of alcohol despite adverse consequences, and distortions of thinking, most notably denial. Each of these symptoms may be continuous or periodic."[13] In this chapter, alcoholism and alcohol dependence are generally used synonymously.

PATHOPHYSIOLOGY

Alcohol affects every organ of the body, manifesting itself in a wide array of pathology. Most critical to the problem of alcoholism are the effects of alcohol on the brain itself. It has been known for millennia that alcohol ingestion creates a pleasurable state of mind. However, after heavy drinking it leads to confusion, incoordination, sedation, and coma. How alcohol produces intoxication is only now beginning to be understood. The brain adapts to long-term exposure to alcohol and eventually functions more normally in its presence (tolerance). When alcohol is withdrawn suddenly, this adaptive state becomes nonadaptive and tremors, hallucinations, and convulsions may ensue (physical dependence).

With repeated drinking, susceptible individuals develop a craving for alcohol that becomes the dominating motivational force, sustaining long-term drinking in the face of loss of family, job, and personal dignity (psychological dependence). After years of heavy use, an alcoholic may suffer nutritional deficiency, repeated episodes of trauma, liver failure, and lesions on the brain due to the toxic effects of alcohol and its breakdown products. In many alcoholics, these accumulated insults result in social deterioration, inability to walk, and severely disabling disorders of memory and cognition and, with continued drinking, culminate in death.[14]

Alcohol abuse can lead to a variety of chronic health disorders. Liver disease, the most prominent of these disorders, is the leading cause of death in alcoholics.[15, 16] Not only is all-cause mortality elevated in alcoholics, but these deaths occur at younger ages.[6] Heavy alcohol consumption and gallstones are the two leading causes of acute pancreatitis.[17] Approximately three-quarters of the patients with chronic pancreatitis have a history of heavy alcohol consumption.[18] Chronic alcohol consumption may also lead to degenerative changes of the heart and skeletal muscle. Reproductive disorders in both men and women are associated with alcohol. In women, they include anovulation, amenorrhea, and early menopause.[15] Alcohol-related testicular atrophy may contribute significantly to sexual problems in male alcoholics.[15] Alcohol consumption is a major risk factor for high blood pressure and contributes to diabetes and neurologic disorders.[19] Alcohol abuse is associated with increased risk of cancer of the liver, esophagus, nasopharynx, and larynx.[20-22] Although the evidence is less conclusive, some studies suggest that alcohol consumption may play a role in cancer of the stomach, large bowel, and female breast.[19, 23] It is clear that alcohol use is a risk factor for many of the chronic diseases discussed elsewhere in this text.

In keeping with the chronic disease epidemiology focus of this book, this chapter concentrates on the primary disease of alcoholism and the chronic disease consequences of alcohol consumption. This does not imply that the acute negative health consequences are not serious. Alcohol-related traffic crashes, the largest single alcohol-related cause of death, represent a public health problem of major proportions against which public health professionals have rallied.[24] A whole separate literature exists for the interested reader (see Suggested Reading section). Equally important but also excluded is discussion of the health impact of behavioral consequences of alcohol use. It has long been known that alcohol lessens inhibitions. Alcohol consumption may lead to sexual risk taking, resulting in pregnancy and sexually transmitted diseases, including HIV/AIDS.

DESCRIPTIVE EPIDEMIOLOGY

In 1994, estimated alcohol consumption in the United States, based predominantly on alcoholic beverage sales data, was as follows:[25]

beer	5 788 229 000 gallons
wine	456 899 000 gallons
spirits	332 743 000 gallons

This results in an estimated per capita alcohol consumption in gallons of ethanol of 1.26 gallons for beer, 0.29 gallons for wine, and 0.66 gallons for distilled spirits (2.21 gallons ethanol total) for each individual aged 14 and older. This is approximately equivalent to 299 12-ounce cans of beer, 58 5-ounce glasses of wine, and 137 shots (1.5 ounces) of 80-proof distilled spirits. Although age 14 is well below the legal drinking age, people aged 14 and over were included in the population used in this calculation because survey data suggest that many youths begin consuming alcohol about this age.

Data from national surveys provide more complete data on drinking patterns and problems. For example, the National Longitudinal Alcohol Epidemiologic Survey (NLAES) is a nationwide household survey of the civilian noninstitutionalized population of the United States that provides information regarding patterns and levels of alcohol consumption as well as prevalence and population estimates of alcohol abuse and dependence. The 1992 NLAES, which featured a complex multistage design, was developed by the National Institute on Alcohol Abuse and Alcoholism (NIAAA) and fielded by the Bureau of the Census, which conducted face-to-face interviews with 42 862 individuals, 18 years of age and older living in the coterminous United States and the District of Columbia. The household response rate was 91.9% and the person-response rate was 97.4%.[3] For this survey, abstainers were defined as people who had had fewer than 12 drinks in the past year (an average of less than 0.01 ounce of ethanol daily in the past year). If desired, this category can be further subdivided into lifetime abstainers, former drinkers, and current but very infrequent drinkers. Drinkers are categorized as follows: *light*, 0.01 to 0.21 ounces average daily ethanol, or roughly 1 to 13 drinks per month; *moderate*, 0.22 to 1.00 ounces, or about 4 to 14 drinks per week; and *heavy*, more than 1.00 ounce, or more than 14 drinks per week.[26] A drink is defined as 12 ounces of beer, 5 ounces of wine, or 1.5 ounces of 80-proof distilled spirits.

The 10% of drinkers who drink most heavily account for half of all alcohol consumed.[27] Using DSM-IV criteria, 13 760 000 individuals aged 18 and older (7.4% of the population) met the criteria for a current 1-year diagnosis of alcohol abuse and/or dependence.[3]

High-Risk Groups

Adolescents. Alcohol is by far the drug most often used by 1995 high school seniors.[28] Although most high school seniors cannot legally buy alcohol, nearly all (79%) have tried it, compared with 64% who have tried cigarettes. Over half (51%) have used alcohol in the past month, and 30% have had five or more drinks in a row at least once in the previous 2 weeks. Even more alarming, 55% of 8th graders and 72% of 10th graders have tried alcohol. Over a quarter of 8th graders and 40% of 10th graders reported having consumed alcohol in the past 30 days. Consuming five or more drinks on one occasion was reported by 16% of 8th graders and 25% of 10th graders. The average age at first use for seniors in the class of 1995 was 12.6 years, with the peak period for initiating alcohol use being between the 7th and 9th grades.[28]

As mentioned earlier, injury is the most frequent health consequence of teenage alcohol use. At present, there is a serious lack of empirical data on the biomedical consequences of alcohol use during adolescence. Alcohol can affect the uptake, storage, and use of vitamins and minerals, and alcohol abuse also has been associated with bulimia and anorexia nervosa. Adolescents who use alcohol have been found to have increased levels of iron in the blood. In adult drinkers, enhanced deposition of iron in the liver may be one precursor to liver damage. Acute and chronic consumption of alcohol suppresses the levels of growth hormones important for bone and muscle development.[29]

Older Americans. Alcohol abuse, dependence, and adverse consequences appear to be less prevalent among individuals aged 65 and older compared with younger individuals.[30] However, among older individuals who drink, the proportion of heavy drinkers is just as high as among younger age groups.[31] One reason for the lower prevalence may be underreporting. Instruments for detecting alcoholism were largely designed and validated on younger individuals. For example, a retired widower who is no longer driving will report no alcohol-related marital or job problems or arrests for drunk driving, regardless of how much alcohol he consumes.

Analysis of hospital discharge data by age group showed that the 65 and older age group consistently had the highest proportion (about 60%) of alcohol-related diagnoses that were not primary diagnoses.[32] In other words, more alcohol-related morbidity was found in older patients than in younger ones after they had been hospitalized for other, non–alcohol-related reasons. These findings suggest that considerable alcohol-related morbidity in older individuals may go undetected and untreated and that clinicians should be alert to the possibility that health problems in older patients may be related to alcohol. Most older individuals with drinking problems began to abuse alcohol earlier in life. However, the risk for new cases continues through the later years even as overall prevalence declines. Late-onset heavy drinking may begin in response to stressful life experi-ences such as bereavement, poor health, economic changes, or retirement.[33] Sensitivity to alcohol increases with age. In addition, many older individuals are taking one or more prescription and over-the-counter medications that may interact negatively with alcohol.

Gender. As shown in Table 6.1, men in the United States are more likely to be drinkers than are women.[26] For alcohol-abusing and -dependent individuals, the overall ratio of men to women is roughly 2.5:1 and the gender differences become more pronounced with increasing age. The male-to-female ratio for prevalence of alcohol dependence varies as a function of age, with the rates for younger women (aged 18 through 29) much closer to those of their male counter-parts.[3] On the whole, women have

Table 6.1—Average Alcohol Consumption for Noninstitutionalized People 18 Years and Older, by Sex, United States, 1992

Category	Men, %	Women, %
Lifetime Abstainer (<12 drinks in life)	21.7	45.3
Former drinker (<12 drinks past year; more previously)	22.5	20.8
Light drinker (>1 per month to < 3 per week)	19.2	17.1
Moderate drinker (3–14 drinks per week)	22.8	12.7
Heavy drinker (more than 14 drinks per week)	13.8	4.2

Note: Data from 1992 National Longitudinal Alcohol Epidemiologic Survey, Grant et al.[3]

fewer alcohol-related problems and dependence symptoms than do men.[27, 34, 35] However, among the heaviest drinkers, women equal or surpass men in the number of problems that result from their drinking.

The interval between onset of drinking-related problems and entry into treatment appears to be shorter for women than for men.[36] Studies of women alcoholics in treatment further suggest that they often experience greater physiological impairment earlier in their drinking careers, despite having consumed less alcohol than men.[37] These findings suggest that the development of consequences associated with heavy drinking may be accelerated or "telescoped" in women. This is particularly true for alcoholic liver disease,[38] alcoholic cardiomyopathy,[39] and alcoholic cognitive impairment.[40]

The enhanced effect of alcohol on women can be explained by several physiologic conditions. First, because a woman has lower total body water content than a man of comparable size, she will achieve a higher concentration of alcohol in her blood than a man after consuming an equivalent amount of alcohol. Second, diminished activity of the enzyme alcohol dehydrogenase in the stomachs of women may also contribute to gender-related differences in blood alcohol concentration

as well as women's heightened vulnerability to the physiological consequences.[41] Finally, fluctuation in gonadal hormone levels during the menstrual cycle may affect the rate of alcohol metabolism, making women more susceptible to elevated blood alcohol concentrations at certain points in the cycle.[42]

Data from a national longitudinal follow-up of women indicate that onset of problem drinking is more likely among women with nontraditional lifestyles (including cohabitation and nontraditional sexual behavior), low self-esteem, a history of childhood sexual abuse, and prior experience using drugs other than alcohol. Persistence of problem drinking is more likely among women with sexual dysfunction, depression, and lack of stable social roles (eg, unemployed, employed part-time, never married). Other risk factors included working in male-dominated occupations and having partners who were frequent drinkers. Women who were problem drinkers at baseline and who divorced or separated during the interim were more likely to show remission of their problem drinking than similar women who stayed in their relationships.[43, 44]

Blacks. Differences in alcohol consumption and problems with and across race/ethnic minorities have become increasingly important as the proportion of race/ethnic minorities in the population of the United States has increased. Past studies of alcohol dependence and adverse consequences of drinking among racial and ethnic minorities have been criticized for assuming that a given group is homogeneous.[45] Intraethnic variations, such as self-assessment of ethnic identification, culture retention, incorporation of mainstream culture, and whether individuals are foreign-born or native-born, must be taken into consideration when examining alcohol-related questions.

Black men have higher rates of abstention than White men (43% versus 30%). The same pattern is found among women, with more Black women than White women abstaining (67% versus 50%).[31] Among Whites, heavy drinking peaks in youth and decreases with age. Among Blacks, on the other hand, prevalence of heavy drinking among the young is quite low, peaking in middle age before declining with age. These age-related differences in heavy drinking were paralleled by similar age-related differences in rates of reported alcohol problems, abuse, and dependence.[46]

Compared with Whites, mortality from cirrhosis is markedly higher among Black men and peaks at a later age.[46] Researchers have speculated that the high levels of health problems among Black men may be related to the later onset of heavy drinking. This late onset may be associated with a more sustained pattern of heavy drinking, whereas among Whites, heavy drinking may be a more short-term, youthful phenomenon. Drinking among Blacks represents two extremes, with abstinence on the one hand and heavy use or abuse on the other. As a result of heavy drinking by a small segment of the population (often those who also have limited financial resources, health care, and insurance), Black adults are disproportionately represented in morbidity and mortality statistics and in data from public treatment centers.[46] Differences in sociodemographic correlates of drinking among Black and White men and women suggest that cultural and social values within these groups influence drinking patterns differently.

Hispanic-Americans. As in the general population, Hispanic men drink more than Hispanic women, and drinking increases with income and education in both sexes. Heavy drinking and adverse consequences are highest for Hispanic men in their 20s and 30s and remain problems through the mid-40s.[47] The prevalence of alcohol dependence among Hispanic men in their 20s also is higher than that among Black or White men.[47]

Hispanics are not a homogeneous population. Most Hispanics in the United States trace their origins to

Mexico. Although Mexican-American men are more likely to abstain than other Hispanic men, they are also more likely to drink heavily and to have more alcohol-related problems. Cuban men are least likely to abstain or drink heavily and report the fewest problems. Puerto Rican and other Latin American men are intermediate on these measures. Among Hispanics, Cuban women are least likely to abstain, Mexican-American and Puerto Rican women are intermediate, and other Latin American women are most likely to abstain. Few foreign-born women drink heavily. First generation US-born men and women drink more than other Hispanics, although they do not experience more alcohol-related problems.

Asian-Americans. Asian-Americans have a lower prevalence of alcohol problems than any other racial or ethnic group of Americans. However, racial differences in alcohol sensitivity between Oriental and Caucasian populations have been well documented.[48] One of the primary manifestations of alcohol consumption is a highly visible facial flushing accompanied by other symptoms of discomfort. These symptoms occur in 45% to 85% of Orientals, compared with 3% to 30% of Caucasians.[48] Grouping Asian-Americans misrepresents their true heterogeneity. Studies in Hawaii indicate that alcohol use by Cauca-sians and Native Hawaiians are comparable but that both of these groups drink more heavily than the Japanese, the Chinese, and the Filipinos. The Chinese and the Filipinos rank lower than the Japanese in most drinking prevalence and alcohol abuse estimates.[49] Asian-American women drink far less alcohol than men, and these sex differences hold across all of the Asian-American subgroups.

American Indians and Alaska Natives. In 1993, the death rate for alcoholism for American Indians and Alaska Natives was 5.6 times that of the general population.[50] The death rate for cirrhosis and other chronic liver disease was 3.8 times that of the general population, for accidents the rate was 2.8 times higher, for suicide 1.5 times higher, and for homicide 1.4 times higher.[50]

Perhaps even more than with other minorities, it is inappropriate to generalize about alcohol abuse and adverse consequences of drinking among American Indians and Alaska Natives. They make up less than 1% of the total population in the United States, yet the federal government recognizes more than 300 different tribes.[51] Social, economic, and educational customs and conditions vary tremendously, even in tribes residing in geographic proximity. These differences extend to attitudes toward alcohol use, drinking patterns, and the prevalence of alcohol-related problems. There are tribes whose members drink moderately with few problems as well as tribes with high rates of heavy drinking and highly visible alcohol-related problems.

Homelessness. Although the prevalence of homelessness is difficult to ascertain, on any given night in the United States at least 250 000 persons are homeless, and as many as 3 million may experience some type of homelessness each year.[52] Estimates of the prevalence of current alcohol abuse or dependence among the homeless range from 20% to 45%,[53] and estimates of lifetime prevalence reach as high as 63%.[52] The homeless are at high risk for health problems in general, and this risk is increased by alcohol abuse and dependence. In a Los Angeles study, 57% of homeless alcohol abusers reported chronic health problems compared with 43% among homeless nonabusers.[54] Alcohol abusers were at least one and a half times more likely to have hypertension, gastrointestinal disorders, trauma, drug abuse, eye disorders, anemia, seizures, nutritional disorders, and liver disease.

Personality. While no evidence suggests that alcoholics have a unique personality type, alcoholism and risk for alcoholism most consistently have been associated with two broad dimensions of personality.[55] The first is behavioral disinhibition (also called behavioral undercontrol or deviance proneness), which refers to an individual's inability or unwillingness to inhibit behavioral responses to cues of impending punishment. Indicators include impulsivity, unconventionality, overactivity, and aggression. The second dimension, negative emotionality or neuroticism, refers to an individual's propensity to experience negative mood states or psychological distress. Indicators of this dimension include emotionality, neuroticism, depression, and anxiety. Current research is aimed at characterizing the process by which personality factors influence drinking behavior and ascertaining how the effects of these personality factors interact with other known risk factors for alcoholism.[55]

Genetics. The observation that alcoholism runs in families is an ancient one, but does a child learn to become an alcoholic from parents and the home environment, or does a child inherit genes that create an underlying predisposition to alcoholism? Research is burgeoning in this area, and dramatic progress is being made in understanding genetic vulnerability. In 1989 the National Institute on Alcohol Abuse and Alcoholism (NIAAA) initiated the collaborative Study on the Genetics of Alcoholism (COGA), a multidisciplinary, multicenter study to identify and analyze the genetic factors contributing to a person's risk for alcoholism. Extensive information including genetic material has now been collected from nearly 3000 individuals in 900 families with multigenerational alcohol problems. To date, several "hot spots" or promising chromosomal locations have been identified and the race is on to find the genes themselves.[55] Unlike single gene disorders such as sickle cell anemia or cystic fibrosis, alcoholism is quite likely a complex genetic disorder, that is, multiple genes are responsible for this vulnerability. It now must be determined what these genes are and whether they are specific for alcoholism or define something more general, such as differences in temperament or personality. Once the genes are identified, researchers will be better able to tease out the impact of the interaction between environment and genetics on vulnerability to alcoholism. This is not a trivial issue; there are approximately 28 million children of alcoholics in the United States today, including 21 million adults and 7 million children under 18.[56] In other words, children of alcoholics represent one of the most prevalent high-risk groups for alcohol abuse. More than one kind of alcohol dependence may exist, with genetic influences more prominent in some subtypes. Studies of families indicate that first degree relatives of alcoholics are 2 to 7 times more likely than the general population to develop alcohol problems sometime during their lifetime.[55] Twin and adoption studies have confirmed that genetic determinants play a critical role in an individual's increased risk for developing the disease.[55] Many people who are at risk for developing alcoholism, however, never develop the disease, suggesting that some factors may be protective or may make some individuals more resilient. Researchers have found that high levels of parental support, close monitoring of adolescent activity by parents and positive adolescent-parent communication may all serve to modify the effects of parental alcohol abuse on adolescent alcohol use.[55]

A separate issue is genetic vulnerability to organ damage. Approximately 10% of detoxified alcoholics are severely impaired as a result of alcohol-induced chronic brain disorders.[57] An aberrant form of the enzyme transketolase may be the underlying agent for this alcoholic brain damage. Current studies are examining the gene that determines the structure of transketolase, and results will be used in family studies to assess the association between forms of transketolase and alcoholic organic brain disease. Studies also are under way to investigate the genetics of differential susceptibility to alcoholic liver disease.

Geographic Distribution

Total per capita consumption in gallons of ethanol by state for 1994 is shown in Figure 6.1.[25] In 1994, the states with the highest decile of per capita consumption were Nevada (4.15 gallons of ethanol), New Hampshire (4.14), the District of Columbia (3.89), Alaska (3.03), and Delaware (2.79). States in the lowest decile for 1994 were Kansas (1.75), Kentucky (1.74), Arkansas (1.68), West Virginia (1.64), and Utah (1.28). Distribution of consumption by region and beverage type are shown in Table 6.2.[25]

As mentioned earlier, per capita consumption calculations are based on the total population of a given state or region. Such data underestimate average consumption for actual drinkers because the percentage of people who abstain varies considerably from state to state. The Behavioral Risk Factor Surveillance System (BRFSS), conducted by individual states and coordinated by the Centers for Disease Control and Prevention, provides annual percentage estimates of the abstainers in those states that participate in the BRFSS. In 1990, 44 states and the

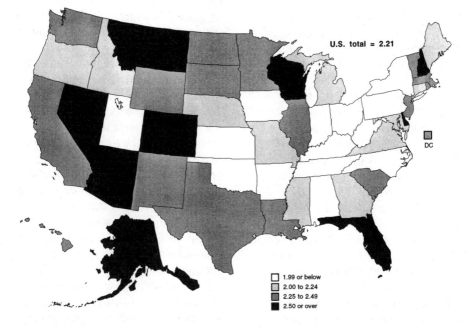

Figure 6.1—Total per capita consumption in gallons of ethanol by state, 1994

Table 6.2—Distribution of Annual Per Capita Ethanol Consumption by Region and Beverage Type, United States, 1994

| | Gallons of Ethanol | | | |
Region	Beer	Wine	Spirits	Total
West	1.22	0.41	0.70	2.33
Northeast	1.12	0.34	0.68	2.14
Midwest	1.32	0.22	0.63	2.17
South	1.33	0.22	0.65	2.19
US total	1.26	0.29	0.66	2.21

Note: Data from Williams et al.[25]

District of Columbia participated.[58] Table 6.3 shows the per drinker average ethanol consumption for participating states. A striking effect can been seen among several states in the South, whose historically low levels of per capita consumption are due, in large part, to high percentages of abstainers. The per drinker estimates in these states are more in line with the estimates in other states. Since the BRFSS now employs a rotating core of questions, state data on non-drinkers were available for only 11 states in 1994. Therefore, calculations of more recent figures for adjusted per capita alcohol consumption per drinker by state are not possible.[25]

Regional and state estimates of the prevalence of alcohol abuse and dependence and morbidity due to the chronic health consequences of alcohol abuse do not exist. In response to needs for data assessing alcohol problems and for planning prevention and treatment programs in small geographic areas, an assessment methodology was developed by the National Institute on Alcohol Abuse and Alcoholism (NIAAA).[59] This methodology, called "County Alcohol Problem Indicators," presents three basic types of data: (1) mortality rates for eight selected causes of death that are commonly regarded as reflecting the extent of alcohol abuse, based on classification of underlying cause of death; (2) mortality rates for each and any of five alcohol-related causes of death, based on classification of multiple causes of death; and (3) estimates of alcohol involvement based on mortality rates and relative state and county rankings based on these estimates. The fourth edition of the County Problem Indicators is currently available.NIAAA, which has also recently published *State Trends in Alcohol-Related Mortality, 1979–1992,* which provides the most

Table 6.3—Per Drinker Average Ethanol Consumption for Selected States, 1990

State	Per Capita Ethanol Cponsumption	Percentage of Abstainers	Average Consumption per Drinker
Alabama	1.94	66.2	5.73
Alaska	*	*	*
Arizona	2.77	48.6	5.39
Arkansas	*	*	*
California	2.79	39.1	4.58
Colorado	2.40	37.2	3.81
Connecticut	2.47	33.5	3.71
Delaware	2.98	43.5	5.27
District of Columbia	4.17	62.5	11.14
Florida	2.97	50.1	5.96
Georgia	2.33	63.7	6.41
Hawaii	2.86	50.8	5.82
Idaho	2.28	54.1	4.96
Illinois	2.64	47.7	5.04
Indiana	2.11	53.5	4.55
Iowa	2.07	48.1	4.00
Kansas	*	*	*
Kentucky	1.85	66.1	5.45
Louisiana	2.57	50.5	5.20
Maine	2.36	48.9	4.61
Maryland	2.52	46.6	4.71
Massachusetts	2.64	34.0	4.01
Michigan	2.43	46.7	4.56
Minnesota	2.57	36.9	4.07
Mississippi	2.11	64.0	5.86
Missouri	2.31	50.0	4.61
Montana	2.68	45.8	4.94

current available information on alcohol-related mortality for individual States as well as the United States as a whole.[4] It is the first uniform source of state-level trends in overall alcohol-related mortality and is the first to employ the alcohol attributable fraction (AAF) method described by Stinson and Proudfit at the state level to calculate such mortality figures. In addition, this document provides national trends in mortality rates from several specific alcohol-related causes of death, including cirrhosis, alcoholic psychoses, and alcohol poisoning.[4]

Table 6.3—Per Drinker Average Ethanol Consumption for Selected States, 1990(*Continued*)

State	Per Capita Ethanol Cponsumption	Percentage of Abstainers	Average Consumption per Drinker
Nebraska	2.26	46.1	4.19
Neveada	*	*	*
New Hampshire	4.33	33.8	6.55
New Jersey	*	*	*
New Mexico	2.65	51.2	5.43
New York	2.31	49.9	4.62
North Carolina	2.09	64.0	5.82
North Dakota	2.59	43.1	4.54
Ohio	2.10	60.8	5.35
Oklahoma	1.81	63.5	4.97
Oregon	2.52	48.4	4.89
Pennsylvania	2.16	45.8	3.99
Rhode Island	2.55	38.6	4.16
South Carolina	2.64	59.8	6.56
South Dakota	2.35	44.3	4.22
Tennessee	1.98	70.1	6.60
Texas	2.48	47.8	4.76
Utah	1.40	69.8	4.65
Vermont	2.82	33.4	4.23
Virginia	2.19	48.8	4.28
Washington	2.50	42.2	4.33
West Virginia	1.73	69.5	5.66
Wisconsin	3.08	30.6	4.44
Wyoming	*	*	*

Note: Based on estimates of abstention among population aged 18 and older from the Behavioral Risk Factor Surveillance System, Centers for Disease Control and Prevention.
*State did not participate in the Behavioral Risk Factor Surveillance System that year.

Time Trends

Beginning in 1934, following Prohibition, per capita alcohol consumption generally increased (excluding fluctuations during and immediately following World War II), reaching a peak of 2.76 gallons of ethanol in 1980, plateauing in 1981, and declining in the remainder of the 1980s. Apparent overall per capita alcohol consumption in 1990 increased by 1.2% from 1989 ending a decline that lasted through the 1980s. This 1990 increase, however, was an anomaly caused by a late surge in sales in the last quarter of 1990, a result of the new federal excise tax increases on alcoholic beverages.[25] In 1991, per capita alcohol consumption dropped 6.1%, increased marginally in 1992, and then continued to decline in 1993 and 1994. For the first half of the 1990s (1990–1994), overall per capita alcohol consumption has declined almost 10%. Beer consumption has remained relatively stable over the past 20 years and in 1994 comprised 57% of the per capita alcohol consumption from all alcoholic beverages combined. Wine consumption increased throughout the 1980s, peaked in the late 1980s, and has since leveled off. Therefore, per capita wine consumption was the same in 1994 as it was in 1977.[25] In 1994, wine represented 13.1% of the per capita alcohol consumption from all alcoholic beverages.[25] In 1994, spirits consumption, which accounted for 29.9% of per capita alcohol consumption, reached its lowest level in 51 years.

Figure 6.2 presents a map of percentage increases or decreases between 1977 and 1994 in overall per capita alcohol consumption among the 50 states and the District of Columbia. Between 1977 and 1994, the 50 states and the District of Columbia averaged a decrease of 16.3% in overall per capita alcohol consumption. Only one state (Arkansas) showed an increase over the 17-year period, 36 states had decreases

of 0.01 to 19.99% and 13 States and the District of Columbia had a 20% or greater decrease.[25] Analyses of national survey data from 1983 and 1988 illustrate further declines in alcohol consumption. In 1988, among both men and women, there were significantly more abstainers and fewer heavy drinkers compared with 1983.[31]

Long-term time trend data on the prevalence of alcohol abuse and dependence in the United States do not exist. Trends in treatment utilization statistics are not a useful surrogate, because as alcohol treatment has become increasingly available and alcoholism has been destigmatized, the numbers of individuals seeking help have mushroomed. Statistics from the Uniform Facility Data Set (UFDS), formerly called the National Drug and Alcohol Treatment Utilization Survey (NDATUS), reveal that from 1979 to 1995, the number of individuals in treatment on a given day during the year has nearly tripled from a point prevalence of about 293 000 people in treatment on April 30, 1979 to about 773 000 on October 2, 1995.[61] Membership in Alcoholics Anonymous (AA) has increased in an equally dramatic manner, going from about 445 000 members in 1979 to 1 133 795 in 1996.[62, 63] A strong association has been reported between increases in AA membership and declines in

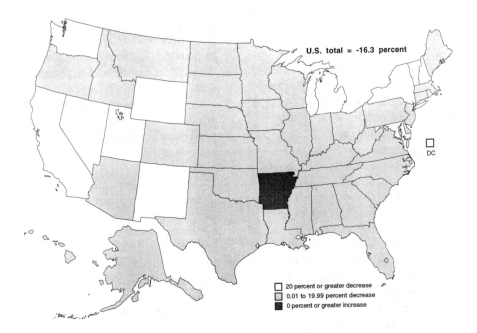

Figure 6.2—Percent change in total per capita ethanol consumption by state, 1977–1994.

cirrhosis mortality on a state-by-state basis.[64]

Long-term time trend data for all-cause alcohol-related mortality do not exist. However, there are trend data on the two largest causes of alcohol-related deaths. In 1973, cirrhosis mortality peaked at a 40-year high and has declined by well over one-third since then.[16] During the 1980s and first half of the 1990s, alcohol-related traffic death rates have declined as well. In 1994, the proportion of traffic crash fatalities that were alcohol-related reached an 18-year low of 33.6%.[66]

Magnitude of Risk Factors

As a discipline, alcohol epidemiology is in its infancy relative to other areas of chronic disease epidemiology. For many areas of interest, baseline data remain to be collected. The state of the art is such that at present it is impossible to quantify the magnitudes of particular risk factors except in the broadest terms.

Age is a modifiable risk factor in that early onset of drinking poses an increased risk for lifetime alcohol-related problems.[67] Some studies have argued that the onset of drinking is an integral part of adolescent development. More recent research indicates that the age at which one starts drinking relates to whether alcohol problems will develop later in life. In addition, a delay in drinking until 20 to 21 years of age significantly reduces the risk of developing alcohol-related problems.[67]

Children of alcoholics are at extremely high risk for developing alcohol problems themselves. On average, one-third of people in a sample of alcoholics will have at least one parent who is alcoholic.[68] Daughters with both parents alcoholic report more alcohol problems than any other group.[68] Knowledge of this increased risk allows children of alcoholics to modify their behavior accordingly.

Population-Attributable Risk

Estimates of the proportion of alcohol use in the population related to various modifiable risk factors cannot be made. These estimates are not possible because precise relative risk estimates for these factors are not available, and no data are available on the proportion of the population exposed to many of these risk factors.

PREVENTION AND CONTROL MEASURES

Prevention

Prevention measures aim to reduce alcohol abuse and its conse-quences through multiple strategies employed at the individual and community level. Such measures include policies regulating alcohol-related behavior on the one hand and community and educational interventions seeking to influence drinking behavior on the other. Most programs are focused on immediate goals, such as decreasing heavy drinking among youth or preventing driving after drinking. If successful, however, these programs also could affect long-term health consequences such as cirrhosis incidence and mortality.

Examples of policy measures implemented in recent years include regulation of the price of alcoholic beverages, increases in the minimum drinking age, zero-tolerance and other blood alcohol concentration (BAC) laws, administrative license revocation laws, server liability, warning labels and limitations on numbers, types, hours of operation, and locations of outlets that sell alcoholic beverages.

Researchers find that alcohol taxes and prices affect alcohol consumption and associated consequences. Studies have demonstrated, for example, that increased beer prices lead to reductions in the levels and frequency of drinking and heavy drinking among youth.[68] Higher taxes on beer are associated with lower traffic crash fatality rates, especially among young drivers,[69, 70] and with reduced incidence of some types of crime.[71] Research suggests that the heaviest-drinking 5% of drinkers do not reduce their consumption significantly in response to price increases, unlike individuals who drink at lower levels.[72] In one study, heavy drinkers who were uninformed as to the negative health consequences of heavy drinking were less responsive to price changes than either moderate drinkers or better informed heavy drinkers.[73] Numerous studies and reviews indicate that raising the price of alcoholic beverages by imposing local, state, or federal excise taxes is one of the most effective strategies for reducing alcohol consumption.[74, 75] A recent study estimated that current excise taxes on alcohol cover only about half the financial burden imposed on others by those who drink heavily.[76] It is also important to note that alcohol taxes are usually imposed for revenue enhancement rather than prevention purposes.

Raising the minimum legal drinking age to 21 has been accompanied by reduced alcohol consumption, traffic crashes, and related fatalities among those under age 21.[74, 77, 78] A nationwide study found a significant decline in single-vehicle nighttime fatal crashes—those most likely to involve alcohol—among drivers under 21 following increases in the minimum legal drinking age.[79] The National Highway Systems Act

provides incentives for all states to adopt "zero-tolerance laws" that set maximum BAC limits for drivers under 21 to 0.02% or lower beginning October 1, 1998.[80] An analysis of the effect of zero-tolerance laws in the first 12 States enacting them found a 20% relative reduction in the proportion of single-vehicle nighttime crashes among drivers under 21, compared to nearby States that did not pass zero-tolerance laws.[78, 81] Seventeen states have lowered BAC limits from 0.10% to 0.08% to reduce alcohol-related traffic crashes. One study found that states with the reduced limit experienced a 16% decline in the proportion of fatal crashes involving fatally injured drivers whose BAC's were 0.08 or above compared with nearby States in which the limit had not been reduced.[82] In separate analyses of this same data, it was found that the states with lower BAC limits also experienced an 18% decline in the proportion of fatal crashes involving fatally injured drivers having BAC's of 0.15 or higher, relative to comparison states.[82]

Mixed results have been reported, however, from studies designed to evaluate the effectiveness of other measures that limit availability. In some instances, control measures might alleviate one alcohol-related problem while exacerbating another.[83] In California, for instance, a study found that limiting on-premises availability was associated with a decrease in cirrhosis mortality but an increase in highway fatalities.[84]

Administrative license revocation laws (laws that permit the withdrawal of driving privileges without court action) have been adopted by 38 states to reduce traffic crashes due to unsafe driving practices including driving with a BAC over the legal limit. These laws have been associated with a 5% to 9% decline in nighttime fatal crashes.[85]

The warning label on containers of alcoholic beverages (mandated in 1988) aims to inform and remind drinkers that alcohol consumption can result in birth defects, impaired ability to drive or operate machinery, and health problems. Research reveals that pubic support for warning labels is extremely high; that awareness of the label's content has increased over time[86]; and that the perception of the described risks was high before the label appeared and has not increased much since.[87] Overall the labels have not had important effects on hazardous behavior, although certain effects may be indicative of the early stages of behavioral change.[86] One study of pregnant women found that after the label appeared, alcohol consumption declined among lighter drinkers but not among those drinking more heavily.[88]

Alcohol servers are increasingly being held liable for injuries and deaths from traffic crashes following the irresponsible selling and serving of alcohol. Researchers in Texas found that single-vehicle nighttime fatal crashes decreased 6.5% after the filing of a major server liability court case in 1983 and decreased an additional 5.3% after a 1984 case was filed.[89] As a result, server training has become mandatory in some states and aims to educate alcohol servers to alter their serving practices, especially with underage customers and those who show obvious signs of intoxication. Such training explains the effects of alcohol, applicable laws, how to refuse service to obviously intoxicated patrons and how to assist customers in obtaining alternate transportation instead of driving. Most studies to date have found more interventions after training than before. One evaluation of the impact of Oregon's mandatory server-training policy reported a decrease in the incidence of single-vehicle nighttime crashes in that state as a result.[90]

Among the community interventions is the "Saving Lives Program." Implemented in 6 communities in Massachusetts, it was designed to reduce drinking and driving and to promote safe driving practices. The program involved the media, businesses, schools and colleges, citizens' advocacy groups, and the police in activities such as high school peer-led education, college prevention programs, increased liquor-outlet surveillance, and other efforts. Participating communities reduced fatal crashes by 25% during the program years compared to the rest of Massachusetts with the decline in alcohol-related fatal crashes being 46% greater in the study communities.[85]

Life skills training teaches students in grades 7 to 9 skills to resist social influences to use alcohol and other drugs and to enhance general competence and self-esteem. Such training has been found to increase students' knowledge of the negative consequences of drinking and to promote realistic, not inflated, perceptions of drinking prevalence. Analysis of long-term effects among 12th grade students who had received a relatively complete version of the program showed significantly lower rates of weekly drinking, heavy drinking, and getting drunk than did control students.

Project Northland is a multicomponent school- and community-based intervention to delay, prevent, and reduce alcohol use and related problems among adolescents. It includes social-behavioral curricula, peer leadership, parental involvement/education, and community wide task force activities.[91] The first 3 years of the intervention conducted in grades 6 to 8, resulted in significantly lower prevalence of past-month and past-week alcohol use among students in the intervention communities compared with controls. Effects were especially dramatic among students who had not yet begun to experiment with alcohol when the program began.[91] These students are now being followed through their high school years. The Alcohol Misuse Prevention Study (AMPS) curriculum for students in grades 5 to 8, focuses mainly on teaching peer-resistance skills and on clarifying students misperceptions of their peers' alcohol use. Among adolescents at greatest risk for escalating alcohol misuse—those engaged in early unsupervised use of alcohol—the AMPS intervention had a modest but lasting, statistically significant effect of slowing the increase in alcohol misuse through grade 8 and into grade 12.[92] Replication of this research also demonstrated a significant effect for the highest risk subgroup. Drug Abuse Resistance Education (DARE), typically taught to 5th and 6th graders by police officers, aims to inform about alcohol and other drugs and to teach social and decision making skills to help students resist their use. Studies to date have found that DARE has essentially no impact on alcohol use.[93] Programs attempting to persuade students not to use alcohol by arousing fear do not work to change behavior and in fact may attract those who tend to be risk takers. Programs providing information about the pharmacological effects of alcohol may arouse curiosity and lead to drinking.[94]

Prevention strategies are typically expensive and labor intensive. Prevention research has made great strides in the last two decades utilizing rigorous and cutting edge scientific methodology. As responsible stewards of scarce resources, it behooves public health officials to employ prevention programs that have been rigorously evaluated and found to be effective.

Screening and Early Detection

Preventive health services include early intervention programs that focus on identifying people who are beginning to experience adverse effects caused by excessive alcohol use and who are modifying their drinking patterns. Preliminary findings are promising, although these programs are relatively new. People targeted by these programs include those with first convictions for driving under the influence as well as those identified through employee assistance programs, routine inquiries by medical providers, or self-referral.

Recent studies suggest that minimal interventions that include discussion of screening and assessment results, brief counseling sessions, and provision of self-help manuals can be effective in moderating drinking habits among those who drink excessively but are not yet alcohol dependent. The effectiveness of these minimal interventions for individuals identified at an early stage may be comparable to more costly and prolonged clinical interventions.[95-97]

Screening all patients for alcohol problems, particularly in primary health care settings, is a medical necessity. The US Preventive Services Task Force recommends that clinicians routinely ask all adults and adolescents to describe their use of alcohol and other drugs.[95]

Structured interviews and self-report instruments are useful for screening. Both are rapid, inexpensive, noninvasive, and relatively accurate tools. However, it is important to note that no "gold standard" exists for evaluating the accuracy of screening instruments. A specific screening instrument should be selected on the basis of staff experience and training, available testing time, and characteristics of the patient population, and the screening instrument should be used consistently.

The CAGE questionnaire (Table 6.4), derives its name from a mnemonic for attempts to cut down on drinking, annoyance with criticisms about drinking, guilt about drinking, and using alcohol as an eye-opener. It is a self-report screening instrument that appears to be suited to a

Table 6.4—CAGE Questions[100]

---

1. Have you ever felt you should Cut down on your drinking?
2. Have people Annoyed you by criticizing your drinking?
3. Have you ever felt bad or Guilty about your drinking?
4. Have you ever taken a drink first thing in the morning (Eye opener) to steady your nerves or get rid of a hangover?

---

busy medical setting when there is limited time for patient interviews.[98] The CAGE questionnaire can be self-administered or conducted by a clinician; it poses four overt yes-no questions. Since it takes less than a minute to administer, the CAGE can be woven into a standard brief clinical history.

In one study, the CAGE questionnaire was used to screen 518 patients in a community teaching hospital.[99] At a cutoff score of 2 (in this case, meaning two "yes" answers), the investigators found that the test correctly identified 75% of alcoholics (sensitivity) and 96% of nonalcoholics (specificity). For routine health screening, the test may identify individuals with alcohol problems who might have been missed otherwise. If at least two questions are answered affirmatively, the probability of alcoholism is high; however, in the elderly, even one affirmative response is strongly suggestive.

The Michigan Alcoholism Screening Test (MAST) is a formal 25-item questionnaire that requires approximately 25 minutes to complete. The MAST focuses on the consequences of problem drinking and on the subjects' own perceptions of their alcohol problems. Recent studies have reported that a cutoff score of 12 or 13 achieves balanced rates of false positives and false negatives. Two shortened forms of the MAST, a 13-item Short MAST (SMAST) and a 10-item brief MAST (b-MAST), have been constructed using items from the original test that are highly discriminating for alcoholism. A cutoff score of 3 is suggested for the SMAST; a cutoff score of 6 is suggested for the b-MAST.[98] A new instrument for use with geriatric patients (MAST-G) has several elder-specific items such as "after drinking have you ever noticed an increase in your heart rate or beating in your chest?" and "does alcohol make you so sleepy that you often fall asleep in your chair?"[101] This instrument is highly reliable among older problem drinkers and can be given as paper and pencil self-administered assessment or by interview and takes about 10 minutes.

The Self-Administered Alcoholism Screening Test (SAAST) is a 35-item questionnaire or interview with a yes-no format. A score of 10 or greater denotes probable alcoholism. A researcher who evaluated the use of the test with patients undergoing general examinations recommended the instrument as an adjunct to physician interview and examination. A more recent study reported that the original SAAST and an abbreviated nine-item version are useful for screening medical patients for alcoholism.[98]

The Alcohol Dependence Scale (ADS) is a self-report questionnaire designed to measure elements of one of the definitions of the alcohol dependence syndrome. The test, which yields an index of severity of alcohol dependence, addresses core features of dependence, including an individual's compulsion to drink excessively, repetitive experiences of withdrawal symptoms, and loss of control over drinking.

Clinical laboratory tests frequently are used to corroborate results from physicians' interviews and self-administered questionnaires. Biochemical markers of heavy alcohol consumption can provide objective evidence of problem drinking, especially in patients who deny any drinking problem. However, the sensitivities and specificities of these markers can be modified by nonalcoholic liver injury, drug use, metabolic disorders, or individual metabolic differences.[98]

Several clinical tests may be useful in detecting harmful alcohol use.

Increased activity of serum gamma glutamyl transferase (GGT) is a relatively sensitive index of liver damage in heavy drinkers. However, this test lacks diagnostic specificity because all types of liver damage and a wide variety of diseases also cause elevated serum activity of this enzyme. Results may be more discriminating when interpreted in conjunction with additional tests, such as the measure of mean corpuscular volume (MCV). MCV, an index of red blood cell volume, increases with excessive alcohol intake. Although this test has a high correlation with alcohol consumption, MCV alone is not a useful screening marker. The liver enzyme aspartate aminotransferase (AST) can be a useful marker for alcohol abuse. The ratio of levels of mitochondrial AST to total AST has been found effective in differentiating alcoholics from other patients and in detecting chronic excessive drinking.[98]

In the last several years, considerable interest has been generated in the potential utility of carbohydrate deficient transferrin (CDT) as a marker for heavy drinking. Research findings have confirmed that CDT elevation is highly specific to heavy alcohol consumption, defined as 50 grams (about 4 drinks) of alcohol daily for at least a week.[102] Few other known disorders can elevate CDT, and they tend to occur in relatively few patients. Initial optimism regarding the usefulness of CDT in detecting heavy drinkers in large heterogeneous drinking populations such as hospitalized patients or general health screening participants has lessened.[102] Recent studies have reported that CDT detection rates range from 26% to 71%, results comparable to more widely available and less expensive markers such as GGT and MCV.[102] A major concern now is that CDT appears to be less sensitive in women than in men, possibly because in women CDT levels are generally considerably higher than in men.[102]

Although research on potential biological markers is currently very active, it is important to note that at this time self-report interviews and questionnaires remain more sensitive and specific than routine blood tests. Laboratory tests may be used most effectively in conjunction with self-report instruments to enhance objectivity.

Treatment, Rehabilitation, and Recovery

Many people abuse alcohol without being dependent on it. While many alcohol abusers do not require intensive therapy, they make respond well to "brief intervention." Brief intervention differs from most other treatments for alcohol problems because it is generally restricted to four or fewer sessions; it is usually

performed in a treatment setting not specific for alcoholism, typically a primary care context; it is commonly performed by personnel who have not specialized in addiction treatment; it is usually provided to individuals who are not yet alcohol dependent; and its goal may be moderate drinking rather than total abstinence. Many people who are not dependent on alcohol nevertheless drink at hazardous levels or appear to be in the early stages of developing problems with alcohol. Brief interventions are inexpensive; can readily be incorporated into many settings; and are reasonably effective. Brief interventions in no way preclude subsequent application of more intensive intervention. People who do not respond well can be referred for further treatment. Six active ingredients have been associated with the effectiveness of brief intervention. They include the following: feedback on personal risk; responsibility of the patient for changing behavior; advice to reduce consumption; menu of choices for reducing drinking; empathetic counseling style; and self-efficacy or patient optimism regarding the possibility of making changes.[102]

Unfortunately, a number of barriers impede implementation of brief intervention, particularly in the primary care setting. Among them are resistance by family physicians toward engaging in preventive activities, inattention to screening for alcohol problems, lack of confidence concerning how to intervene if problems are discovered, concern that patients may be offended and seek care elsewhere, and doubts that intervention will be successful. Perhaps the most critical factor may be that many reimbursement systems do not provide incentives for brief intervention.[102]

The primary goal of alcoholism treatment, as in all areas of medicine, is to help the patient to achieve and maintain long-term remission of disease. For people who are alcohol dependent, remission means the continuous maintenance of sobriety. There is continuing and growing concern among clinicians about the high rate of relapse among their patients, and the increasingly adverse consequences of continuing disease. For this reason, preventing relapse is, perhaps, the fundamental issue in alcoholism treatment today.[103]

Both biological and behavioral studies have explored leads in the quest to prevent relapse. Some of the most exciting advances are being made in the realm of medications development. In December 1994, naltrexone (trade name ReVia), originally developed as an opioid antagonist, was approved by the US Food and Drug Administration for the treatment of alcoholism. This was the first approval of a drug for the treatment of alcoholism in the nearly

50 years since disulfiram (Antabuse) was approved in 1948. Double-blind clinical trials demonstrated that naltrexone decreased alcohol craving and drinking days among patients participating in psychosocial treatments. Naltrexone prevented relapse to heavy drinking among patients who resumed drinking. Among placebo-treated patients, the risk for relapse was more than twice that of naltrexone-treated individuals.[102]

The selections of treatment type and setting are governed by the condition and the expectations. Chronic alcoholics with unstable social supports who are in danger of harm require referral to supportive living environments that will deal simultaneously with their detoxification from alcohol and their immediate social and safety needs. Socially stable alcoholics require treatment in outpatient or inpatient settings with modalities selected based on clinical judgment and treatment availability.

To build on studies of patient-treatment matching that had already been conducted and to make recommendations about appropriate patient-treatment matches, NIAAA initiated Project MATCH (Matching Alcoholism Treatment to Client Heterogeneity) in late 1989.[104] A total of 1726 patients were recruited at treatment facilities throughout the United States, making this the largest clinical trial of psychotherapies for alcoholism undertaken to date. The findings of this study have challenged the notion that patient-treatment matching is a prerequisite for effective alcoholism treatment. In addition to knowledge gained about matching, the trial also demonstrated that compared with their status before treatment, both drinking and negative consequences declined regardless of which of the three carefully controlled treatments the patients received.[104]

The availability of alcoholism treatment services varies, with more services available in urban areas. Where available, assessment and referral services can provide a recommendation for treatment intensity and location that is not influenced by the treatment service's own perception of client needs. Criteria for determining levels of care and discharge readiness have been adopted by the American Society of Addiction Medicine as a guide to providers, health insurers, and managed-care companies.

Intervention and treatment of alcohol-dependent individuals is vital. Patients who refuse treatment or who want to "cut down" on drinking rather than quit entirely must be empathetically reminded that the average alcoholic successfully cuts back hundreds of times but that sooner or later drinking escalates again.[105]

Although alcoholism is a chronic disease with all the attendant re-

lapses and patient compliance issues, as the results of Project MATCH so eloquently demonstrate, the prognosis is not as grim as sometimes painted. At entry to Project MATCH almost all patients reported very heavy drinking and resulting recurring problems. One year after treatment only about 50% reported such problems.[104] Results from the 3-year follow up of these patients will be reported soon.

Abstinence is critical not only to recovery from alcoholism itself, but it also has a significant positive impact on other chronic health consequences. For example, although cirrhosis is an irreversible condition, abstinence plays a key role in length and quality of life. In cirrhosis patients without serious complications, 5-year survival is 89% for patients who abstain compared with 68% for those who continue to drink. In cirrhosis patients with serious complications, 5-year survival was 60% for abstainers versus 34% for continuing drinkers.[82]

Abstinence from alcohol may lead to the alcohol withdrawal syndrome, which is a cluster of symptoms observed in people who stop drinking alcohol following continuous heavy consumption. Milder manifestations of alcohol withdrawal include tremulousness, seizures, and hallucinations, typically occurring within 6 to 48 hours after the last drink. Much more serious is delirium tremens (DTs), which includes profound confusion, hallucinations, and severe autonomic nervous system over activity, typically beginning 48 to 96 hours after the last drink. Many withdrawal symptoms appear to result in part from over activity of the sympathetic nervous system. Thus, the preferred medications are benzodiazepines that help to brake the racing sympathetic nervous system while also preventing seizures. Ongoing research indicates potential deleterious effects of repeated, unmedicated alcohol withdrawal episodes for increasing seizure risk during detoxification.[102]

According to the Uniform Facility Data Set collected by the Office of Applied Studies (OAS) at the Substance Abuse and Mental Health Services Administration (SAMHSA) approximately 772 986 clients having alcohol problems were enrolled in 10 746 treatment facilities in the United States on the point prevalence date of October 2, 1995, with about 13% in inpatient rehabilitation programs, 84% in outpatient units, and the remaining 3% receiving care for detoxification alone.[61] Because of recent changes in the way the above-mentioned data are collected, it is no longer possible to examine individual demographic characteristics by type of problem (alcohol versus other drug).[61] Data from the 1995 State Alcohol and Drug Profile

(SADAP), also funded by OAS and collected by the National Association of State Drug and Alcohol Abuse Directors (NASADAD), reveal that the great majority of alcoholism clients (73%) were male. The single largest age grouping was 25 through 34 years, which represented nearly one-third of the population in treatment. The next largest age group was 35 through 44 years, representing 28.5% of the clients.[107] This 1995 data from 7218 programs receiving support from funds administered by state drug and alcohol agencies indicate that 57% of total alcohol treatment admissions were for outpatient care, continuing the trend away from inpatient care. The total number of admissions for clients with the primary problem of alcoholism numbered just over 1 029 081 people for the entire year. Not included in this number are people in treatment who may be alcoholic but whose primary drug of abuse was other than alcohol. It should be noted that the data provided by SADAP do not include information on those programs that did not receive any funding from a State Alcohol and Drug Agency in fiscal year 1995. Excluded programs include most private for-profit programs, some private not-for-profit programs, some county and local government programs and most Federal programs such as those operated by the Department of

Veterans Affairs. Therefore, the financial information provides a conservative estimate of actual expenditures.[107]

EXAMPLES OF PUBLIC HEALTH INTERVENTIONS

Multiple successful prevention and intervention strategies that could serve as effective components of a public health effort have been outlined in earlier sections of this chapter.

Education of primary health care providers is an evolving public health intervention. Tobacco, alcohol, and other drug use must be a routine part of every medical history. The American Medical Association has established guidelines that allow physicians to fulfill their responsibility to meet the needs of alcohol and other drug abuse patients by providing care at one of three levels: (1) diagnosis and referral (designated as the minimum acceptable level of care), (2) acceptance of limited responsibility for treatment (ie, restoring the patient to a point of being capable of participating in a long-term treatment program), or (3) acceptance of responsibility for long-term treatment and follow-up care. The guidelines further specify the actions and knowledge required at each level of involvement.[108]

Health care providers for population subgroups at high risk should be made more aware of the need for increased use of alcohol abuse screening and intervention. Hospitalized trauma patients represent one such population. The American Medical Association and the American Society of Addiction Medicine recommend that blood alcohol concentrations be ascertained in all such patients and, when positive, that individuals be evaluated and treated for their alcohol problems as well as the traumatic injury.

Public health officials strengthen and magnify their impact in addressing alcohol problems when they work in collaboration with other health care professionals, designated public officials and community groups dedicated to the prevention and treatment of alcohol abuse. All too often, public health practitioners in chronic disease control and alcohol and drug abuse professionals are located in different state or local agencies and may not even know each other.

AREAS OF FUTURE RESEARCH DEMONSTRATION

Alcohol research is progressing at an unprecedented pace. Exciting advances in neuroscience are contributing significant new insights. Utilization of new imaging techniques has permitted alcohol neuroscientists to study alcohol's effects on the brain in ways not even possible just a decade ago. As the mechanisms of alcohol's impact on the brain become elucidated, medication development is proceeding apace. Treatment research is focused not only on discovering the most effective psychosocial therapies but also on clinical trials to ascertain the best combinations of psychosocial and pharmacotherapy. Progress in the genetics of alcoholism has been explosive. Several promising chromosomal locations or "hot spots" where genes associated with alcoholism are likely to be found are currently under investigation. When actual genes are identified and their functions explicated, not only will we be in a better position to identify individuals at increased genetic risk, but we will also be in a better position to clarify environmental factors that further increase risk or that confer protection. Important advances are being made in our understanding of exactly how alcohol damages the body, particularly understanding of the mechanisms involved in alcoholic liver damage. We are also gaining a much clearer understanding of alcohol's protective effects against coronary artery disease and in possibly protecting postmenopausal women against osteoporosis. Results of all of this research will more fully inform public health policy makers and practitioners. Issues under investigation of particular interest to public health professionals include:

- Better quantifying the magnitude and modifiability of specific risk and protective factors including quantifying the risks and benefits of various levels of alcohol consumption across the life span.
- Identifying individuals susceptible to alcoholism and specific chronic health consequences so that interventions may be made before irreversible damage is done.
- Developing additional, more effective pharmacologic agents to diminish craving or other factors that result in relapse.
- Developing more precise biological measurements of alcohol use, abuse, and dependence to improve diagnosis, intervention, and treatment.
- Determining the most effective, cost-effective and user-friendly screening procedures, and further refining screening tools for special populations, including women, minorities, adolescents, and older individuals.

REFERENCES

1. Rubin E, Thomas AP. Effects of alcohol on the heart and cardiovasculr system. In: Mendelson JH, Mello NK, eds. *Medical Diagnosis and Treatment of Alcoholism.* New York: McGraw-Hill, Inc., 1992:263–287.
2. *Diagnostic and Statistical Manual of Mental Disorders:*

DSM-IV. 4th ed. Washington DC: American Psychiatric Association,1994.

3. Grant BF, Harford TC, Dawson DA, Chou P, Dufour M, Pickering R. Prevalence of DSM-IV alcohol abuse and dependence United States, 1992. Alcohol Health and Research World 18(3):243–248, 1994.

4. National Institute on Alcohol Abuse and Alcoholism. *State Trends in Alcohol-Related Mortality, 1979-92. U.S. Alcohol Epidemiologic Data Reference Manual,* Vol 5, 1st ed., Bethesda, Md, 1996.

5. National Center for Health Statistics. *Health, United States, 1995.* Hyattsville, Md: Public Health Service, 1996;14.

6. Taylor JR, Combs-Orme T, Taylor DA. Alcohol and mortality: diagnostic considerations. *J Stud Alcohol.* 1983;44:17–25.

7. Alcohol Health Services Research. *Ninth Special Report to Congress on Alcohol and Health.* Bethesda, Md: National Institute on Alcohol Abuse and Alcoholism; 1997. NIH publication 97-4017.

8. Umbricht-Schneiter A, Santora P, Moore RD. The impact of alcohol-associated morbidity in hospitalized patients. *Substance Abuse.* 1991;12:145–155.

9. Holder HD. Alcoholism treatment and potential health care cost savings. *Medical Care.* 1987;25:52–71.

10. Klatsky AL, Armstrong MA, Friedman GD. Alcohol and mortality. *Ann Intern Med.* 1992;117:646—654.

11. World Health Organization. *The International Classification of Diseases, Tenth Revision: Clinical Descriptions and Diagnostic Guidelines.* Geneva: 1992.

12. Edwards G, Gross MM. Alcohol dependence: provisional description of a clinical syndrome. *Br Med J.* 1976;1:1058–1061.

13. Morse RM, Flavin DK. The definition of alcoholism. *JAMA.* 1992;268:1012–1014.

14. Charness ME. Alcohol and the brain. *Alcohol Health & Res World.* 1990;14:85–89.

15. Rubin E. How alcohol damages the body. *Alcohol Health & Res World.* 1989;13:322–333.

16. DeBakey SF, Stinson FS, Grant BF, Dufour MC. *Cirrhosis Mortality in the United States, 1970-1993.* Surveillance Report #41. Bethesda, Md: National Institute on Alcohol Abuse and Alcoholism; 1996.

17. Fuller RK. The laboratory diagnosis of pancreatic diseases. *Medical Rounds.* 1987;1:197–205.

18. Van Thiel DH, Lipsitz HD, Porter LE, Schade RR, Gottleib GP, Graham TO. Gastrointestinal and hepatic manifestations of chronic

alcoholism. *Gastroenterology.* 1981;81:594–615.

19. Medical consequences. In: *Seventh Special Report to Congress on Alcohol and Health.* Rockville, Md: Alcohol Drug Abuse and Mental Health Administration; 1990. DHHS publication ADM 90-1656.

20. Driver HE, Swann PF. Alcohol and human cancer (review). *Anticancer Res.* 1987;7:309–320.

21. Tuyns A. Epidemiology of alcohol and cancer. *Cancer Res.* 1979;39:2840–2843.

22. Decker J, Goldstein J. Risk factors in head and neck cancer. *N Engl J Med.* 1982;306:1151–1155.

23. Gapstur SM, Potter JD, Sellers TA, Folsom AR. Increased risk of breast cancer with alcohol consumption in postmenopausal women. *Am J Epidemiol.* 1991;136:1221–1231.

24. Effects of Alcohol on Behavior and Safety. In: *Ninth Special Report to Congress on Alcohol and Health.* Bethesda, Md: National Institute on Alcohol Abuse and Alcoholism; 1997. NIH publication 97-4017.

25. Williams GD, Stinson FS, Lane JD, Tunson SL, Dufour M. *Apparent Per Capita Alcohol Consumption: National, State, and Regional Trends, 1977–1994.* Surveillance Report #39. Bethesda, Md: National Institute on Alcohol Abuse and Alcoholism, 1996.

26. Dawson DA, Grant BF, Chou PS. Gender differences in alcohol intake. In: *Research Monograph No. 29. Stress, Gender, and Alcohol-Seeking Behavior.* Hunt WA, Zakhari S (eds). Bethesda, Md: National Institute on Alcohol Abuse and Alcoholism; 1995. NIH publication 95-3893.

27. Malin H, Coakley J, Kaelber C, Munch N, Holland W. An epidemiologic perspective on alcohol use and abuse in the United States. In: *Alcohol and Health Monograph 1: Alcohol Consumption and Related Problems.* Rockville, Md: Alcohol, Drug Abuse and Mental Health Administration; 1982. DHHS publication ADM 82-1190.

28. Johnston LD, O'Mally PM, Bachman JG. *National Survey Results on Drug Use from Monitoring the Future Study, 1975-1995. Volume 1, Secondary School Students.* Rockville, Md: National Institute on Drug Abuse; 1996. NIH publication 96-4139.

29. Arria AM, Tarter RE, Van Thiel DH. The effects of alcohol abuse on the health of adolescents. *Alcohol Health & Res World.* 1991;15:52–57.

30. Dufour MC, Colliver JC, Grigson MB, Stinson FS. Use of alcohol and tobacco. In: Cornoni-Huntley JC, Huntley RR, Feldman JJ, eds. *Health Status and Well-*

Being of the Elderly, National Health and Nutrition Examination Survey-I Epidemiologic Followup Study. New York, NY: Oxford University Press Inc; 1990:172–183.

31. Williams GD, DeBakey SF. Changes in levels of alcohol consumption: United States, 1983–1988. *Br J Addict*. 1992; 87:643–648.

32. Stinson FS, Dufour MC, Bertolucci D. Alcohol-related morbidity in the aging population. *Alcohol Health & Res World*. 1989;13:80–87.

33. Atkinson RM. Alcoholism in the elderly population. *Mayo Clin Proc*. 1988;63:825–828.

34. Wilsnack RW, Wilsnack SC, Klassen AD Jr. Women's drinking and drinking problems: patterns from a 1981 national survey. *Am J Public Health*. 1984;74:1231–1238.

35. Williams GD, Stinson FS, Parker DA, Harford TC, Noble J. Demographic trends, alcohol abuse and alcoholism 1985–1995. *Alcohol Health & Res World*. 1987;11:80–83,91.

36. Piazza NJ, Vrbka JL, Yeager RD. Telescoping of alcoholism in women alcoholics. *Int J Addict*. 1988;23:437–448.

37. Hill SY. Vulnerability to the biomedical consequences of alcoholism and alcohol-related problems among women. In: Wilsnack SC, Beckman LJ, eds. *Alcohol Problems in Women. Antecedents, Consequences and Intervention*. New York, NY: Guilford Press; 1984:121–154.

38. Morgan MY, Sherlock S. Sex-related differences among 100 patients with alcoholic liver disease. *Br Med J*. 1977;1(6066): 939–941.

39. Urbano-Marquez A, Estruch R, Fernandez-Sola J, Nicolas JM, Pare JC, Rubin E. The greater risk of alcoholic cardiomyopathy and myopathy in women compared with men. *JAMA*. 1995;274(2):149—154.

40. Nixon SJ. Cognitive deficits in alcoholic women. *Alcohol Health & Res World*. 1994;18(3):228–232.

41. Frezza M, DiPadova C, Pozza G, Terpin M, Boraona E, Leiber CS. High blood alcohol levels in women: the role of decreased gastric alcohol dehydrogenase and first pass metabolism. *N Engl J Med*. 1990;322:95–99.

42. Marshall AW, Kingstone D, Boss M, Morgan MY. Ethanol elimination in males and females: relationships to menstrual cycle and body composition. *Hepatology*. 1983;3:701–706.

43. Wilsnack RW, Cheloha R. Women's roles and problem drinking across the lifespan. *Soc Problems*. 1987;34:231–248.

44. Wilsnack SC, Wilsnack RW. Drinking and problem drinking

among U.S. women: patterns and recent trends. In: Galanter M ed. *Recent Developments in Alcoholism. Vol 12: Alcoholism and Women: The Effects of Gender.* New York: Plenum Press; 1995;29–60.

45. Epidemiology of Alcohol Use and Alcohol-Related Consequences. In: *Ninth Special Report to Congress on Alcohol and Health.* Bethesda, Md: National Institute on Alcohol Abuse and Alcoholism; 1997. NIH publication 97-4017.

46. Herd D. The epidemiology of drinking patterns and alcohol-related problems among US blacks. In: Spiegler D, Tate D, Aitken S, Christian C, eds. *Alcohol Use among US Ethnic Minorities: Proceedings of a Conference on the Epidemiology of Alcohol Use and Abuse among Ethnic Minority Groups. NIAAA Research Monograph 18.* Rockville, Md: National Institute on Alcohol Abuse and Alcoholism; 1989:3–50. DHHS publication ADM 89-1435.

47. Caetano R. Drinking patterns and alcohol problems in a national sample of US Hispanics. In: Spiegler D, Tate D, Aitken S, Christian C, eds. *Alcohol Use among US Ethnic Minorities: Proceedings of a Conference on the Epidemiology of Alcohol Use and Abuse Among Ethnic Minority Groups. NIAAA Research Monograph 18.* Rockville, Md: National Institute on Alcohol Abuse and Alcoholism; 1989: 147–162. DHHS publication ADM 89-1435.

48. Chan AWK. Racial differences in alcohol sensitivity. *Alcohol & Alcoholism.* 1986;21:93–104.

49. Ahern F. Alcohol use and abuse among four ethnic groups in Hawaii: Native Hawaiians, Japanese, Filipino and Caucasians. In: Spiegler D, Tate D, Aitken S, Christian C, eds. *Alcohol Use among US Ethnic Minorities: Proceedings of a Conference on the Epidemiology of Alcohol Use and Abuse Among Ethnic Minority Groups. NIAAA Research Monograph 18.* Rockville, Md: National Institute on Alcohol Abuse and Alcoholism; 1989:315–328. DHHS publication ADM 89-1435.

50. Indian Health Service. *1996 Trends in Indian Health.* Rockville, Md: Indian Health Service; 1996:57.

51. May PA. Alcohol abuse and alcoholism among American Indians: an overview. In: Watts TD, Wright R Jr, eds. *Alcoholism in Minority Populations.* Springfield, Ill: Charles C Thomas; 1989:95–119.

52. Ropers RH, Boyer R. Homelessness as a health risk.

Alcohol Health & Res World. 1987;11:38–41.

53. Fisher PJ, Breakey WR. Profile of the Baltimore homeless with alcohol problems. *Alcohol Health & Res World.* 1987;11:36–37,61.

54. Wright JD, Knight JW, Weber-Burdin E, Lam J. Ailments and alcohol: health status among the drinking homeless. *Alcohol Health & Res World.* 1987;11:22–27.

55. Genetic, Psychological, and Sociocultural Influences on Alcohol Use and Abuse. In: *Ninth Special Report to Congress on Alcohol and Health.* Bethesda, Md: National Institute on Alcohol Abuse and Alcoholism; 1997.NIH publication 97-4017,

56. Woodside M. *Children of Alcoholics: A Report to Hugh L. Carey, Governor, State of New York for Joseph Califano Jr, Special Counselor for Alcoholism and Drug Abuse.* New York, NY: Children of Alcoholics Foundation; 1982:12.

57. Eckardt MJ, Martin PR. Clinical assessment of cognition in alcoholism. *Alcohol Clin Exp Res.* 1986;10:123–127.

58. Williams GD, Stinson FS, Clem D, Noble J. *Apparent Per Capita Alcohol Consumption: National, State, and Regional Trends, 1977–1990.* Surveillance Report #23. Rockville, Md: National

Institute on Alcohol Abuse and Alcoholism; 1992.

59. *US Alcohol Epidemiologic Data Reference Manual.* Volume 3, 3rd ed. County Problem Indicators. Rockville, Md: National Institute on Alcohol Abuse and Alcoholism; 1991.

60. *National Drug and Alcoholism Treatment Utilization Survey 1979: Comprehensive Report.* Rockville, Md: National Institute on Alcohol Abuse and Alcoholism; 1979.

61. Office of Applied Studies. *Uniform Facility Data Set (UFDS): Data for 1995 and 1980–1995.* Rockville, Md: Substance Abuse and Mental Health Services Administration; 1997. DHHS publication (SMA) 97-3161.

62. *Comments on AA's Triennial Survey.* New York, NY: General Services Board of Alcoholics Anonymous, Inc; 1991.

63. Alcoholics Anonymous website at http://www.alcoholics-anonymous.org

64. Mann RE, Smart RG, Anglin L. Reduction in cirrhosis deaths in the United States: associations with per capita consumption and AA membership. *J Stud Alcohol.* 1991;52:361–365.

65. Campbell KE, Stinson FS, Zobeck TS, Bertolucci D. Surveillance Report #38. *Trends in Alcohol-Related Fatal Traffic Crashes,*

United States: 1977-1994. Bethesda, Md: National Institute on Alcohol Abuse and Alcoholism; 1996.

66. Chou SP, Pickering R. Early onset of drinking as a risk factor for lifetime alcohol-related problems. *Br J Addict.* 1992;87:1199–1204.

67. Harford TC, Haack MR, Spiegler DL. Positive family history for alcoholism. *Alcohol Health & Res World.* 1987/88(winter):138–143.

68. Grossman M, Coate D, Arluck GM. Price sensitivity of alcoholic beverages in the United States: youth alcohol consumption. In: Holder H, ed. *Control Issues in Alcohol Abuse Prevention: Strategies for States and Communities.* Greenwich CT: JAI Press, 1987;169–198.

69. Ruhm CJ. Alcohol policies and highway vehicle fatalities. *J Health Econ.* In press.

70. Saffer H, Grossman M. Beer taxes, the legal drinking age, and youth motor vehicle fatalities. *J Legal Stud.* 16(2):351–374.

71. Cook PJ, Moore MJ. Economic perspectives on reducing alcohol-related violence. In: Martin SE, ed. *Alcohol and Interpersonal Violence: Fostering Multidisciplinary Perspectives. Monograph No. 24.* National Institute on Alcohol Abuse and Alcoholism Research Rockville, Md: 1993;193–212. NIH publication 93-3496.

72. Manning WG, Blumberg L, Moulton LH. The demand for alcohol: the differential response to price. *J Health Econ.* 1995; 14(2):123–148..

73. Kenkel DS. New estimates of the optimal tax on alcohol. *Econ Inquiry* 1996;XXIV(2):296—319.

74. Rankin JG, Ashley MJ. Alcohol-related health problems. In: Last JM, Wallace RB, eds. *Maxcy-Rosenau-Last Textbook of Public Health and Preventive Medicine.* 13th ed. Norwalk, Conn: Appleton & Lange; 1992;741–767.

75. Cook P, Tauchen G. The effect of liquor taxes on heavy drinking. *Bell J Econ.* 1982;13:379–390.

76. Manning WG, Keeler EB, Newhouse JP, Sloss EM, Wasserman J. The taxes of sin: do smokers and drinkers pay their way? *JAMA.* 1989;261:1604–1609.

77. Waganaar AC. Minimum drinking age and alcohol availability to youth: issues and research needs. In: Hilton ME, Bloss G, eds. *Economics and the Prevention of Alcohol-Related Problems. Research Monograph No. 25.* National Institute on Alcohol Abuse and Alcoholism Rockville, Md: 1993;175–200. NIH publication 93-3513.

78. Hingson R, Heeren T, Winter M. Lower legal blood alcohol limits for young drivers. *Public Health Rep.* 1994;109(6):738–744.

79. O'Malley PM, Waganaar AC. Effects of minimum drinking age laws on alcohol use, related behaviors and traffic crash involvement among American youth: 1976–1987. *J Stud Alcohol.* 1991;52(5):478—491.

80. *Alcohol Alert No. 31: Drinking and Driving. PH 362.* Bethesda, Md: National Institute on Alcohol Abuse and Alcoholism; 1996.

81. Martin SE, Voas R, Hingson R. Zero tolerance laws: effective public policy? *Alcoholism Clin Exp Res.* In press.

82. Hingson R, Heeren T, Winter M. Lowering state legal blood alcohol limits to 0.08%: the effect on fatal motor vehicle crashes. *Am J Public Health.* 1996; 86(9):1297–1299.

83. Smith DI. Effect on liver cirrhosis and traffic accident mortality of changing the number and type of alcohol outlets in Western Australia. *Alcohol Clin Exp Res.* 1989;13:190–195.

84. Colon I, Cutter HSG. The relationship of beer consumption and state alcohol and motor vehicle policies to fatal accidents. *J Safety Res.* 1983; 14:83–89.

85. Hingson R. Prevention of alcohol-impaired driving. *Alcohol Health Res World* 1993;17(1):28–34.

86. MacKinnon DP. Review of the effects of the alcohol warning label. In: Watson RR, ed. *Alcohol, Cocaine, and Acci-* dents. Totowa, NJ: Humana Press; 1995.

87. Hilton ME. An overview of recent findings on alcoholic beverage warning labels. *J Public Policy Market.* 1993;12(1):1—9.

88. Hankin JR, Firestone JI, Sloane JJ et al. The impact of the alcohol warning label on drinking during pregnancy. *J Public Policy Market.* 1993;12(1):10—18.

89. Waganaar AC, Holder HD. Effects of alcoholic beverage server liability on traffic crash injuries. *Alcoholism Clin Exp Res.* 1991;15(6):942—947.

90. Holder HD, Waganaar AC. Mandated server training and reduced alcohol-involved traffic crashes: a time series analysis of the Oregon experience. *Accident Anal Prevent.* 1994;26(1):89—97.

91. Perry CL, Williams Cl, Veblen-Mortenson S, et al. Project Northland: outcomes of a communitywide alcohol use prevention program during early adolescence. *Am J Public Health.* 1996;86:956–965.

92. Dielman TE. School-based research on the prevention of adolescent alcohol use and misuse: Methodological issues and advances. In: Boyd G, Howard J, Zucker R. eds. *Alcohol Problems among Adolescents: Current Directions in Prevention Research,* Hillsdale, NJ: Lawrence Earlbaum Associates; 1995.

93. Ennett ST, Tobler NS, Ringwalt CL, et al. How effective is drug abuse resistance education? A meta-analysis of Project DARE outcome evaluations. *Am J Public Health*. 1994;84:1394–1401.

94. Botvin GJ. Principles of prevention. In: Coombs RH, Ziedonis DM, eds. *Handbook on Drug Abuse Prevention: A Comprehensive Strategy to Prevent the Abuse of Alcohol and Other Drugs*. Boston, Mass: Allyn and Bacon; 1995.

95. Screening for alcohol and other drug abuse. In: Fisher M, Eckhart C, eds. *Guide to Clinical Prevention Services: An Assessment of the Effectiveness of 169 Interventions*. US Prevention Services Task Force. Baltimore, Md: Williams & Wilkins; 1989:277–286.

96. Chapman Walsh D, Hingson RW, Merrigan DM, et al. The impact of a physician's warning on recovery from alcoholism treatment. *JAMA*. 1992;267:663–667.

97. Nathan PE. Alcohol dependency prevention and early intervention. *Public Health Rep*. 1988; 103:683–689.

98. *Alcohol Alert No. 8: Screening for Alcoholism*. Rockville, Md: National Institute on Alcohol Abuse and Alcoholism; 1990.

99. Bush B, Shaw S, Cleary P, Delbanco TL, Aronson MD. Screening for alcohol abuse using the CAGE questionnaire. *Am J Med*. 1987;82:231–235.

100. Mayfield D, McLeod G, Hall P. The CAGE questionnaire: validation of a new alcoholism instrument. *Am J Psychiatry* 1974;131:1121–1123.

101. Blow FC, Beresford TP, Demo-Dananberg L, Singer K. The Michigan alcoholism screening test-geriatric version (MAST-G). *Am J Psychiatry*. In press.

102. Treatment of Alcoholism and Related Problems. In: *Ninth Special Report to Congress on Alcohol and Health*. Bethesda, Md: National Institute on Alcohol Abuse and Alcoholism; 1997. NIH publication 97-4017.

103. *Alcohol Alert No. 6: Relapse and Craving*. Rockville, Md: National Institute on Alcohol Abuse and Alcoholism; 1989.

104. Project MATCH Research Group. Matching alcoholism treatments to client heterogeneity: Project MATCH Posttreatment drinking outcomes. *J Stud Alcohol* 1997;58(1):7—29.

105. Schuckit MA. Alcohol and alcoholism. In: Wilson JD, Braunwald E, Isselbacher KJ, et al, eds. *Harrison's Principles of Internal Medicine*. 12th ed. New York, NY: McGraw-Hill Inc; 1991;2146–2151.

106. Powell W, Klatskin G. Duration of survival in patients with

Laennec's cirrhosis. *Am J Med.* 1968;44:406–420.

107. Gustafson JS, Reda JL, McMullen H, Sheehan K, McGencey S, Rugaber C, Anderson R, DiCarlo M. *State Resources and Services Related to Alcohol and Other Drug Problems Fiscal Year 1995.* Washington DC; National Association of State Alcohol and Drug Abuse Directors, Inc; 1997.

108. Wilford BB. AMA: stopping silent losses. *Alcohol Health & Res World.* 1989;13:70–72.

SUGGESTED READING

National Institute on Alcohol Abuse and Alcoholism. *Ninth Special Report to the US Congress on Alcohol and Health.* Washington, DC: Supt. of Docs., US Govt. Print. Off., 1997.

Recent issues of *Alcohol Health and Research World* (a quarterly scientific publication for educated lay readers):

volume 20(3) 1996—Drinking Over the Life Span

volume 20(4) 1996—Alcohol Research and Social Policy

volume 21(1) 1997—Alcohol's Effect on Organ Function

volume 21(2) 1997—Neuroscience: Pathways of Addiction

Alcoholism: getting the facts (A brochure for lay readers)

The Physician's Guide to Helping Patients with Alcohol Problems -a 12-page booklet for primary health care providers which outlines the steps for alcohol screening and brief intervention, including specific suggestions for how to word questions to patients

State Trends in Alcohol-Related Mortality, 1979–92. U.S. Alcohol Epidemiologic Data Reference Manual Vol 5, Bethesda, Md: 1996.

Recent Surveillance Reports

Surveillance Report #38. *Trends in Alcohol-Related Fatal Traffic Crashes, United States: 1977–1994.* Bethesda, Md: National Institute on Alcohol Abuse and Alcoholism; 1996.

Surveillance Report #39. *Apparent Per Capita Alcohol Consumption: National, State, and Regional Trends, 1977–1994.* Bethesda, Md: National Institute on Alcohol Abuse and Alcoholism; 1996.

Surveillance Report #40. *Trends in Alcohol-Related Morbidity Among Short-Stay Community Hospital Discharges, United States, 1979–1994.* Bethesda, Md: National Institute on Alcohol Abuse and Alcoholism; 1996.

Surveillance Report #41. *Cirrhosis Mortality in the United States, 1970–1993.* Bethesda, Md: National Institute on Alcohol Abuse and Alcoholism; 1996.

Data Reference Manual, Volume 3, 4th ed. *County Alcohol Problem Indicators 1986-1990*. Rockville, Md: National Institute on Alcohol Abuse and Alcoholism; 1994.

All of the above-mentioned publications are available from the NIAAA Scientific Communications Branch. Many are also available online (see below).

NIAAA Website address: http://www.niaaa.nih.gov

Website includes the following:
• Welcome
• Publications and Databases

NIAAA publications including the *Alcohol Alert* bulletin, the quarterly scientific journal *Alcohol Health and Research World*, pamphlets/brochures, surveillance reports, research monographs, manuals, and online databases (ETOH and Quick Facts)—

ETOH—Search the ETOH database online. The most comprehensive online resource covering alcohol-related biomedical and behavioral research. Currently includes abstracts of over 100 000 references.

Quick Facts—An electronic bulletin board that provides data on a number of alcohol topics, both national and international, such as per capita alcohol consumption by beverage type, cirrhosis mortality, etc.

• News and Events
• Grants/Contracts Information
NIAAA Extramural Program Descriptions Handbook, NIH grant application policies, NIAAA research program announcements, peer-review committee membership rosters, etc.
• Other Resources

Referrals and links to other organizations and associations

RESOURCES

Alcohol Epidemiologic Data System
CSR, Incorporated
Suite 200
1400 Eye Street, NW
Washington, DC 20005
(202) 842-7600

American Society of Addiction Medicine
5225 Wisconsin Avenue, NW, Suite 409
Washington, DC 20015

National Association of State Alcohol and Drug Abuse Directors
444 North Capitol Street, NW
Washington, DC 20001
(202) 783-6868

National Council on Alcoholism and Drug Dependence
12 West 21st Street
New York, NY
(212) 206-6770

National Institute on Alcohol Abuse
and Alcoholism
Office of Scientific Affairs
Scientific Communications Branch

6000 Executive Boulevard Suite 409
MSC 7003
Bethesda, MD 20892-7003
(301) 443-3860

7

PHYSICAL INACTIVITY

Physical inactivity is a term used to classify people who achieve less than the recommended amounts of regular physical activity. In 1996, the Report of the Surgeon General on Physical Activity and Health summarized the many health benefits associated with physical activity and suggested that the minimum level of physical activity required to achieve health benefits was a daily expenditure of 150 kilocalories in moderate or vigorous activities.[1] This recommendation is consistent with a 1995 consensus statement issued by the Centers for Disease Control and Prevention (CDC) and American College of Sports Medicine (ACSM) and a 1996 consensus statement from the National Institutes of Health recommending that every adult should accumulate at least 30 minutes of moderate activity most days of the week.[2, 3] According to the 1996 Surgeon General's Report, more than 60% of US adults are not physically active at levels associated with decreased risk of premature mortality and chronic disease morbidity.[1]

SIGNIFICANCE

The consequences of physical inactivity (defined as no regular leisure time, physical activity) are felt among many dimensions of health including physical, physiological, psychological, and societal. Regular physical activity performed on most days of the week reduces the risk of dying prematurely, dying from coronary heart disease, and developing diabetes and colon cancer.[2] Regular activity also reduces blood pressure among people with hypertension,[4] promotes psychological well being, and builds and maintains healthy bones, muscles, and joints so that older adults can avoid falls and maintain functional independence.[1]

Physical inactivity is a major risk factor for coronary heart disease mortality with a relative risk of 1.9, similar to risks associated with cigarette smoking, increased systolic

Barbara E. Ainsworth, PhD, MPH, FACSM
Caroline A. Macera, PhD, FACSM

blood pressure, and elevated serum cholesterol.[5] In 1990, approximately 300 000 US deaths were attributed to physical inactivity and poor nutrition, while 400 000 were attributed to tobacco.[6] A 1986 mortality analysis found that over 350 000 deaths were attributable to tobacco and about 250 000 were attributable to physical inactivity.[7] One reason for the major impact this risk factor has on mortality is its prevalence. While only about 30% of adults use tobacco, twice that many are physically inactive.

Using available estimates of the prevalence of physical inactivity and the coronary heart disease risk associated with physical inactivity, it has been suggested that approximately 35% of coronary heart disease mortality is due to physical inactivity.[8, 9] This is particularly important because coronary heart disease is the leading cause of death in the United States with over 700 000 deaths annually, which represents 34% of all deaths.[6] Furthermore, for every person who dies of coronary heart disease, many others are disabled.

The major economic impact of physical inactivity is felt through a loss of income and productivity associated with disease and disability. On the basis of 1989 all-cause mortality statistics, physical inactivity was estimated to cost the nation $5.7 billion in hospital, physician and nursing services, medicines, and lost productivity.[6] A cost-benefit analysis concluded that $4.3 billion per year could be saved if all sedentary adults (about 40% of the population) participated in a walking program.[10]

The high prevalence of physical inactivity is a significant public health problem that affects various populations, is multidimensional in its scope, and is interdependent on other factors that may compound its effects. Actions are needed at the personal, social, economic, scientific, legal, and policy levels to reduce the prevalence of physical inactivity in the United States.

DEFINITIONS

Several terms, shown in Table 7.1, are used to characterize human movement. *Physical activity* refers to any bodily movement that increases energy expenditure.[11] This is contrasted with the term *exercise*, which is planned, structured and repetitive physical activity done to improve or maintain one or more of the components of physical fitness.[11-13] *Physical fitness* is a set of attributes that allows individuals to carry out daily tasks without undue fatigue. Components of health-related fitness include cardiorespiratory, muscular, metabolic, morphological, and motor.[11] The terms *frequency, duration,* and *intensity* of an activity are used to measure the *activity dose,* or the threshold

Table 7.1—Definitions Used to Characterize Human Movement

Term	Definition
Physical activity	Bodily movement that is produced by the contraction of skeletal muscle and that substantially increases energy expenditure[11] • Occupational • Nonoccupational (leisure, family, transportation, household, other activities)
Exercise	Planned, structured, and repetitive bodily movement done to improve or maintain one or more components of physical fitness[11]
Physical fitness	A set of attributes that people have or achieve that relates to the ability to perform physical activity[11] The ability to carry out daily tasks with vigor and alertness, without undue fatigue and with ample energy to enjoy leisure-time pursuits and to meet unforseen emergencies[12] The ability to perform moderate to vigorous levels of physical activity without undue fatigue and the capability of maintaining such ability throughout life[13] Components of health-related fitness[14] • *Cardiorespiratory:* submaximal exercise capacity, maximal aerobic power, heart and lung functions, blood pressure • *Muscular:* power, strength, endurance • *Metabolic:* glucose tolerance, insulin sensitivity, lipid and lipoprotein metabolism, substrate oxidation characteristics, motor • *Morphological:* body mass for height, body composition, subcutaneous fat distribution, abdominal visceral fat, bone density, flexibility • *Motor:* agility, balance, coordination, speed of movement, reaction time
Frequency	The times an activity is performed in a selected period (eg, 1 week)[13,17]
Duration	The minutes or hours one engages in physical activity[13, 17]
Intensity	The energy cost of performing an activity[2, 13, 15, 17] • *METs:* The activity metabolic cost divided by the resting metabolic rate • *MET-minutes:* The activity MET level + minutes of participation • *Kilocalories:* Met-minutes + (body weight in kilograms/60 kg) • *Light intensity:* Physical activities < 3 METs • *Moderate intensity:* Physical activities from 3 to 6 METs • *Vigorous intensity:* Physical activities > 6 METs
Activity dose	A threshold for physical activity associated with health benefits. It is generally expressed in terms of energy expenditure, frequency, intensity, or duration[2, 17]
Leisure	Activities done in a setting that include the elements of free choice, freedom from constraints, intrinsic motivation, enjoyment, relaxation, personal involvement, and self-expression.[16]

level of physical activity associated with health benefits.[12–15]

Another term that is often used concerning physical activity is *leisure*, as in leisure-time physical activity. This term applies to physical activities that include the elements of free choice, freedom from constraints, intrinsic motivation, enjoyment, relaxation, personal involvement, and self-expression.[16] Incorporating physical activity during leisure time is a behavior that should be encouraged, as these activities are likely to become habits that endure throughout life.

PATHOPHYSIOLOGY

Physical activity affects all body systems associated with energy production, metabolism, and bodily movement. Table 7.2 shows the acute and chronic changes in body systems and associated disease risks following moderate amounts of physical activity. Acute changes refer to the immediate adaptations in body systems during a physical activity period. Chronic changes refer to long-term adaptations in body systems resulting from regular participation over time.[14, 17] The time required for physical activity participation to produce chronic changes in the body may range from 1 week (in the neuromuscular system) to several years (some metabolic hormones and enzymes).

Regular physical activity reduces risk factors for coronary heart disease by raising high-density lipoprotein-cholesterol, lowering triglycerides, lowering resting and exercise blood pressures, and increasing blood clot dissolving mechanisms. Among people with coronary heart disease, regular physical activity can reduce the threshold for angina pectoris during physical activity and reduce the risks for sudden death. Regular physical activity is inversely associated with obesity and glucose-insulin intolerance and is positively associated with immune function, muscular strength, mobility, psychological well-being, and increased bone mass. Through modifications of these intermediate factors, regular physical activity can reduce the risks for diabetes mellitus, depression, injuries, osteoporosis, and some forms of cancer associated with immune deficiencies and excess body fat.[1–3]

The disease risk reducing and health enhancing effects of regular, moderate physical activity involve the integration of many body systems. Adaptations to body systems are specific to the imposed demands of the physical activity stress.[17] This is called the SAID principle (Specific Adaptations to Imposed Demands). Types of physical activities that impose the greatest stress on most systems

Table 7.2—Acute and Chronic Changes Associated with Disease Risk Following Moderate Amounts of Physical Activity

System	Acute Changes	Chronic Changes
Cardiovascular ↓CHD risk ↓Stroke risk ↑CHD rehabilitation ↓Symptoms of claudication	↑Heart rate ↑Stroke volume ↑Cardiac output ↑Systolic blood pressure	↓Resting heart rate ↑Maximal Stroke Volume ↑Maximal cardiac output ↑Hemoglobin ↑Blood volume ↓Blood pressure in hypertensives ↑Blood clot lysis ↓Thrombosis
Pulmonary ↑Pulmonary rehabilitation	↑Breath rate and depth ↑Oxygen diffusion ↑Dialation of airways	↓Breath rate for submax activity
Neuromuscular ↑Mobility ↑Strength ↑Functional independence	↑Rate of nerve impulses ↑Oxygen utilization ↑Mitochondria ↑Anerobic enzymes ↑Aerobic enzymes	↑Size of motor nerves ↑Size of muscle fibers ↑Aerobic capacity ↑Fat and carbohydrate utilization ↑Muscle flexibility
Skeletal ↓Osteoporotic Bone Loss ↓Risk of Joint Injury		↑Bone mass and density ↑Tendon and ligament strength
Endocrine ↓Diabetes ↑Psychological well being	↑Release of hormones from Pituitary (most), adrenal, thyroid, parathyroid, kidney, ovaries, testes, pancreas (Glucagon) and endorphins ↓Insulin	↑Sensitivity of muscles to insulin ↓Release of glucose during activity ↓Adrenaline release during rest
Metabolic ↓Obesity ↓Cancer		↓Body fat stores ↑Muscle mass ↑Ratio of lipid: carbohydrate oxidation ↑HDL-cholesterol ↓Triglycerides
Immune ↓Cancer ↓Acute illness ↓Atherosclerosis & CHD		↑Resistance to illness ↑Leukocyte distribution ↑Lymphocyte proliferation ↑Innate immunity ↑Humoral immunity ↑Cytokines and cytotoxicity

Note. Adapted from Bouchard et al.[14] and Ainsworth et al.[17] CHD indicates coronary heart disease.

simultaneously are aerobic (moderate or vigorous intensity), weight bearing, and resistance activities. These activities include brisk walking, gardening, home repair, most sports and conditioning activities, manual labor occupations, and vigorous house cleaning.[15]

Figure 7.1 shows a model proposed by Bouchard et al.[14] describing the relationships among habitual physical activity, health-related fitness, and health status. Health-related fitness refers to changes in morphological, muscular, motor, cardiorespiratory, and metabolic systems due to regular physical activity. Components in the health-related fitness model are modified by levels of physical activity, health status, heredity, and other factors, such as lifestyle behaviors, personal attributes, physical and social environments. Regular physical

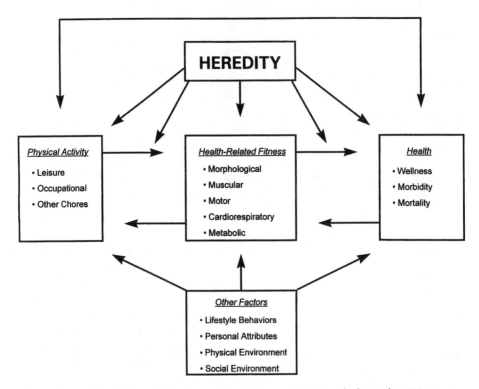

Figure 7.1—A model describing the relationship among habitual physical activity, health-related fitness, and health status. (Reprinted with permission from Bouchard et al.[14])

activity can provide a direct effect on health-related fitness, as observed in Table 7.2, or may indirectly modify health-related fitness levels through other changes in health status. (See Bouchard et al.[14] for more discussion of the model).

Descriptive Epidemiology

Three major population-based surveys measure leisure-time physical activity among US adults. The *National Health Interview Survey* (NHIS) is a household interview conducted by the National Center for Health Statistics on a representative sample of noninstitutionalized adults aged 18 and older.[18] Questions on physical activity were included in 1985, 1990, and 1991. These questions include the type, frequency, intensity, and duration of the activity over the past 2 weeks.

The *Behavioral Risk Factor Surveillance System* (BRFSS) is a telephone-administered survey conducted monthly by participating states in collaboration with CDC.[19] National estimates are developed from state-specific data. The BRFSS included physical activity items from 1986 through 1992 and in even numbered years afterward. Questions include the type, intensity, frequency, and duration of leisure-time physical activity during the past month.

The *Third National Health and Nutrition Examination Survey* (NHANES III) is a household interview survey conducted by the National Center for Health Statistics in two 3-year phases.[20] From each phase, national estimates can be obtained for noninstitutionalized adults aged 18 and older. Data on the type and frequency of physically active hobbies, sports, and exercises during the past month are available from the first phase (1988 to1991).

High-Risk Groups

In spite of different modes of administration, wording of the questions, and the 2-week versus 1-month time frames, results from these surveys are consistent in reporting that about 25% of US adults report no physical activity in their leisure time, and about 60% do not get the recommended amount of daily activity to prevent chronic diseases.[21–23] Further, only 20% of adults are regularly active at levels recommended to improve cardiorespiratory endurance.[22, 23]

Results from these surveys are also consistent in reporting that the prevalence of physical inactivity increases with age and is higher among women and ethnic minorities as compared with men and Caucasian populations.[1, 21] In Table 7.3, the prevalence of physical inactivity is shown for adult men and women by ethnicity and age. More than one-

Table 7.3—Self-Reported Levels of Leisure-Time Physical Inactivity by Demographic Characteristics, Adults, United States, 1992

	Men	Women
Overall	26.5	30.7
Race/Ethnicity:		
White (non-Hispanic)	25.3	28.2
Black (non-Hispanic)	33.1	42.7
Hispanic	30.2	39.0
Other	27.6	35.8
Age (years):		
18-29	18.9	25.4
30-44	25.0	26.9
45-64	32.0	32.1
65-74	33.2	36.6
75+	38.2	50.5

Note. Adapted from US Dept of Health and Human Services.[1]

fourth of all men and nearly one-third of all women age 18 and older were physically inactive in 1992.[1] For both men and women, physical inactivity is higher among Blacks, Hispanics, and other ethnic groups as compared with Whites. Among men, physical inactivity levels increase from about 20% to 40% between the ages of 18 and 75 years. Among women, physical inactivity levels increase from about 25% to 50% between the ages of 18 and 75 years.

Although most of the national physical activity surveys focus on adults, physical inactivity among adolescents is of increasing concern.

An expert panel, convened in 1994 to examine physical activity requirements for adolescents, developed two guidelines: (1) adolescents should be physically active daily or nearly every day as part of their lifestyles, and (2) adolescents should engage in three or more sessions per week of moderate-vigorous activities that last at least 20 minutes.[24]

There are two national surveys to obtain information on the physical activity patterns of adolescents. The *Youth Risk Behavior Survey* (YRBS) is self-administered through schools (9th through 12th grade) and in 1991, 1993, and 1995 included questions about physical activities done in the past 7 days.[25] The *National Health Interview Survey— Youth Risk Behavior Survey* (NHIS-YRBS) is household-administered via audiotape and self-completed answer sheets, conducted in 1992, and includes information about physical activity for adolescents in and out of school between the ages of 12 and 21 years.[18] The question that assessed vigorous physical activity asked how many days in the past 7 did they exercise or take part in sports that made them sweat or breathe hard. The question to assess moderate physical activity asked how many days in the past 7 did they ride a bicycle or walk for 30 minutes at a time.

These surveys suggest that about 75% of young men and about 50% of young women meet the guideline regarding vigorous physical activity.[25, 26] Similar to findings among adults, the percentage of adolescents engaging in vigorous physical activity decreases with increasing age and is higher among boys than girls at all ages. Overall, White students report more vigorous physical activity than Black students and vigorous physical activity is positively related to the socioeconomic status of the parents.[25–27] Contributing to the overall problem is the lack of required physical education classes. In 1995, less than 60% of students nationwide were enrolled in a physical education class, and only 25% attended physical education classes daily.[25] Furthermore, among those enrolled in physical education classes, about 30% did not exercise 20 or more minutes during an average class.[25]

Geographic Distribution

The 1994 BRFSS survey found that the prevalence of leisure-time physical inactivity among adults 18 years and older ranged from a low of 18.3% in the state of Washington, to a high of 49.3% in the District of Columbia.[22] Comparison by region of the country shows the highest proportion of physically inactive adults in the southern states (27.0%) and lowest proportion among adults in the western (22.5%) and north central (20.8%) states.[1]

Time Trends

From a baseline level of 24% in 1985, national objectives call for a reduction in the prevalence of leisure-time physical inactivity to 15% by the year 2000.[28] BRFSS data suggest very little change between the mid-1980s and the mid-1990s in the percentage of adults who participate in no leisure-time physical activity.[1] Older individuals can gain enormous benefits by increasing physical activity levels. While the prevalence of physical inactivity has declined slightly between 1987 and 1992 among those, aged 65 and older, at this rate it is unlikely that this age group will meet their year 2000 objective of 22%.[28–30]

Monthly variation is seen in the prevalence of leisure-time physical inactivity. During 1994, 29% of adults engaged in no leisure-time activity for the entire year, ranging from 35% in January to 25% in June.[31] Analysis of these seasonal patterns showed that monthly rates of inactivity were higher and more stable among older persons, Hispanics, and residents of southern states.[31]

RISK FACTORS

Populations at Risk

Data from national surveys identify US adults who are at risk for low levels of physical activity. These are the physically disabled,[1, 32] people with injuries that limit movement,[1] older adults,[1, 29] adolescents,[29] adults who are overweight,[33] women,[1, 34] ethnic minorities, and people with low incomes.[1]

Determinants of Physical Activity

Identifying factors associated with a physically active lifestyle (also called determinants of physical activity) is important for the development of effective interventions. Although much work remains to be done, several investigators have suggested that determinants of behavior involve personal (ie, age), psychological (ie, motivation), confidence in the ability to exercise (self-efficacy), social and cultural factors, and the physical environment.[35] As for adults, determinants of physical activity behavior among youth and adolescents are not well identified but include confidence in one's ability to engage in exercise, perceptions of competence in sports, and enjoyment of physical activity.[27] Among youth, developmental factors could also play an important role in physical activity participation.[36]

Barriers to Physical Activity

Common barriers to physical activity are lack of time, motivation, social support, facilities, and knowledge of ways to become more physically active.[35] Certain lifestyle characteristics may promote physical inactivity. These include commuting long distances to work, sedentary

jobs, watching television, and using computers during leisure time.[37] However, more research is needed to understand lifestyle behaviors associated with physically inactive lifestyles.

Among women, fear of assault, cultural expectations, obligations to family care and others are also cited as common barriers to being physically active.[16] Women who work full time and have home and family responsibilities report less physical activity than working women without family care responsibilities.[38] Among minority women, additional barriers may include differences in native languages, acculturation issues, and economic status.[39]

For some individuals, other health conditions may contribute to physical inactivity. Overweight status, chronic and infectious disease, injury, and physical disability may increase the energy cost of physical activity. The conditions may also prohibit being physically active. Often, inactivity due to existing health conditions may create a positive feedback response by which the condition may worsen with decreased physical activity.

PREVENTION AND CONTROL

National

As with any public health problem, prevention works best when operating at many levels: personal, medical, work site, school, and community. To guide prevention efforts and to measure the improvement in the risk profiles of the US population, the Public Health Service routinely develops national health objectives. The most recent document, Healthy People 2000,[28] lists over 300 objectives in 22 priority areas. These objectives provide baseline prevalence data and set 10-year targets for each objective. Table 7.4 shows the detail of objective 1.5, which relates to physical inactivity. On the basis of 1995 national surveillance data, it appears as if these targets will not be met by the year 2000.[30]

Besides the Healthy People 2000 initiative, the Surgeon General's Report on Physical Activity and Health was published in 1996.[1] This work is a major compilation of all the scientific evidence linking physical activity and health. Incorporated into this report are specific suggestions for obtaining at least 150 kilocalories per day of moderate or vigorous physical activity. These suggestions include doing 15 to 20 minutes of vigorous activities (such as running) or 30 to 45 minutes of

Table 7.4—Healthy People 2000 Risk Reduction Objective Related to Physical Activity

Objective No.		Baseline	Target	1991
1.5	Reduce to no more than 15% the proportion of people aged 6 and older who engage in no leisure-time physical activity	24% (18+ years)	15%	24%
1.5a	People aged 65 and older	43%	22%	29%
1.5b	People with disabilities	35%	20%	30%
1.5c	People with lower income (<$20 000 annual)	32%	17%	32%
1.5d	Blacks aged 18 and older	—	20%	28%
1.5e	Hispanics aged 18 and older	—	25%	34%
1.5f	American Indians/Alaska Natives aged 18 and older—		21%	29%

Note. Adapted from Healthy People 2000 Review.[30]

moderate activities (such as walking) each day.

The Guide to Clinical Preventive Services[40] is a report of the US Preventive Services Task Force that provides updated counseling information for clinicians. This guide contains recommendations for prevention based on a review of over 100 interventions to prevent 60 different illnesses and conditions. In the 1996 edition, counseling on the health benefits of physical activity is recommended for all children and adults. Current recommendations for physical activity focus on consistently performed moderate rather than vigorous intensity activity for sedentary patients. Examples of moderate physical activities that can be used to increase overall physical activity levels include walking or cycling to work, taking the stairs, and raking leaves.

Surveillance

A comprehensive surveillance system is essential to monitor levels of physical activity among the general population and to develop and evaluate interventions. The national surveys already in place provide a framework from which to collect data regularly. However, physical activity surveillance systems must be updated regularly to provide sufficient information on a variety of activities to assure that prevalence data on physical activity patterns and trends are meaningful and complete. Current systems focus on sports, conditioning, and leisure-time activities. More information is needed on occupation, transportation, gender-, and ethnic-specific activities.[39, 41] Such activities may include walking, lifting and carrying activities during work, walking and cycling to and from work, family care and household activities, and activities relating to religious and cultural traditions.

Environmental and Policy Factors

Changes in public policy to promote physical activity often arise from grass roots community organizations designed to affect change at local, state, and national levels. Activities may be focused on removing environmental barriers, de-emphasizing automation, building more accessible facilities to enhance movement, requiring school physical education, or subsidizing parks and recreational facilities to provide physical activity programs for people of all ages.[42] An example of an environmental policy is to require architects to design buildings with open, well-lit, safe, and accessible stairways placed in visible locations, such as in the lobby of buildings. This provides an alternative to elevators and escalators. Other environmental interventions can be developed at community levels, within work sites, at schools, and in recreation centers.[42, 43] For example, community developers and city councils could be encouraged to install bicycle trails, walking trails, and sidewalks in developments. Employers could provide safe and convenient exercise facilities as well as flexible work schedules to promote increased activity during the work day. Other examples of environmental opportunities for promoting physical activity include building bicycling paths and sidewalks along busy streets and providing access to shopping malls and schools as safe, heated or air-conditioned walking and exercise spaces. See King et al.[42, 43] and Brownson et al.[44] for excellent reviews in this area.

Efforts to encourage state and local school boards to require school physical education with a focus on activities that can be practiced throughout life should be part of the overall physical activity promotion plan for young adults.[45] Similarly, schools and recreation facilities could be subsidized to serve as after school day care centers for children with working parents. By opening these facilities to seniors to help care for the children, physical activity messages could be targeted to both children and seniors.

EXAMPLES OF PUBLIC HEALTH INTERVENTIONS

Many programs conducted over the past decade provide insight as to strategies for behavior change through community interventions and initiatives. Applying theories of behavior change allows interventions to target groups with messages appropriate to their readiness to modify their behaviors. The Stages of Change, also called the Transtheoretical model, describes five stages to behavior change: *precontemplation,* one is not thinking about behavior change; *contemplation,* one is thinking about changing a behavior but has not done anything about it; *action,* one has adopted a new behavior for less than 6 months; *maintenance,* one has practiced a new behavior for longer than 6 months; and *relapse,* one has stopped the new behavior but plans to resume the behavior change.[46] The Stages of Change approach has been used to promote physical activity in individual and physician-based interventions.

Individual-based projects focus on the individual as the target for behavior change. An example of a program that compared the effects of a lifestyle (home-based) exercises intervention with a traditional (a health club) exercise intervention on cardiovascular risk factors is Project

Active.[47] The lifestyle exercise intervention consists of advising each participant to accumulate at least 30 minutes of moderate intensity physical activity on most days of the week, in a way unique to each participant's lifestyle. The traditional exercise intervention offers structured exercise programs in a health club setting. Activity programs and motivational messages are targeted to participants based on their level of readiness to change their physical activity behaviors. After 6 months, both groups had similar reductions in cardiovascular disease risk factors such as total cholesterol, the ratio of total to high-density lipoprotein cholesterol, diastolic blood pressure, and percentage body fat.[47]

Physician-based programs have great potential for increasing physical activity among all age groups. A community study of White and Black adults found that the strongest determinant for increasing physical activity after 4 years was whether or not a physician had recommended increasing physical activity.[48] The problem is that very few physicians have specific training in physical activity promotion. Although guidelines for prescribing physical activity for patients are available,[40] this counseling takes valuable time and may not be appropriate for every patient.

Several projects are underway that use physicians as agents of behavior change.[49, 50] These projects are well received by clinical practices who want to provide more support to their sedentary patients but are constrained by time and resources. The PACE project (Physician-Based Assessment and Counseling for Exercise) provides a guide for the appropriate level of intervention depending on a person's stage of behavior change with respect to physical activity.[50] This targeted intervention allows the physician or the office staff to provide materials geared to the patient's level of acceptance. This approach has also been used effectively among elderly patients.[51]

Other important settings for physical activity intervention programs are work sites, schools, and assisted-living facilities. Work site physical activity promotion can operate at many levels. Some companies are large enough to provide exercise facilities including showers and changing rooms. Other companies can support physical activity by allowing time off during the day for regular exercise. Still other companies may incorporate physical activity education into their health promotion program along with smoking cessation and nutritional education. Providing a supportive work site environment will help employees to recognize the importance of physical activity and to participate in social interaction as well as physical activity. Work site physical activity may be especially important for adults with family responsibilities that constrain physical activity at home.[16]

An important approach to increasing physical activity in communities involves public policy and environmental changes. A partnership between physical activity and public health policy experts provides an important opportunity to increase physical activity among community residents. The Intermodal Surface Travel Efficiency Act (ISTEA) is an example of a collaboration that has resulted in legislation to make environmental changes that promote physical activity.[52] An outcome of ISTEA is the "Rails to Trails" program where unused railways are converted to walking and cycling paths.

Examples of public health approaches to promoting physical activity include several national and state campaigns.

National Coalition for Promotion of Physical Activity (NCPPA). The NCPPA coordinates the efforts of sports medicine, public health, and corporate agencies to increase physical activity in the United States. The goal of the Coalition is to unite the strengths of public and private efforts into a collaborative partnership to inspire Americans to lead physically active lifestyles to enhance their health and quality of life. The NCPPA is open to nonprofit organi-

zations that are membership-based and have identified physical activity and health as a primary mission.

President's Council on Physical Fitness and Sport (PCPFS). The PCPFS was established in 1956 to promote physical activity, fitness, and sports for all Americans. Members of the PCPFS are national leaders in physical activity, fitness, and sport. The PCPFS supports community, state, and national organizations to promote active lifestyles. Types of activities supported include holding physical activity and fitness clinics and writing public service advertising campaigns. In addition, the PCPFS provides grassroots support to educators, parents, physicians and health professionals, youth sport coaches and recreation workers, employers, public officials, and community leaders interested in promoting physical activity, fitness, and sport.

State Governor's Councils for Physical Fitness. State Governor's Councils for Physical Fitness are an extension of the PCPFS at the state and community levels. The Chairs of Governor's Councils are generally employed by the State Health Department or the Governor's Office. Council members are state leaders in physical activity and are appointed to the Council by the Governor. Physical activity and fitness promotion efforts vary by state. However, they generally include regular meetings of the Council, newsletters, awareness campaigns, conferences, and participation on policy decisions.

State Health Department Physical Activity Initiatives and Campaigns. Under the leadership of state and local health departments, physical activity initiatives and campaigns are designed to promote physical activity. Examples of initiatives are walking and bicycling events, work site challenges, and physical activity marketing efforts.

AREAS OF FUTURE RESEARCH AND DEMONSTRATION

Although the health effects of physical activity have been studied for several decades, it has been only recently that the emphasis has shifted from performance and cardiorespiratory fitness benefits to the myriad of health benefits that we now know accompany even small increases in moderate activity. The future directions for research are outlined below.

Lifestyle Activity Versus Structured Physical Activity

Results from Project Active suggest that health benefits and compliance with a lifestyle approach to increasing physical activity is as effective as more structured personal approaches to increasing physical activity.[47, 53] Additional research and demonstra-

tion projects are needed to confirm these results and to answer many questions about the appropriate types and amounts of physical activity required for health benefits.[54, 55] Further studies are also needed on the health benefits of lifestyle activities such as walking for exercise.[56]

Measurement of Physical Activity

In the past 10 years, there has been considerable progress in validating and determining the reliability of physical activity surveys.[57] Most surveys used in major epidemiological studies measure continuous, vigorous physical activity.[58] However, participation in moderate intensity and intermittent physical activities are seldom measured. When such activities are included in physical activity surveys, validation studies yield low correlations when compared with objective measures of physical activity.[57] An inability to measure participation in moderate activities may reflect a lack of sensitivity in survey questions, especially for women and ethnic minorities.[39, 41] Studies are ongoing to develop physical activity surveys that reflect patterns of activity in these groups.

Strength Versus Aerobic Conditioning for Older Adults

There has been considerable discussion on whether programs for older adults should focus on strength or aerobic conditioning. Although both are necessary for independent living, many frail, older individuals would benefit more from a strength program than from aerobic conditioning, at least until they are able to perform the basic activities of daily living. Research and demonstration projects are needed to identify optimal activities for maintaining and improving strength and balance in middle and early old age to provide functional independence in later life.

Adolescent Physical Activity

Adoption of guidelines to promote physical activity in schools[45] and out of school settings[59] provide a framework to address the decline in physical activity among adolescents. However, additional research and demonstration projects are needed to identify effective strategies to encourage youth, especially girls and young women, to remain active during adolescence and to balance activity levels with adequate nutrition needed for growth and development.[1]

Physician-Delivered Health Messages

Physician-delivered programs are effective in increasing physical activity and are well received by patients, at least in short-term studies.[47, 49] Future work needs to be done to assess the long-term effects of physician counseling. In general, physicians are recognizing the importance of physical inactivity as a risk factor and the proportion who discuss physical activity with their patients is increasing. However, many physicians are not confident in their ability to change this behavior.[60] Programs such as PACE need to be adapted to different populations (older adults, ethnic minorities, persons with disabilities) and different settings (eg, physician's office, health provider clinic) to provide physicians with an important tool to help modify this unhealthy behavior.

Environmental and Policy Changes

Continued efforts are needed by coalitions, educators, and community residents to effect environmental and policy changes that promote physical activity among people of all ages. These efforts may take the form of working with neighborhood coalitions to adopt residential policies conducive to being physically active, writing letters to the editor of local newspapers, writing position statements for local agencies, and lobbying legislators and city planners to pass laws to require environmental changes that promote physical activity. Additional funding is needed for research into the effectiveness of environmental and policy changes in decreasing the prevalence of physical inactivity.

REFERENCES

1. US Dept of Health and Human Services. *Physical Activity and*

Health: A Report of the Surgeon General. Atlanta, Ga: US Dept of Health and Human Services, Centers for Disease Control and Prevention, National Center for Chronic Disease Prevention and Health Promotion; 1996.

2. Pate RR, Pratt M, Blair SN, et al. Physical activity and public health: a recommendation from the Centers for Disease Control and Prevention and the American College of Sports Medicine. *JAMA.* 1995;273:402–407.

3. NIH Consensus Conference. Physical activity and cardiovascular health. *JAMA.* 1996;276:241–246.

4. Ainsworth BE, Keenan NL, Strogatz DS, Garrett JM, James SA. Physical activity and hypertension in Black adults: The Pitt County Study. *Am J Public Health.* 1991;81:1477–1479.

5. Powell KE, Thompson PD, Caspersen CJ, Kendrick JS. Physical activity and the incidence of coronary heart disease. *Annu Rev Public Health.* 1987;8:253–287.

6. McGinnis JM, Foege WH. Actual causes of death in the United States. *JAMA.* 1993;270:2207–2212.

7. Hahn RA, Teutsch SM, Rothenberg RB, Marks JS. Excess deaths from nine chronic diseases in the United States, 1986. *JAMA.* 1990;264:2654–2659.

8. Centers for Disease Control. Physical activity and the prevention of coronary heart disease. *MMWR.* 199342:669–672.

9. Powell KE, Blair SN. The public health burdens of sedentary living habits: theoretical but realistic estimates. *Med Sci Sports Exerc.* 1994;26:851–856.

10. Jones TF, Eaton CB. Cost-benefit analysis of walking to prevent coronary heart disease. *Arch Family Med.* 1994;703–710.

11. Caspersen CJ. Physical activity epidemiology: concepts, methods, and applications to exercise science. *Exerc Sport Sci Rev.* 1989;17:423–473.

12. President's Council on Physical Fitness and Sports. *Physical Fitness Research Digest.* Series 1, No. 1. Washington, DC; 1971.

13. American College of Sports Medicine. The recommended quantity and quality of exercise for developing and maintaining cardiorespiratory and muscular fitness in healthy adults. *Med Sci Sports Exerc.* 1990;22:265–274.

14. Bouchard C, Shephard RJ, Stephens T. *Physical Activity, Fitness, and Health: International Proceedings and Consensus Statement.* Champaign, Ill: Human Kinetics; 1994.

15. Ainsworth BE, Haskell WL, Leon AS, et al. Compendium of physical activities: classification of energy costs of human

physical activities. *Med Sci Sports Exerc.* 1993;25:71–80.

16. Henderson KA, Bialeschki MD, Shaw SM, Freysinger VJ. *Both Gains and Gaps: Feminist Perspectives on Women's Leisure.* State College, Pa: Venture; 1996.

17. de Vries HA, Housh TJ. *Physiology of Exercise.* 5th ed. Dubuque, Iowa: Brown & Benchmark Publishers; 1994.

18. National Center for Health Statistics, Benson V, Marano MA. *Current Estimates From the National Health Interview Survey, 1992.* Vital and Health Statistics, Series 10, No. 189. Hyattsville, Md: US Dept of Health and Human Services. Public Health Service, Centers for Disease Control and Prevention, National Center for Health Statistics; 1994. DHHS publication (PHS) 94-1517.

19. Remington PL, Smith MY, Williamson DF, Anda RF, Gentry EM, Hogelin GC. Design, characteristics, and usefulness of state-based behavioral risk factor surveillance: 1981–1987. *Public Health Rep.* 1988;103:366–375.

20. National Center for Health Statistics. *Plan and Operation of the Third National Health and Nutrition Examination Survey, 1988–94.* Vital and Health Statistics, Series 1, No. 32. Hyattsville, Md: US Dept of Health and Human Services,

Public Health Service, Centers for Disease Control and Prevention, National Center for Health Statistics; 1994. DHHS publication (PHS) 94-1308.

21. Crespo CJ, Keteyian SJ, Heath GW, Sempos CT. Leisure-time physical activity among US adults: results from the Third National Health and Nutrition Examination Survey. *Arch Intern Med.* 1996;156:93–98.

22. US Dept of Health and Human Services, Public Health Service. State-specific prevalence of participation in physical activity—Behavioral Risk Factor Surveillance System, 1994. . *MMWR.* 1996;45(31):673–675.

23. Jones DA, Ainsworth BE, Croft JB, Macera CA, Lloyd EE, Yusuf HR. Moderate leisure-time physical activity: Who is meeting the public health recommendations? *Arch Fam Med.* 1998;7:285–289.

24. Sallis JF, Patrick K. Physical activity guidelines for adolescents: consensus statement. *Pediatric Exerc Sci.* 1994;6:302–314.

25. Centers for Disease Control and Prevention. Youth risk behavior survey, United States, 1995. *MMWR.* 1996;45:1–25.

26. Lowry R, Kann L, Collins JL, Kolbe LJ. The effect of socioeconomic status on chronic disease risk behaviors among US adolescents. *JAMA.* 1996;276:792–797.

27. Zakarian JM, Hovell MF, Hofstetter CR, Sallis JF, Keating KJ. Correlates of vigorous exercise in a predominantly low SES and minority high school population. *Prev Med.* 1994;23: 314–321.

28. US Dept of Health and Human Services. Public Health Service. *Healthy People 2000: National Health Promotion and Disease Prevention Objectives.* Washington, DC: US Dept of Health and Human Services, Public Health Service, 1991. DHHS publication 91-50212.

29. Centers for Disease Control. State-specific changes in physical inactivity among persons aged 65 years or older —United States, 1987–1992. *MMWR.* 1995;44:663–673.

30. National Center for Health Statistics. *Healthy People 2000 Review, 1997.* Hyattsville, Md: Public Health Service; 1997.

31. Centers for Disease Control. Monthly estimates of leisure-time physical inactivity—United States, 1994. *MMWR.* 1997;44: 393–397.

32. Centers for Disease Control. Prevalence of leisure-time physical activity among persons with arthritis and other rheumatic conditions —United States, 1990–1991. *MMWR.* 1997;46:389–393.

33. Centers for Disease Control. Prevalence of physical inactivity during leisure time among overweight persons—Behavioral Risk Factor Surveillance System, 1994. *MMWR.* 1996;45:185–188.

34. Centers for Disease Control. Prevalence of recommended levels of physical activity among women—Behavioral Risk Factor Surveillance System, 1992. *MMWR.* 1995;44:105–107, 113.

35. Dishman RK, Sallis JF. Determinants and interventions for physical activity and exercise. In: Bouchard C, Shepard RJ, Stephens T, eds. *Physical Activity, Fitness, and Health: International Proceedings and Consensus Statement.* Champaign, Ill: Human Kinetics; 1994.

36. Sallis JF, Simons-Morton BG, Stone EJ, et al. Determinants of physical activity and interventions in youth. *Med Sci Sports Exerc.* 1992;24:s248–s257.

37. President's Council on Physical Fitness and Sports and Sporting Goods Manufacturers Association. *American Attitudes Toward Physical Activity and Fitness: A National Survey.* Washington, DC: President's Council on Physical Fitness and Sports; 1993.

38. Verhoef MJ, Love EJ. Women's exercise participation: the relevance of social roles compared to non-role-related determinants. *Can J Public Health* 1992;83:367–370.

39. Mâsse LC, Ainsworth BE, Tortolero S, et al. Measuring physical activity in mid-life, older, and minority women: issues from an expert's panel meeting. *J Womens Health*. 1998;7:57–67.

40. US Preventive Services Task Force. *Guide to Clinical Preventive Services*, 2nd ed. Baltimore: Williams & Wilkins; 1996.

41. Ainsworth BE, Richardson M, Jacobs DR Jr., Leon AS. Gender differences in physical activity. *Women Sport Phys Act*. 1993;2:1–16.

42. King AC, Jeffery RW, Fridinger F, et al. Environmental and policy approaches to cardiovascular disease prevention through physical activity: issues and opportunities. *Health Educ Q*. 1995;22:499–511.

43. King AC. Community and public health approaches to the promotion of physical activity. *Med Sci Sports Exerc*. 1994;26:1405–1412.

44. Brownson RC, Newschaffer CJ, Ali-Abarghoui F. Policy research for disease prevention: Challenges and practical recommendations. *Am J Public Health*. 1997;87:735–739.

45. Centers for Disease Control. Guidelines for school and community programs to promote lifelong physical activity among young people. *MMWR*. 1997;46:1–36.

46. Marcus BH, Simkin LR. The transtheoretical model: applications to exercise behavior. *Med Sci Sports Exerc*. 1994;26:1400–1404.

47. Dunn AL, Marcus BH, Kampert JB, Garcia ME, Kohl HW, Blair SN. Reduction in cardiovascular disease risk factors: 6-month results from Project Active. *Prev Med*. 1997;26:883–892.

48. Macera CA, Croft JB, Brown DR, Ferguson J, Lane MJ. Predictors of adoption of leisure-time physical activity in a biracial community sample. *Am J Epidemiol*. 1995;142:629–635.

49. Marcus BH, Pinto BM, Clark MM, DePue JD, Goldstein MG, Silverman LS. Physician-delivered physical activity and nutrition interventions. *Med Exerc Nutr Health*. 1995;4:325–334

50. Calfas KJ, Long BJ, Sallis JF, Wooten WJ, Pratt M, Patrick K. A controlled trial of physician counseling to promote the adoption of physical activity. *Prevent Med*. 1996;25:225–233.

51. Wenger NK. Physical inactivity and coronary heart disease in elderly patients. *Clin Geriatr Med*. 1996;12:79–88.

52. US Dept of Transportation, Zehnpfenning G. *Measures to Overcome Impediments to Bicycling and Walking: The National Bicycling and Walking*

Study, Case Study No. 4. Washington, DC: US Dept of Transportation, Federal Highway Administration; 1993. FHWA publication PD-94-031.

53. Phillips WT, Pruitt LA, King AC. Lifestyle activity: current recommendations. *Sports Med.* 1996; 22:1–7.

54. Blair SN, Connelly JC. How much physical activity should we do? The case for moderate amounts and intensities of physical activity. *Res Quart Exerc Sport.* 1996;67:193–205.

55. Slattery ML. How much physical activity do we need to maintain health and prevent disease? Different diseases—different mechanisms. *Res Quart Exerc Sport.* 1996;67:209–212.

56. Hakim AA, Petrovitch H, Burchfiel CM, et al. Effects of walking on mortality among nonsmoking retired men. *New Engl J Med.* 1998;338:94–99.

57. Jacobs DR, Ainsworth BE, Hartman TJ, Leon AS. A simultaneous evaluation of 10 commonly used physical activity questionnaires. *Med Sci Sports Exerc.* 1993;25:81–91.

58. Ainsworth BE, Montoye HJ, Leon AS. Methods of assessing physical activity during leisure and work. In: Bouchard C, Shephard RJ, Stephens T., eds. *Physical Activity, Fitness, and Health: International Proceedings and Consensus Statement.* Champaign, Ill: Human Kinetics; 1994:146–159.

59. Centers for Disease Control. Health risk behaviors among adolescents who do and do not attend school—United States, 1992. *MMWR.* 1994;43:129–132.

60. Yeager KK, Donehoo RS, Macera CA, Croft JA, Heath GW, Lane M. Physician health promotion practice patterns. *Am J Prev Med.* 1996;12:238–241.

SUGGESTED READING

Calfas KJ, Long BJ, Sallis JF, Wooten WJ, Pratt M, Patrick K. A controlled trial of physician counseling to promote the adoption of physical activity. *Prev Med.* 1996;25:225–233.

Centers for Disease Control and Prevention. Guidelines for school and community programs to promote lifelong physical activity among young people. *MMWR.* 1997;46:1–36.

King AC, Jeffery RW, Fridinger F, et al. Environmental and policy approaches to cardiovascular disease prevention through physical activity: issues and opportunities. *Health Educ Q.* 1995;22:499–511.

King AC. Community and public health approaches to the promotion of physical activity. *Med Sci Sports Exerc.* 1994;26:1405–1412.

Pate RR, Pratt M, Blair SN, et al. Physical activity and public health: a recommendation from the Centers for Disease Control and Prevention and the American College of Sports Medicine. *JAMA*. 1995;273:402–407.

US Dept of Health and Human Services. *Physical Activity and Health: A Report of the Surgeon General.* Atlanta, Ga: US Dept of Health and Human Services, Centers for Disease Control and Prevention, National Center for Chronic Disease Prevention and Health Promotion; 1996.

RESOURCES

American College of Sports Medicine
401 West Michigan Street
Indianapolis, IN 46202
317-637-9200

American Heart Association
7272 Greenville Avenue
Dallas, TX 75231-4596
214-373-6300

Division of Nutrition and Physical Activity
Centers for Disease Control and Prevention
4770 Buford Highway, NE (Mailstop K-46)
Atlanta, GA 30341
770-488-5692

President's Council on Physical Fitness and Sports
Hubert H. Humphrey Building, Room 738H
200 Independence Avenue, SW
Washington, DC 20201
202-690-9000

8

DIET AND NUTRITION

Dietary behavior is influenced by many factors. These include culture, cuisine, and agriculture; sociodemographics, lifestyle, and the proportion of women in the workplace; consumerism and economics; food manufacturing, advertising, and retailing; and health and nutrition.[1-3] Changing dietary habits in the population is not easy, as the US food system accounted in 1989 for at least 1 in every 10 jobs, over $600 billion in consumer sales, and over $30 billion in advertising.[3] This chapter will focus on the dietary factors associated with major chronic diseases, policy recommendations for healthy eating, and public health initiatives to promote dietary change.

Apart from Ancel Keys' early research and the American Heart Association's landmark dietary guidelines of the mid-1950s, it was not until the hearings held in the mid-1970s of the US Senate Select Committee on Nutrition and Human Needs that policy attention began to expand beyond problems of undernutrition to include those of chronic disease prevention. Since the issuance in 1977 of the then-controversial Dietary Goals for the United States,[4] a number of scientific reports have linked the typical US diet to coronary heart disease, cancer, stroke, diabetes, osteoporosis, and obesity.[5-20]

In recognition of the role that dietary factors play in the etiology of these major chronic diseases, the US Department of Agriculture and the US Department of Health and Human Services have issued and periodically updated the Dietary Guidelines for Americans; the fourth edition was published in 1995.[21] These guidelines are summarized in Table 8.1. Although these guidelines do not explicitly recommend a specific dietary pattern, they are generally interpreted to suggest that diets that emphasize a variety of plant foods, including whole grains, beans, vegetables, and fruits, and that minimize animal foods, especially red meat such as beef, pork, or

Lawrence H. Kushi, ScD
Susan B. Foerster, MPH, RD

Table 8.1—Dietary Guidelines for Americans, 1995

1. Eat a variety of foods
2. Balance the food you eat with physical activity; maintain or improve your weight
3. Choose a diet with plenty of grain products, vegetables, and fruits
4. Choose a diet low in fat, saturated fat, and cholesterol
5. Choose a diet moderate in sugars
6. Choose a diet moderate in salt and sodium
7. If you drink alcoholic beverages, do so in moderation

Note: Adapted from US Department of Agriculture.[21]

lamb, are healthful and likely to carry a lower risk of chronic disease in comparison with typical US dietary patterns. This was recently outlined explicitly in the recent revision of the American Cancer Society (ACS) dietary guidelines for cancer prevention.[13] Among the four ACS guidelines, the first two were "Choose most of the foods you eat from plant sources" and "Limit your intake of high-fat foods, particularly from animal sources."

SIGNIFICANCE

In 1990, it was estimated that 300 000 to 580 000 deaths were attributable to poor diet and physical inactivity in the United States.[22] These two lifestyle factors are the second most common "actual" cause of death (after tobacco use) and responsible for 14% of US deaths. Indeed, among the large majority of Americans who do not smoke, unhealthy diet and exercise patterns are the major cause of death and disability. Improvements in dietary intake have been slow, even though healthy eating is likely to benefit agriculture.[23, 24] Appreciable changes in a nation's disease statistics would be expected after 5 years of change in a population's diet.[7] Research on large-scale methods to promote healthy eating is growing but as yet relatively sparse.[25-28]

PATHOPHYSIOLOGY AND ANALYTIC EPIDEMIOLOGY

The pathophysiologic effects on diet and nutrition relate to numerous disease processes in a large body of literature. Because of this diverse literature and varied chronic diseases affected, the most important diet-disease relationships are described below, with pertinent details on their pathophysiology.

The primary base for a recommendation to consume diets that are abundant in plant foods comes from the large and consistent literature linking vegetable and fruit intake with risk of various cancers and from studies that have examined the association of antioxidant vitamins and dietary fiber with heart disease. Evidence from other areas that also supports these recommendations includes associations of folic acid and related nutrients with risk of neural tube defects[29, 30] and cardiovascular disease,[31, 32] and associations of carotenoids with diseases such as cataracts[33] and age-related macular degeneration,[34] among other disorders. Since the primary motivations for these recommendations come from associations with cancer and heart disease, however, an overview of these areas is presented here.

Vegetables, Fruits, and Cancer

Numerous studies demonstrate an inverse association between vegetable and fruit intake and cancer risk, and these associations have been seen across a wide variety of cancer sites. One recent review noted that there have been at least 20 cohort studies and 174 case-control studies examining the association of vegetables and fruits and cancer.[35] Among the 20 cohort studies, 12 demonstrated statistically significant inverse associations of some measure of vegetable or fruit intake and cancer risk, and the majority of others also demonstrated inverse associations. The overwhelming majority of the case-control studies also reported inverse associations of vegetables and fruits with cancer risk, with studies most consistent for cancers of the stomach, lung, esophagus, oral cavity and

pharynx, larynx, rectum, bladder, cervix, and endometrium.

The inverse association of vegetable and fruit intake with lung cancer is strong and consistent.[36–45] These studies uniformly indicate that those who consume vegetables or fruit more frequently are at decreased risk of lung cancer, with relative risks of about 0.3 to 0.5 comparing frequent with infrequent consumers. There has been some focus on the role of β-carotene as a protective factor, both for its antioxidant capabilities and as a precursor of vitamin A, which is required for cellular differentiation.[46] Although most of the epidemiologic studies are not able to disentangle the effects of β-carotene separately from other phytochemicals that may play a role in cancer prevention, one additional cohort study did find a protective effect for β-carotene, but not retinol, in relation to lung cancer[47]; this study did not report effects of foods on lung cancer risk. Recent evidence from the United States and Finland indicates that attribution of the observed protective effect of vegetables and fruit on lung cancer to specific components such as β-carotene was premature.[48–50] In addition, some studies, such as the Iowa Women's Health Study, show stronger inverse associations with vegetables and fruits than with micronutrients such as β-carotene.[45]

Vegetable and fruit intake is also inversely associated with cancers of the esophagus, stomach, and pancreas. For example, in a recent review of stomach cancer, inverse associations of vegetable or fruit intake were seen in 18 of 20 case-control studies that examined this association.[51] Among the five cohort studies identified in this review, inverse associations were reported in two of the studies; the others failed to find a significant association with vegetable or fruit intake. For esophageal cancer, a recent review indicated that inverse associations of vegetable or fruit intake with esophageal cancer were observed in 22 of 25 case-control studies[52]; this review also noted that the two cohort studies that were identified also observed inverse associations of vegetable intake with esophageal cancer risk. For pancreatic cancer, a recent review noted that 10 of 11 case-control studies and both cohort studies that reported information related to vegetable or fruit intake were supportive of an inverse association.[53]

The evidence from case-control studies of colon cancer is generally supportive of a protective association of vegetable intake, with the vast majority of case-control studies[54] and some cohort studies reporting an inverse association.[55,56] Findings for dietary fiber in particular are also reasonably consistent.[57,58] For ex-

ample, in a combined analysis of data from 13 case-control studies, there was a direct, inverse association between dietary fiber and colon cancer risk,[58] with study subjects in the highest quintile of dietary fiber intake having approximately one-half the risk of developing colon cancer as those in the lowest quintile of dietary fiber intake.

Several mechanisms have been proposed for a potential anticarcinogenic effect of fiber intake.[59,60] These include mechanical effects such as decreasing transit time and increasing stool bulk, thereby decreasing exposure to and concentration of carcinogens in the gut; and biochemical effects including the binding of bile acids that may act as promoters of carcinogenesis, or the production of short chain fatty acids such as butyrate that may alter carcinogen metabolism.

In addition to dietary fiber, there are numerous other compounds that may account for the anticancer effects seen for vegetable and fruit intake.[59,60] Vitamin C, vitamin E, and selenium, as well as previously mentioned carotenoids, have antioxidant effects that may provide protection against oxidative damage. Vitamin C may also block formation of nitrosamines through its ability to scavenge and reduce nitrite and is required for collagen synthesis and therefore the integrity of the intercellular matrix. Other compounds found in vegetables also provide antioxidant protection; examples include flavonoids such as quercetin and kaempferol that are widely distributed in plant foods.[61] Various phytochemicals appear to induce enzymatic detoxification systems, including mixed function oxidase systems and glutathione-S-transferase. Examples of such phytochemicals include indoles[62] and dithiolthiones,[63] abundant in cruciferous vegetables; allium compounds such as diallyl sulfide, abundant in vegetables such as garlic, onions, and leeks; limonene, found in citrus fruit oils; and phenolic compounds such as caffeic acid,[64] found in many fruits and vegetables. Other phytochemicals may have antiestrogenic or weak estrogenic effects and may therefore be antagonists of endogenous estrogens.[65] Examples include lignans that are found in whole grains and isoflavones such as genistein and daidzein that are particularly abundant in soybeans and certain other legumes.[66] Overall, the inverse association of vegetable and fruit intake and cancer risk is among the most consistent diet-disease associations observed in epidemiologic studies.

Plant Foods and Coronary Heart Disease

Evidence supporting a role for plant foods in the prevention of atherosclerotic heart disease comes primarily from several studies that have examined the effects of dietary fiber on blood cholesterol or coronary heart disease. Studies that have investigated the role of antioxidants on lipoprotein oxidation, atherogenesis, and heart disease are also generally supportive of dietary patterns that emphasize consumption of plant foods. In contrast with the research on cancer, relatively few studies of heart disease have focused on the role of foods such as vegetables or fruits per se, although these studies tend to support an inverse association between intake of these foods and cardiovascular disease.[67]

Dietary Fiber and Heart Disease. Although the major focus of most epidemiological studies of diet and heart disease has been the role of dietary lipids, there is a substantial research literature on dietary fiber. After the initial observations of Trowell,[68] there have been several prospective cohort studies that have investigated the association of dietary fiber with heart disease. The earliest of these, a 10 to 20 year follow-up of 337 British mail, bank, and bus employees, reported a striking inverse association of total and cereal fiber intake with incident coronary heart disease.[69, 70] Findings from several other cohort studies published through the early 1990s are also generally consistent with inverse associations of dietary fiber or carbohydrates from sources other than sugar or starch with coronary heart disease.[71-76]

In 1996, two large prospective investigations of dietary fiber intake and heart disease risk were published.[77, 78] In the first of these, a 6-year follow-up of 43 757 male US health professionals, it was observed that men in the highest quintile of dietary fiber intake had a relative risk of myocardial infarction of 0.64 (95% confidence interval 0.47 to 0.87) compared with men in the lowest quintile of intake.[77] In further analyses, this association was found to hold primarily for cereal fiber than for fiber from vegetables or fruit. The second study was a follow-up of participants in the Alpha-Tocopoherol, Beta-Carotene Cancer Prevention Study.[78] In this study, dietary fiber was inversely associated with coronary heart disease incidence; this association was stronger for soluble fiber and vegetable fiber sources but present for insoluble fiber and cereal and fruit fibers as well. Preliminary analyses from the Iowa Women's Health Study, a prospective cohort study of 34 487 women, also suggest an inverse association of dietary fiber, especially from cereals, with risk of death from coronary heart disease.[79]

The influence of dietary fiber on coronary heart disease risk factors such as blood lipids and blood pressure has been examined in numerous studies. A number of studies examined the effects of oat bran or oatmeal, relatively rich sources of soluble fiber, on blood lipid levels; several of these were reviewed in a meta-analysis by Ripsin et al.[80] These and similar studies formed the basis for the recent approval of a food label health claim by the US Food and Drug Administration for oat products related to its effect on lowering blood cholesterol levels.[81] In the review by Ripsin et al.[80] a clear majority of studies demonstrated that oat bran feeding in comparison with control diets resulted in decreases in total cholesterol levels. Of the 19 studies reviewed, only one suggested a cholesterol-raising effect, and the summary effect size across the studies suggested that a dose of about 2 g of soluble fiber (corresponding to about 50 g of oat bran) lowers total blood cholesterol by about -0.13 mmol/L (-5.9 mg/dL). Studies that have examined the effects of oat bran on lipoproteins indicate that the cholesterol-lowering effects appear to be greatest for low-density lipoprotein (LDL) cholesterol, with minimal effects on high-density lipoprotein (HDL) cholesterol (eg, Refs. 82 and 83).

Other foods with a high-soluble fiber content also appear to have cholesterol-lowering effects similar to oat bran. For example, one of the initial studies to report an effect of soluble fiber on cholesterol lowering noted that beans lower blood cholesterol levels.[84] The cholesterol-lowering influence of beans has been seen in other studies as well.[85] Other soluble fiber sources also appear to lower blood cholesterol levels.[86-89] These effects probably result from binding of bile acids by soluble fibers, thereby preventing their reabsorption; cholestyramine, a cholesterol-lowering medication demonstrated to lower blood cholesterol levels,[90, 91] exerts its effects through similar mechanisms. There also may be other effects of dietary fiber on cardiovascular disease risk aside from its effects on blood lipid profiles. For example, some (eg, Refs. 92 and 93), but not all (eg, Refs. 94 and 95) studies have suggested there is a blood-pressure-lowering effect of dietary fiber; a high vegetable and fruit intake dietary pattern has also been demonstrated to lower blood pressure levels.[20] Increased dietary fiber intake may be related to decreased glycemic response.[96, 97] Dietary fiber intake appears to be inversely associated with blood insulin levels,[98] which may have consequences for development of insulin resistance (see Chapter 14). In addition, low dietary fiber intake and high intake of foods with a high glycemic load may increase the risk of development of diabetes mellitus[99, 100] and may influence coronary heart disease risk as well.

Antioxidants. There is growing recognition that oxidation of LDL particles may be a key step in the development of atherosclerotic plaques and that dietary antioxidants may inhibit this process.[101, 102] Epidemiologic studies in this area were spurred by observations of an inverse association of plasma vitamin E levels and coronary heart disease mortality across 16 European populations.[103] Observations indicating inverse associations of plasma total and LDL cholesterol with dietary antioxidants also serve to support a role for antioxidants in the prevention of atherosclerotic disease.[104, 105] Feeding studies indicate that vitamin E supplementation may also improve resistance of LDL to oxidation.[106]

In recent years, several prospective epidemiologic studies have reported associations of dietary antioxidants and risk of heart disease. Higher intakes of dietary antioxidants, such as vitamin C and particularly vitamin E, appear to be associated with lower risk of coronary heart disease mortality.[107-109] Other studies have also found inverse associations between vitamin E intake, whether from foods[110] or supplements,[111, 112] and risk of coronary heart disease.

The role of dietary antioxidants in the prevention of atherosclerotic heart disease is supported by an additional prospective cohort study that examined the influence of flavonoids, another class of dietary antioxidants.[113] Examples of flavonoids include quercetin, kaempferol, and myricetin. In this study, the relative risk of coronary heart disease death after 5 years of follow-up for those in the highest third of flavonoid intake compared with those in the lowest third was 0.32; the relative risk for both fatal and nonfatal heart disease was 0.52. Unlike vitamin E, which may be widely ingested in supplemental form, relatively few people as yet take flavonoids as supplements. Thus, the primary sources of flavonoids in this population were food sources, including tea, onions, apples, and other vegetables.[114] Similar findings were observed in a cohort study in Finland.[115] However, in a study of male health professionals, no association was observed between the antioxidant flavonoid intake and coronary disease.[116]

Saturated Fat, Dietary Cholesterol, Red Meat, and Heart Disease

The association of dietary fat with heart disease has been an area of active investigation for several decades. While initial observations of international differences in coronary disease rates and correlates with dietary fat intake differences laid the foundation for the now generally accepted association of high saturated fat and cholesterol intake with increased risk of heart disease, these

associations came to be accepted in large part because of consistent demonstrations that manipulations of dietary lipids in the diet result in predictable alterations in the levels of total and LDL cholesterol in the blood.[117, 118] Generally, altering dietary lipid patterns to decrease saturated fatty acids and cholesterol and increase polyunsaturated fatty acids will result in decreases in total and LDL cholesterol levels.

In recent years, feeding studies have demonstrated that monounsaturated fatty acids may also result in decreases in LDL cholesterol but will minimize reductions in HDL cholesterol.[119] Thus, diets that are not necessarily low in monounsaturated fatty acids or total fat but are still low in saturated fat and cholesterol may result in a lipoprotein profile with lower atherogenic risk than a low-fat diet per se. These observations are among the bases for recent interest in traditional Mediterranean dietary patterns.[120] *Trans* fatty acids, much of which are formed through the commercial process of hydrogenation, also appear to result in less favorable lipoprotein profiles.[121, 122] The replacement of other fatty acids by *trans* fatty acids appears to result in an increase in LDL and a decrease in HDL cholesterol levels.

There have been several prospective epidemiologic studies that have investigated the association of dietary lipids with coronary heart disease risk. Early studies in this area have generally not observed an association[123]; however, most of these were based on relatively imprecise dietary assessment methods or short-term follow-up and therefore may not have provided the best setting for examination of this association. One of the first prospective studies to demonstrate associations of dietary lipids with coronary mortality was the Western Electric Study.[124] In this study, the Keys dietary score, a summary of saturated fatty acid, polyunsaturated fatty acid, and dietary cholesterol intake,[125] was significantly and positively associated with increased risk of death from coronary heart disease. Since then, several other studies have demonstrated positive associations of dietary cholesterol or saturated fatty acids with coronary heart disease.[74, 126–130] Some studies suggest *trans* fatty acids may increase risk of coronary disease.[129–131] These observations and the effect of *trans* fatty acids on blood lipoprotein profiles[121, 122] have led some investigators to advocate food labels that identify *trans* fatty acid content.[132]

It has generally been recognized that regular meat consumption, because of its high saturated fat and cholesterol content, will increase the risk of death from coronary heart disease. For example, it has been demonstrated that regular consumption of beef when added to a vegetar-ian diet will increase blood cholesterol, especially LDL levels, and increase systolic blood pressure.[133] In studies of Seventh Day Adventists, regular meat eaters are at increased risk of heart disease compared with those who eat meat infrequently.[134, 135] Other studies have also indicated that vegetarians have a substantially reduced risk of heart disease than nonvegetarians.[136, 137] In addition to its effects on blood cholesterol levels, red meat intake may increase heart disease risk in other ways. For example, it has been suggested that body iron stores may be directly associated with risk of coronary heart disease.[138] A Finnish study demonstrated a positive association of serum ferritin levels and dietary iron intake with risk of acute myocardial infarction.[139] Although subsequent studies have been inconsistent in regards to this hypothesis,[140–142] it was observed in the Health Professionals Follow-up Study that dietary intake of heme iron increased risk of coronary heart disease, whereas dietary intake of nonheme iron was unrelated to coronary heart disease risk[143]; red meat is the primary source of heme iron in the diet. This distinction may be important as absorption of non-heme iron is better regulated than that of heme iron; in the presence of adequate iron stores, nonheme iron is poorly absorbed.

There is also growing interest in the role of homocysteinemia in the pathogenesis of atherosclerosis and coronary heart disease. A review of studies that had examined the association between blood homocysteine levels and atherosclerotic disease demonstrated that 16 of 21 such studies reported significantly higher homocysteine concentrations among cases than controls.[144] Since the majority of these studies examined homocysteine levels in blood samples collected after diagnosis, this consistent finding may have been a result of disease on blood levels. However, a prospective study of participants in the Physicians Health Study demonstrated that elevated plasma homocysteine may be an independent risk factor for myocardial infarction.[145] While blood homocysteine levels may be decreased by increased intake of folic acid or vitamin B-6[29, 30, 146] (and hence of vegetables and whole grains), they may also be increased by intake of methionine, the direct metabolic precursor of homocysteine. As red meat is a principal source of methionine in the diet, a higher intake of red meat may increase plasma homocysteine levels. Thus, these observations are consistent with the increased risk of heart disease associated with red meat intake.

Fat, Red Meat, and Cancer

Substantial research has focused on the role of dietary fat intake and cancer risk. Rodent studies almost uniformly indicate that animals fed higher fat diets have greater rates of tumorigenesis,[147, 148] while international correlation studies indicate that countries with higher per capita fat availability have higher rates of colon, breast, prostate, and other cancers.[148–150] These observations were among the bases for the conclusion of the 1982 National Academy of Sciences panel that of all the dietary components it studied, the combined epidemiological and experimental evidence is most suggestive for a causal relationship between fat intake and the occurrence of cancer.[9] Since the 1982 National Academy of Sciences report, there has been substantial epidemiological work on the association of dietary fat with various cancers.

Several prospective cohort studies have been conducted examining the association of fat intake with risk of breast cancer; these have been reviewed recently by Hunter and Willett.[151] Generally, these studies provide little evidence of an association between dietary fat intake and breast cancer risk. Recently, data from six of these cohort studies were pooled to examine this association.[152] In this pooled analysis, the relative risk of breast cancer comparing the highest quintile of fat intake with the lowest quintile was 1.02; even at extremely low fat intakes (less than 20% of calories), there was no evidence of a decreased risk of breast cancer. Although some investigators suggest that there is substantial measurement error that may account for this failure to find an association,[153] it is generally agreed that there is little evidence that changes in total fat intake in adulthood are unlikely to have a major impact on breast cancer risk. The Women's Health Initiative, an ongoing randomized clinical trial, should provide more definitive evidence of whether changes to a low-fat eating pattern may reduce breast cancer risk.[154]

Unlike breast cancer, the evidence that fat intake is associated with increased risk of cancers of the colon and prostate are more consistent.[54, 155] In the case of colon cancer, it is unclear whether the association with fat intake is due to fat or to the intake of red meat, which is more consistently related to risk of colon cancer. Other cancers have been suggested to be associated with fat intake, including cancers of the lung and endometrium.[36, 156]

An association between meat intake and colon cancer incidence or mortality has been observed in most cross-cultural studies that have examined this association. A recent review indicated that 17 of the 29 analytic epidemiology studies published to date that investigated an association of meat intake with colon cancer had shown a positive association.[54] Only one study, a large

prospective cohort study of Japanese adults aged 40 years and older, reported an inverse association.[157] One case-control study found a positive association with beef intake and an inverse association with pork intake.[158] When limited to the better conducted studies, 8 of 12 found positive associations of red meat intake and colon cancer.[54]

Several prospective cohort studies with comprehensive dietary assessment have examined the association of red meat intake with risk of colon cancer. In the Nurses Health Study,[159] a positive association of red meat intake with colon cancer incidence was reported after 6 years of follow-up. Women who reported consuming beef, pork, or lamb as a main dish every day had a relative risk of colon cancer of 2.49 compared with women who reported intake of less than once per month. Two of the other cohort studies in the United States and the Netherlands[160, 161] also reported positive associations of red meat intake with risk of incident colon cancer. Overall, 9 of 12 cohort studies are consistent with this association.

It has been observed consistently that red meat intake is associated with increased risk of pancreatic cancer.[16, 53] The evidence comes primarily from case-control studies; among 13 such studies that had been conducted through 1993, 9 showed evidence of a positive association, and only one showed evidence of an inverse association. A series of five case-control studies conducted under the auspices of the SEARCH program of the International Agency for Research on Cancer also provide evidence that is consistent with the suggestion that animal food intake increases risk of pancreatic cancer.[53] These studies used standardized methods to allow pooling of results while being conducted in several different countries, including Australia, Canada, the Netherlands, and Poland. When results were pooled across these studies, there was an increased risk of pancreatic cancer with increasing cholesterol intake, with the relative risk comparing high with low cholesterol intake of 1.47.

Several studies have focused on the association of fat, animal fat, or meat intake with prostate cancer. As with colon cancer, ecologic studies suggest a positive association of fat or meat intake and prostate cancer. The majority of case-control studies that have examined an association of diet with prostate cancer have seen a positive association with meat intake or animal fat intake; according to one review, eight of nine such studies reported positive associations.[155] Although some cohort studies with crude dietary assessment methods were unable to detect associations of meat intake with prostate cancer,[162-164] more recent cohort studies have observed a positive, significant

association of red meat intake and prostate cancer.[165, 166] In addition, studies in Seventh Day Adventists, in which meat intake varies considerably in the population, support a positive association of meat intake with prostate cancer.[167-169]

The above cancers are not the only ones that have been suggested to be causally associated with increased meat intake. For example, studies have suggested positive associations of meat intake with stomach cancer[170, 171] and breast cancer.[172-174] Much of the focus of potential biological mechanisms of meat intake on cancer has focused on fat intake. Thus, although the evidence for a causal association for some cancers is stronger for red meat intake than for fat per se, dietary recommendations to decrease cancer risk have generally focused on reduction of dietary fat intake.[13] Of relevance to hormone-dependent cancers such as those of the breast or prostate, sex hormone metabolism may be influenced by altering the fat content of the diet.[65] For colon cancer, diacylglycerides, which result from incomplete digestion of triacyl-glycerides, may have mitogenic effects on adenomas and carcinomas, but not on normal cells.[175] Dietary fat also stimulates bile acid production and secretion into the lumen of the small intestine; secondary bile acids, formed by the action of gut bacteria, may be cocarcinogenic.[60] More generally, fat is a more concentrated source of calories than other dietary factors, and excess caloric intake is known to promote carcinogenesis.

The associations seen between meat intake and cancer risk may be due to several additional mechanisms. Some of the carcinogenic potential of meat intake may result from the mutagenic or carcinogenic N-nitroso compounds that may exist in certain types of meat, especially processed meats.[176] Heterocyclic aromatic amines that are formed during the cooking process of meats are also carcinogenic.[177, 178] Dietary iron may act as a prooxidant and increase lipid peroxidation and free radical production.[179, 180] In addition, diets high in red meat tend to be low in plant foods and their numerous associated anticancer compounds.

DESCRIPTIVE EPIDEMIOLOGY

Information on nutrient intake, dietary patterns, and foods that are major contributors to nutrient intake are provided through the National Nutrition Monitoring and Related Research Program (NNMRRP).[181] The NNMRRP includes federal government data sources on food use and nutrient availability at the retail level and food consumption information that is collected on the individual level. Information on food intake patterns are also available from epidemiologic surveys conducted in selected populations around the United States, or for comparison purposes, other regions or countries, and these data can provide important information on the relationship of dietary patterns to risk of chronic diseases.

Food use, or food disappearance data, provide information related to quantities of foods and nutrients that "disappear" into the retail distribution channels of the food supply each year.[182] These data are derived by summing the total quantity of foods produced in this country, inventories from the previous year, and imported food. Subtracted from this sum are current year-end inventories, exported foods, and foodstuffs used for nonfood purposes. The resulting quantities of foods are assumed to be available for human consumption. Nutrient availability estimates are derived from these food disappearance data. As these data refer to foods available for purchase at the retail level, and not foods as actually consumed, they typically will overestimate food actually consumed. However, they can be used to examine trends in food availability.

In the United States, the federal government collects food consumption data in surveys such as the Nationwide Food Consumption Surveys (NFCS) and Continuing Survey of Food Intakes of Individuals (CSFII) conducted by the US Department of Agriculture, and the National Health and Nutrition Examination Surveys (NHANES), conducted by the National Center for Health Statistics of the US Department of Health and Human Services.

High-Risk Groups

Generally speaking, the US population as a whole can be considered to be at relatively high risk of developing chronic diseases that are influenced by dietary patterns characterized by regular consumption of high saturated fat, high red meat diets, and relatively infrequent consumption of vegetables, fruits, and whole grains. Although the US diet is characterized

by abundant availability of a wide variety of foodstuffs, international comparisons clearly indicate that the dietary patterns that are typically consumed in the US carry with it high rates of atherosclerotic diseases[183] and certain cancers, including cancers of the breast, endometrium, prostate, and colon and rectum.[19] Figure 8.1 shows the association of dietary fat availability with breast cancer incidence across various countries. Observations of changing dietary patterns and disease trends as populations migrate from low-disease-rate countries to high-disease-rate countries, or as they become increasingly industrialized, demonstrate that such marked

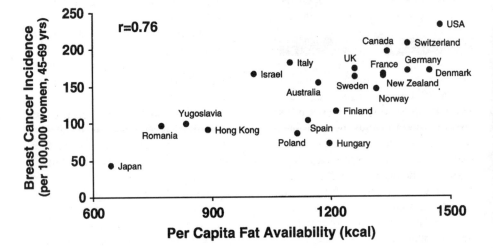

Figure 8.1—Association of per capita fat availability and breast cancer incidence. *Source:* Adapted from Prentice RL, Kakar F, Hursting S, Sheppard L, Klein R, Kushi LH. Aspects of the rationale for the Women's Health Trial. *J Natl Cancer Inst.* 1988;80:802–814.

variations in disease patterns are influenced by environmental factors, including diet, and that these diseases are largely preventable.

Although the US population as a whole can be considered to be at "high risk" of major chronic diseases when compared to much of the rest of the world, within the United States, certain groups tend to consume diets that are relatively higher in fat and saturated fat intake, and lower in whole grains, fresh fruit, and vegetables, than other groups. People who have higher levels of educational attainment and higher incomes tend to consume dietary patterns that carry a lower risk of developing chronic diseases.[181, 184, 185] Somewhat difficult to disentangle from this relationship are observations that racial or ethnic groups that tend to have lower socioeconomic status also may have somewhat different dietary patterns than the majority population.[185, 186] These differences in dietary consumption patterns are also generally mirrored by differences in chronic disease rates, although there are important exceptions to this observation. For example, although Northern Plains Indians consume high-fat and high-saturated fat diets, their coronary disease rates are relatively low; on the other hand, African Americans have substantially higher cardiovascular disease and cancer rates than Whites,[187] but their nutrient intake

patterns indicate somewhat higher vegetable and fruit intake. Differences in fat intake according to selected sociodemographic factors are provided in Table 8.2.

Geographic Distribution

As noted above, there are substantial international differences in dietary patterns and chronic disease rates around the world. Within the United States, there are also important regional differences in consumption of specific food items. For example, grits or corn meal is frequently eaten in the South, but less so in other regions, while seafood is generally consumed more frequently in coastal areas than in the central parts of the country. These patterns reflect longstanding regional differences in culture and food availability, as commercial food distribution has made similar foods, restaurants, etc. available throughout the country regardless of seasonal changes or fluctuations in local agricultural production. Because most staple foods are widely available in the United States, the typical dietary pattern that includes regular consumption of red meat and dairy products, but also of certain grains, vegetables, and fruits, describes food choices for the vast majority of the US population. Thus, dietary patterns and chronic disease rates are generally less varied within the United States than across the globe.

Table 8.2—Percentage of People with Total Fat Intake ≤30% of Calories, >30% to ≤40% of Calories, and >40% of Calories During 3 Days, by Selected Sociodemographic Variables, 1989-1991

Variable	≤30%		>30% to ≤40%		>40%	
	Male	**Female**	**Male**	**Female**	**Male**	**Female**
Age (years)						
6-11	18.2	17.7	64.2	66.9	17.6	15.4
12-19	14.0	17.9	67.5	61.1	18.6	21.0
≥20	20.9	25.2	53.8	53.6	25.3	21.1
Race (age ≥20 years)						
White	20.6	25.3	53.1	53.7	26.3	21.0
Black	17.0	21.3	62.5	55.5	20.5	23.3
Income level (age ≥20 years)						
<131% poverty	21.7	25.9	50.9	53.0	27.4	21.2
131-350% poverty	18.2	26.0	56.0	54.7	25.8	19.3
>350% poverty	22.3	23.6	52.0	53.4	25.7	23.0
Food Stamp Participation (age ≥20 years)						
Participant	21.5	23.5	48.6	52.7	30.0	23.8
Nonparticipant	21.8	26.9	51.5	53.1	26.7	20.0

Note: Adapted from Table ES-1 of Federation of American Societies for Experimental Biology, Life Sciences Research Office. Prepared for the Interagency Board for Nutrition Monitoring and Related Research. Third Report on Nutrition Monitoring in the United States: Executive Summary. Washington, DC: US Government Printing Office; 1995.

Perhaps of equal importance in examining chronic disease rates and dietary patterns in the United States are differences in food availability on a microgeographic scale. In many inner-city neighborhoods in the United States, full-spectrum supermarkets no longer exist, and the only food stores within reasonable distance of many homes are convenience food stores. Meanwhile, supermarkets that offer a wide variety of fresh produce and other foods are located in more affluent neighborhoods and suburbs, and these retail food outlets are increasing the variety of foods they offer. Thus, the opportunity for healthful food choices are limited in poorer neighborhoods, even as variety in the availability of foods increases in the United States as a whole.

Time Trends

Nutrient intake in the United States has generally been fairly stable over the past 2 or 3 decades. There have, however, been incremental and significant changes in intake of key nutrients and food groups that form the basis for dietary guidelines. Fat intake was estimated in the 1965 to 1966 Nationwide Food Consumption Survey at approximately 42% of calories, was approximately 36% of calories in both the 1971 to 1974 NHANES I and 1976-80 NHANES II food consumption, and about 40% of calories in the 1977 to 1978 Nationwide Food Consumption Survey. In 1977, the US Dietary Goals established 30% of calories as a population target,[4] a figure that has since been reiterated in numerous other dietary recommendations, including the Healthy People 2000 objectives.[188] Since then, more recent food consumption surveys suggest a gradual decrease in proportion of food calories from fat, with the 1987

to 1988 Nationwide Food Consumption Survey estimating fat intake at 36% of calories, the 1988 to 1991 NHANES III estimating fat intake at 34% of calories, and the 1994 to 1995 Continuing Survey of Food Intakes of Individuals estimating fat intake at 33% of calories. This apparent trend in decreasing fat intake is shown in Figure 8.2.

Another common dietary recommendation is to increase vegetable, fruit, and whole grain intake. Information from food disappearance data indicates that per capita availability of these foods has been gradually increasing over the past two and a half decades. Between 1970 and 1994, vegetables increased by about 19%, fruits by 22%, and

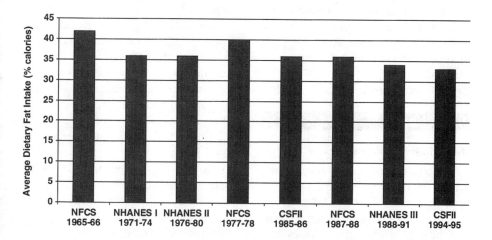

Figure 8.2—Food calories from dietary fat for selected national surveys, 1965–1995. NFCS indicates Nationwide Food Consumption Survey; NHANES, National Health and Nutrition Examination Survey; CSFII, Continuing Survey of Food Intakes of Individuals.

grains by 47%.[182] If one examines food disappearance data since 1909, it is apparent that vegetable and fruit consumption has been increasing steadily throughout this century.[189] On the other hand, consumption of cereals was substantially higher— almost 300 pounds per capita per year in 1909 to 1913.[189] From this level of consumption, availability of cereals decreased to about 150 pounds per capita per year in 1970 and has since increased to about 200 pounds per capita per year in 1994.[182] While the proportion of cereals that are consumed as whole as opposed to refined grains is not readily discernible from food disappearance data, it has been estimated that approximately 11.5 pounds per capita per year of whole wheat and oats were available for consumption in 1994, and that this number has increased in recent decades.[190] Changes in food availability for various commodities from 1970 to 1994 are provided in Table 8.3.

RISK FACTORS

Magnitude of Risk Factors

Although there is substantial work on the relationship of dietary patterns and specific foods and nutrients on chronic disease risk, there is very little epidemiologic work on the determinants of intake of specific foods or dietary patterns. It is generally recognized that dietary habits are established relatively early in life, and major changes in diet are a relatively rare occurrence. Studies indicate that dietary habits and nutrient intake tend to cluster in families, suggesting that familial influences are a major determinant of food intake patterns.[191] There are also societal determinants of food and nutrient intake choices. The food industry plays a major role in the awareness of specific food products and can create demand for food items that did not previously exist. As most food advertising is for snack and convenience foods that are relatively high in sugars and fats, the influence of advertising in the United States can be considered to be a factor that increases the risk of adopting a less healthful dietary pattern.[192]

Legislative and policy initiatives may also affect the availability of foods and the types of foods for certain population groups, in particular low-income populations. The Special Supplemental Feeding Program for Women, Infants and Children (WIC) designates certain food items that may be purchased using vouchers. These food items are selected because they provide adequate nutrient intake that is important for pregnant and lactating women and young children up to 4 years of age. The National School Lunch Program has dictated the mix of foods that can be made available

. . . .

Table 8.3—Average Annual Per Capita Consumption of Major Foods in the United States, Pounds, 1970-1994.[a]

Food	1970-1974	1975-1979	1980-1984	1985-1989	1990-1994	1994
Meat, poultry and fish						
Meat	130.2	128.6	123.8	120.0	113.0	114.8
Poultry	34.1	36.3	42.3	50.0	60.4	63.7
Fish and shellfish	12.1	12.8	13.0	15.4	14.9	15.1
Total	176.5	177.8	179.1	185.4	188.3	193.5
Eggs	38.3	34.9	33.9	32.1	30.3	30.6
Dairy products,						
including butter	554.2	542.3	558.6	586.5	572.0	586.2
Fats and oils						
Animal	13.1	10.8	12.0	11.6	10.4	11.6
Vegetable	39.6	43.7	46.3	51.4	55.0	55.2
Total	52.7	54.5	58.3	63.0	65.4	66.9
Flour and cereal						
products	135.1	141.2	147.0	167.9	191.5	198.7
Selected fruits						
Fresh	93.3	96.9	102.9	113.2	115.4	126.7
Canned	22.4	21.2	18.7	18.3	18.3	18.3
Frozen	3.3	2.9	2.8	3.4	3.4	3.4
Dried	2.5	2.4	2.6	3.1	3.1	3.1
Selected juices	52.4	59.0	64.6	69.4	68.1	75.1
Selected vegetables						
Fresh	80.2	83.2	86.5	99.0	105.0	104.7
Canned	97.4	95.3	94.7	95.3	107.3	104.5
Frozen	17.0	17.5	17.5	19.9	21.6	21.6
Potatoes						
Fresh	53.3	47.5	46.5	46.6	46.3	48.2
Frozen	14.9	20.2	19.8	23.0	26.5	28.9

Note. Adapted from Table 2 in Putnam and Allshouse.[182]

to school children through lunches that are provided through this program. Through most of its history, the primary consideration was the provision of at least one-third of the Recommended Dietary Allowance for selected key nutrients. In 1995, the US Department of Agriculture specified that school lunches would in the future also have to provide meals that were consistent with the Dietary Guidelines for Americans, recognizing the importance of establishing dietary habits consistent with reduction of chronic disease risk.[193]

Population-Attributable Risk

There is virtually no work on the proportion of the population that may be influenced by familial, advertising, policy initiatives, or other determinants in shaping dietary habits. On the other hand, there have been several estimates made of the proportion of various cancers that may be prevented through modification of dietary habits; comparable work for other chronic diseases has generally not been done, although it has been suggested that perhaps 70% of coronary heart disease may be attributed to high serum cholesterol levels and physical inactivity, both factors with dietary antecedents or cofactors.[194]

Regarding cancer, it was estimated by Doll and Peto[195] in 1981 in a report that was commissioned for the Office of Technology Assessment, Congress, that approximately 35% of the cancer burden in the United States may be attributable to dietary factors; there was great uncertainty in this estimate, with the range of reasonable estimates for the impact of diet placed at 10% to 70%. This proportion of cancers was comparable only to that estimated to be attributable to tobacco, which was placed at 30% of cancer, with a range of 25% to 40% of total cancers. This estimate of the contribution of diet to cancer in the United States was comparable to earlier estimates by Wynder and Gori[196] that approxi-mately 40% of male and 57% of female cancers could be attributable to diet.

Most recently, the World Cancer Research Fund and American Institute for Cancer Research esti-mated that approximately 23% of cancers worldwide could be pre-vented by increasing vegetable and fruit intake.[19] They also estimated that between 29% and 40% of cancers could be prevented through dietary means, including modifica-tions in meat and alcohol intake. For cancers that are common in the United States, they estimated that dietary modifications could prevent between 20% and 33% of lung cancers, 33% and 50% of breast cancers, 66% and 75% of colorectal cancer, and 10% and 20% of prostate cancers.

PREVENTION AND CONTROL MEASURES

Since the 1950s, research on chronic diseases has investigated foods and food components that can be harmful when consumed in excess, those that may be consumed in insufficient amounts for good health, and more recently, those that may protect against chronic diseases. Such studies have gradually laid the foundation for fundamental shifts in US dietary guidance policy. In the interim, however, the sometimes conflicting recommendations issued by scientific bodies, voluntary health organizations, and units of the US government have led to confusion and even skepticism. Sodium, fat, saturated fat, cholesterol, and sugar have been the most contentious issues.

In 1990, the National Nutrition Monitoring and Related Research Act eliminated mixed nutrition messages from government by requiring all federal dietary guidelines to pass an interagency approval process that also resulted in more attention to chronic disease prevention. The 1990 Dietary Guidelines for Americans were the first to mention the terms "whole grain," "low fat," and "lean" in official dietary guidance and to shift from the "foundation diet" approach of the Basic 4 Food Groups to a "total diet" for good health.[21] Two years later, the Food Guide Pyramid (Figure 8.3)[197] was released by the USDA. Media attention was drawn by its graphic shift in emphasis from a protein-centered to a plant-based diet. Simultaneously, the Nutrition Labeling and Education Act of 1992 focused on chronic disease factors. It required mandatory nutrition labeling on packaged foods for the first time, with the Nutrition Facts information displaying nutrients important to chronic disease control. It also defined strictly the use of descriptors such as "reduced" or "low fat," and limited health claims that could be made on food.

In the 1980s, the US Department of Health and Human Services developed the nation's first measurable prevention targets. The 1990 Health Objectives for the Nation spelled out 17 objectives for nutrition. They included reduction of high blood cholesterol, obesity, salt/sodium intake; increased knowledge of diet/disease relationships and food selection; and promotion of Dietary Guidelines in work site and school cafeterias, nutrition education in schools, and nutrition assessment by clinicians. In 1990, the *Healthy People 2000: National Health Promotion and Disease Prevention Objectives* expanded nutrition priorities to 27 objectives, all but four of which focused on chronic disease control.[188]

The 1990 nutrition objectives included multiple chronic disease outcomes. The targets for change included children, the food environment and organizational policies, and disparities among demographic subgroups. Compared to 1990, new objectives were added for health status measures for coronary heart disease, cancer, colorectal cancer, stroke, and diabetes; the risk factors of hypertension, fat/saturated fat, fruits/vegetables/grains, milk products and sodium, and use of food labels; and services including low-fat restaurant food, work site nutrition programs, home-delivered meals for seniors, and nutritious food in schools and child care settings.

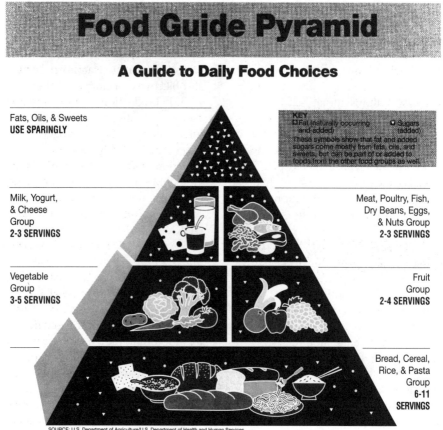

Food Guide Pyramid

A Guide to Daily Food Choices

Fats, Oils, & Sweets
USE SPARINGLY

KEY
☐ Fat (naturally occurring and added) ♥ Sugars (added)
These symbols show that fat and added sugars come mostly from fats, oils, and sweets, but can be part of or added to foods from the other food groups as well.

Milk, Yogurt, & Cheese Group
2-3 SERVINGS

Meat, Poultry, Fish, Dry Beans, Eggs, & Nuts Group
2-3 SERVINGS

Vegetable Group
3-5 SERVINGS

Fruit Group
2-4 SERVINGS

Bread, Cereal, Rice, & Pasta Group
6-11 SERVINGS

SOURCE: U.S. Department of Agriculture/U.S. Department of Health and Human Services

Use the Food Guide Pyramid to help you eat better every day. . .the Dietary Guidelines way. Start with plenty of Breads, Cereals, Rice, and Pasta; Vegetables; and Fruits. Add two to three servings from the Milk group and two to three servings from the Meat group.

Each of these food groups provides some, but not all, of the nutrients you need. No one food group is more important than another — for good health you need them all. Go easy on fats, oils, and sweets, the foods in the small tip of the Pyramid.

Figure 8.3—The food guide pyramid. *Source*: US Department of Agriculture, Human Nutrition Information Service.[197]

In contrast to the 1990 period, when none of the goals were met and over half were considered either unlikely to be met or not assessable, the 1998 midcourse review of Healthy People 2000 showed that 5 nutrition objectives have been met, 13 were progressing, 1 was mixed, 5 were moving away from the target, and only 3 could not be assessed.[198] The objectives moving away from the target were prevalence of overweight, diabetes, iron deficiency, intake of foods rich in calcium, and sound weight loss practices. Salt/sodium intake showed mixed results. For the proportion of calories from fat, there appears to be a trend that some population segments are reaching the goal while others are falling behind, resulting in small changes of the population average.

EXAMPLES OF PUBLIC HEALTH INTERVENTIONS

Sustained public interest in nutrition and the growing presence of health groups in the food arena have led more food marketers to use nutrition as a marketing edge, sometimes with mixed consumer response. At the same time, health groups have recognized the need to build consumer demand for healthy eating and to view social marketing, environmental, and policy approaches as being cheaper and possibly more effective in changing behavior on a large scale than traditional educational or community organizing techniques.[199–202] A growing number of organizations are sponsoring large-scale dietary initiatives (Table 8.4).[203] Four initiatives illustrate the growing interest in using marketing approaches.

The National Cancer Institute/Kelloggs Campaign was the earliest large-scale chronic disease nutrition initiative. The then-controversial partnership between government and industry used a marketing approach that included mass media advertising, information on cereal boxes, in-store merchandising, and other commercial techniques to reach the general adult market and health professionals. The campaign increased consumer awareness of diet/cancer relationships and had a halo effect beyond the Kelloggs brand of cereals into a wide range of bran products.[25]

The more recent National 5 A Day Program uses a more classic social marketing approach of targeting the general population and specific market segments with a communications campaign and social marketing interventions delivered in multiple channels.[27] Its goal is to increase daily fruit and vegetable consumption as part of a low-fat, high-fiber diet. The behavior change theories used to guide its messages and program execution include Social Learning Theory, and the Diffusion of Innovations. A network of national, industry, state, tribal, and armed services partners numbering about 3000 organizations delivers the program in a variety of venues. A feature of the National 5 A Day Program has been its ability to leverage funds, with an estimated

Table 8.4—Chronology of Large-Scale Nutrition Initiatives to Control Chronic Diseases

Year Initiated	Campaign (Principal Sponsor)
1984	NCI, Kelloggs Fiber Campaign (Kelloggs, National Cancer Institute (NCI))
1985	National Cholesterol Education Program (National Heart, Lung and Blood Institute (NHLBI))
	NutriFacts Labeling Initiatives (National Live Stock and Meat Board, Produce Marketing Association)
1987	Changing the Course School Program (American Cancer Society)
1988	National Project LEAN Campaign (Kaiser Family Foundation)
1991	National 5 A Day Program (NCI, Produce for Better Health Foundation)
	National Obesity Initiative (NHLBI)
1993	Food Stamp Nutrition Education Programs (State Extension Services, US Department of Agriculture (USDA))
	Nutrition and Health Campaign for Women (American Dietetic Association (ADA))
1994	Food Certification Program (American Heart Association (AHA))
	Weight Control Information Network (National Institute of Digestive Diseases and Kidney Diseases (NIDDK))
	Shape Up America! (Shape Up American Campaign Foundation)
	Food Stamp Community Nutrition Education Demonstrations (USDA)
	Team Nutrition (USDA)
1995	Heart Power! School Program (AHA)
	1% Or Less Campaign (Center for Science in the Public Interest)
	Milk, Where's Your Mustache? (National Fluid Milk Promotion Board (NFMPB)
	Food Stamp Social Marketing Networks (States, USDA)
	Child Nutrition and Health Campaign (ADA, Kelloggs, National Dairy Council)
1996	Cardiovascular Heart Disease Promotion Project (NHLBI)
	It's All About You! (Dietary Guidelines Alliance)
	Breakfast Matters! (American Health Foundation)
	Sisters Together: Move More, Feel Better! (pilot) (NIDDK)
	CRAVE to Be the Best (Ocean Spray Cranberries)
1997	CATCH (Child and Adolescent Trial for Adolescent Health) Roll-out (NHLBI)
	Drink 3 for the Calcium You Need (NFMPB)
	Calcium! Do You Get It? (Food and Drug Administration)
	Working Together with Managed Care in Worksites (Centers for Disease Control and Prevention (CDC))
	Girl Power and You! (FDA)
	Physical Activity—It's Everywhere You Go! (CDC)
1998	National Diabetes Education Program (NIDDK)

Note. Adapted from Center for Nutrition Policy and Promotion, US Department of Agriculture.[203]

$50 million redirected by industry and governmental partners for every $1 million in intervention spent by NCI. National consumption for persons 2 years of age and older rose from 4.1 servings (1989 to 1991 baseline) to 4.6 servings (1994 to 1996), with 2 to 19 year olds increasing little (3.6 to 4.0 servings) compared to adults aged 20 and over (4.3 to 4.9 servings).[198] Since the previous decade's rate of increase was only 1% per year and the majority of evaluations for smaller 5 a Day interventions have been positive, the 12% increase over the first 4 years suggests a positive program impact.

The 1% Or Less Campaign to promote low-fat milk consumption showed dramatic short-term increases in low-fat milk sales by using paid advertising and public relations, with and without community programs.[204] In contrast, advertising alone, or public relations and community programs alone, showed little change in sales. The intervention study was conducted over a 2-month period in eight small West Virginia towns with follow-up conducted for another 6 months. It is not known how much longer the sales increases would be maintained, but the per capita costs for communities with paid ads were far lower than the cost for community programs only because more people were reached and behavior changed.

An objective of this study was to demonstrate that guaranteed media exposure would change dietary behavior.

Planning for new statewide social marketing "network" campaigns that will begin rolling out in 1998 was initiated by USDA in 1995. The goal was to enhance the Food Stamp Program with a strong nutrition education component. Each state will use a coalition approach, develop state resources, and conduct formative research including consumer focus groups, key informant interviews with intermediaries, and pilot testing of materials and interventions. The 22 state programs will address somewhat different market segments of Food Stamp households with interventions tailored to the available state partners, resources, and research. The Networks are significant because, if states can raise matching funds, leverage them, and sustain the efforts over time, these initiatives may be sufficient in funding and of long enough duration to influence dietary behavior on a large scale. Disparities in nutrition and physical activity among lower income and people of color are believed to be at least partially responsible for higher chronic disease rates experienced by many of these groups.

Given the scope of the food system, it is not surprising that community-level interventions alone have not achieved significant improvements in dietary behavior.[205–207] Further, there has been no unifying framework for organizing large-scale, complex dietary campaigns. However, by combining social marketing techniques with approaches found successful in large-scale anti-tobacco campaigns, it is possible to construct a framework for systematically organizing large-scale dietary initiatives that accommodate factors that shape consumer behavior, including social norms, the media and physical environments, and industry practices (advertising, public relations, promotion, professional education, and research).

This model starts with identifying which demographic or lifestyle segments to target and the channels with the greatest reach and feasibility for conducting interventions. Formative research with consumers and intermediaries then defines the wants, needs, benefits, and barriers specific to each channel to guide development of the message and execution of the campaign. Planners must systematically determine the following:

• Which media would reach the segment the most persuasively, including print, electronic, outdoor, transit, or "small" media like organizational or membership newsletters, and how to work with those media;
• What environmental influences would help or hinder dietary behavior, and how they might be modified;

• What program services, including information and interactive interventions, would stimulate the desired behaviors, then develop and test them;
• What institutional policies help or hinder behavior and how they might be modified;
• The ongoing research with consumers, intermediaries, and intervention channels that would be needed; and,
• How the campaign could be delivered as turnkey and user-friendly as possible.

Large-scale initiatives require a mix of professional disciplines. These include epidemiology, behavioral sciences, public relations/communications, design and creative (art, photography, film, music), nutrition education, recipe development, retail merchandising, marketing, public health law, and resource development. While some of the resources may be made available through public/private partnerships, public health agencies need their own resources for these functions.

AREAS OF FUTURE RESEARCH AND DEMONSTRATION

Around the world, developed countries are grappling with rising rates of chronic disease caused in large measure by changes in diet and physical activity patterns.[28] Many countries report problems such as a

240

lack of policy attention, inadequate surveillance, fragmentation, conflict between the health and agriculture sectors, unrealistic expectations, inadequate intervention research, and a shortage of operational resources. At the same time, the solutions they are finding include clear trends toward using partnerships; conducting longer-term campaigns; expanding activity into media, supermarket and other secular channels, rather than only health care; and establishing clearer, simpler behavioral targets.

In the United States, a chronic disease challenge of the current decade has been to control tobacco use. For the next millennium, the promotion of healthy eating is likely to assume a much more important role, with physical activity also growing in priority.[208, 209] Unlike the field of tobacco control, there are opportunities to develop cooperative rather than confrontational relationships with the food industry. For example, it is possible that a large fraction of the more than $30 billion now spent annually on food advertising and promotion could be redirected toward the promotion of good nutrition and physical activity. Such a massive reorientation of effort and redirection of funds is what will be needed to achieve large-scale dietary improvement, and some public health agencies will find it necessary to develop new skills and

new partnerships. It remains to be seen whether partnerships will work and, if so, what it will take to sustain newly established healthy behavior. Much is still to be learned, but past experience suggests that there is room for cautious optimism.

A special case may also be made for understanding what interventions are effective in improving the diets of children and youth, including the possibility of reducing children's exposure to the advertising and promotion of less healthy foods on television and in school settings.[192, 210-212]

As the science base continues to evolve, controversies about the relationships between food and chronic disease are inevitable.[213-217] However, from a public health perspective, dietary guidance has been constant over the last 20 years and is unlikely to digress substantially. For public health applications, priorities for new research would include further delineation of the etiologic pathways for disease causation and protection; strengthening the descriptive epidemiology of diet-disease relationships, including variability and time trend analysis by geographic and demographic categories; delineating the elements of channel- and population-specific interventions; understanding marketplace factors such as economic incentives and disincentives, mass communications, and food marketing; identifying the mix of elements required for channel-specific interventions to be successful on a large scale; and understanding how organizations on the national, state, regional, and local levels can complement and gain synergy from each others' efforts.

REFERENCES

1. Levenstein H. *Paradox of Plenty: A Social History of Eating in Modern America.* New York, NY: Oxford University Press Inc; 1993.
2. Schor JB. *The Overworked American: The Unexpected Decline of Leisure.* New York, NY: Basic Books, HarperCollins Publishers; 1993.
3. Senauer B, Asp E, Kinsey J. *Food Trends and the Changing Consumer.* St. Paul, Minn: Eagan Press; 1991.
4. US Senate, Select Committee on Nutrition and Human Needs. Dietary Goals for the United States. Washington, DC: US Government Printing Office; February 1977.
5. National Research Council, Committee on Diet, Nutrition, and Cancer. *Diet, Nutrition, and Cancer.* Washington, DC: National Academy Press; 1982.
6. National Cancer Institute. *Cancer Objectives for the Nation: 1985–2000.* Washington, DC: US

Government Printing Office; 1986.
7. World Health Organization Study Group. *Diet, Nutrition and the Prevention of Chronic Diseases..* Geneva, Switzerland: World Health Organization; 1990. WHO Technical Report Series 797.
8. US Department of Health and Human Services, Public Health Service. *The Surgeon General's Report on Nutrition and Human Health.* Washington, DC: US Government Printing Office; 1988. DHHS publication PHS 88-50210.
9. National Research Council, Committee on Diet and Health. *Diet and Health: Implications for Reducing Chronic Disease Risk.* Washington, DC: National Academy Press; 1989.
10. Diabetes Control and Complications Trial Research Group. The effect of intensive treatment of diabetes on the development and progression of long-term complications in insulin-dependent diabetes mellitus. *N Engl J Med.* 1993; 329(14):977–986.
11. American Diabetes Association. Nutrition recommendations and principles for people with diabetes mellitus. *J Am Diet Assoc.* 1994; 94(5):504-506.
12. Franz MJ, Horton ES, Bantle JP, et al. Nutrition principles for the management of diabetes and related complications (Technical

review). *Diabetes Care.* 1994;17:490–518.

13. American Cancer Society 1996 Advisory Committee on Diet, Nutrition, and Cancer Prevention. Guidelines on Diet, Nutrition, and Cancer Prevention: Reducing the Risk of Cancer with Healthy Food Choices and Physical Activity. *CA Cancer J Clin* 1996;46:325–341.

14. Meisler JG, St Jeor S. Summary and recommendations from the American Health Foundation's Expert Panel on Healthy Weight. *Am J Clin Nutr.* 1996;63(3 suppl):474S–477S.

15. American Heart Association. Dietary guidelines for healthy American adults. *Circulation.* 1996;94:1795–1800.

16. Willett WC, Trichopoulos D. Summary of the evidence: Nutrition and Cancer. *Cancer Causes Control.* 1996;7(1):178–180.

17. Harvard Report on Cancer Prevention. Volume 1: Causes of Human Cancer. *Cancer Causes Control.* 1996;7(suppl):S7-18, S55–S58.

18. National High Blood Pressure Education Program. *The Sixth Report of the Joint National Committee on Prevention, Detection, Evaluation and Treatment of High Blood Pressure.* National Institutes of Health, National Heart, Lung and Blood Institute; 1997. NIH publication 98-4080.

19. World Cancer Research Fund/ American Institute for Cancer Research. *Food, Nutrition and the Prevention of Cancer: A Global Perspective.* Washington, DC: American Institute for Cancer Research; 1997.

20. Appel LJ, Moore TJ, Obarzanek E, et al. A clinical trial of the effects of dietary patterns on blood pressure. *N Engl J Med.* 1997;336(16):1117–1124.

21. *Nutrition and Your Health: Dietary Guidelines for Americans.* 4th ed. Washington, DC: U.S. Department of Agriculture; 1995. Home and Garden Bulletin 232.

22. McGinnis JM, Foege WH. Actual causes of death in the United States. *JAMA.* 1993;270(18):2207–2212.

23. Byers T. Dietary trends in the United States. *Cancer.* 1993;72(3 suppl):1015–1018.

24. O'Brien P. Dietary shifts and implications for U.S. agriculture. *Am J Clin Nutr.* 1995;61(suppl):1390S–1396S.

25. Levy AS, Stokes RC. Effects of a health promotion advertising campaign on sales of ready-to-eat cereals. *Publ Health Rep.* 1987;102:398–403.

26. Foerster SB, Kizer KW, DiSogra LK, Krieg BK, Bunch K. California's 5 a Day-for Better

Health! Campaign: an innovative population-based effort to effect large scale dietary change. *Am J Prev Med.* 1995;11(2):124–131.

27. Heimendinger J, Chapelsky D. The National 5 A Day for Better Health Program. *Adv Exp Med Biol.* 1996;401:199–206.

28. Wheelock V, ed. *Implementing Dietary Guidelines for Healthy Eating.* London, England: Chapman & Hall; 1997.

29. From the Centers for Disease Control and Prevention. Recommendations for use of folic acid to reduce number of spina bifida cases and other neural tube defects. *JAMA.* 1993;269(10): 1233.

30. Folic acid for the prevention of recurrent neural tube defects. ACOG Committee Opinion: Committee on Obstetrics: Maternal and Fetal Medicine Number 120—March 1993. *Int J Gynaecol Obstet.* 1993;42(1):75–77.

31. Malinow MR. Hyperhomocyst(e)inenia: a common and easily reversible risk factor for occlusive atherosclerosis. *Circulation.* 1990;81:2004–2006.

32. Brattstrom LE, Israelsson B, Jeppsson JO, Hultberg BL. Folic acid: an innocuous means to reduce plasma homocyst(e)ine. *Scand J Clin Lab Invest.* 1988;48: 215–221.

33. Varma SD, Devamanoharan PS, Morris SM. Prevention of cataracts by nutritional and metabolic antioxidants. *Crit Rev Food Sci Nutr.* 1995;35(1–2):111–129.

34. Seddon JM, Ajani UA, Sperduto RD, et al. Dietary carotenoids, vitamins A, C, and E, and advanced age-related macular degeneration. Eye Disease Case-Control Study Group. *JAMA.* 1994;272(18):1413–1420. (Published erratum appears in *JAMA* 1995 Feb 22;273(8):622.)

35. Steinmetz KA, Potter JD. Vegetables, fruit, and cancer prevention: a review. *J Am Diet Assoc.* 1996;96(10):1027–1039.

36. Ziegler RG, Mayne ST, Swanson CA. Nutrition and lung cancer. *Cancer Causes Control.* 1996; 7(1):157–177.

37. Kvale G, Bjelke E, Gart JJ. Dietary habits and lung cancer risk. *Int J Cancer.* 1983;31:397–405.

38. Long-de W, Hammond EC. Lung cancer, fruit, green salad and vitamin pills. *Chin Med J.* 1985;98:206–210.

39. Hirayama T. Nutrition and cancer: a large-scale cohort study. *Prog Clin Biol Res.* 1986; 206:299–311.

40. Kromhout D. Essential micronutrients in relation to carcinogenesis. *Am J Clin Nutr.* 1987; 45:1361–1367.

41. Fraser GE, Beeson WL, Phillips RL. Diet and lung cancer risk in Seventh-day Adventists. *Am J Epidemiol.* 1991; 133:683–693.

42. Knekt P, Jarvinen R, Seppanen R, et al. Dietary antioxidants and the risk of lung cancer. *Am J Epidemiol.* 1991;134(5):471–479.

43. Shibata A, Paganini-Hill A, Ross RK, Henderson BE. Intake of vegetables, fruits, beta-carotene, vitamin C and vitamin supplements and cancer incidence among the elderly: a prospective study. *Br J Cancer.* 1992;66:673–679.

44. Chow WH, Schuman LM, McLaughlin JK, et al. A cohort study of tobacco use, diet, occupation, and lung cancer mortality. *Cancer Causes Control.* 1992;3(3):247–254.

45. Steinmetz KA, Potter JD, Folsom AR. Vegetables, fruit, and lung cancer in the Iowa Women's Health Study. *Cancer Res.* 1993; 53:536–543.

46. Peto R, Doll R, Buckley JD, Sporn MB. Can dietary beta-carotene materially reduce human cancer rates? *Nature.* 1981; 290:201–208.

47. Shekelle RB, Lepper M, Liu S, et al. Dietary vitamin A and risk of cancer in the Western Electric study. *Lancet* 1981;2(8257):1186–1190.

48. The Alpha-Tocopherol, Beta Carotene Cancer Prevention Study Group. The effect of vitamin E and beta carotene on the incidence of lung cancer and other cancers in male smokers. *N Engl J Med.* 1994;330(15):1029–1035.

49. Omenn GS, Goodman GE, Thornquist MD, et al. Effects of a combination of beta carotene and vitamin A on lung cancer and cardiovascular disease. *N Engl J Med.* 1996;334(18):1150–1155.

50. Hennekens CH, Buring JE, Manson JE, et al. Lack of effect of long-term supplementation with beta carotene on the incidence of malignant neoplasms and cardiovascular disease. *N Engl J Med.* 1996;334(18):1145–1149.

51. Kono S, Hirohata T. Nutrition and stomach cancer. *Cancer Causes Control.* 1996;7(1):41–55.

52. Cheng KK, Day NE. Nutrition and esophageal cancer. *Cancer Causes Control.* 1996;7(1):33–40.

53. Howe GR, Burch JD. Nutrition and pancreatic cancer. *Cancer Causes Control.* 1996;7(1):69–82.

54. Potter JD. Nutrition and colorectal cancer. *Cancer Causes Control.* 1996;7(1):127–146.

55. Thun MJ, Calle EE, Namboodiri MM, et al. Risk factors for fatal colon cancer in a large prospective study. *J Natl Cancer Inst.* 1992;84(19):1491–1500.

56. Steinmetz KA, Kushi LH, Bostick RM, Folsom AR, Potter JD. Vegetables, fruit, and colon cancer in the Iowa Women's Health Study. *Am J Epidemiol.* 1994; 139:1–15.

57. Trock B, Lanza E, Greenwald P. Dietary fiber, vegetables, and colon cancer: critical review and meta-analyses of the epidemiologic evidence. *J Natl Cancer Inst.* 1990;82:650–661.

58. Howe GR, Benito E, Castelleto R, et al. Dietary intake of fiber and decreased risk of cancers of the colon and rectum: evidence from the combined analysis of 13 case-control studies. *J Natl Cancer Inst.* 1992;84:1887—1896.

59. Wattenberg LW. Chemoprevention of cancer. *Cancer Res.* 1985;45:1—8.

60. Steinmetz KA, Potter JD. Vegetables, fruit, and cancer: II. Mechanisms. *Cancer Causes Control.* 1991;2:427–442.

61. Hertog MGL, Hollman PCH, Katan MB. Content of potentially anticarcinogenic flavonoids of 28 vegetables and 9 fruits commonly consumed in the Netherlands. *J Agric Food Chem.* 1992;40:2379–2383.

62. Hocman G. Prevention of cancer: vegetables and plants. *Comp Biochem Physiol.* 1989;93:201–212.

63. Bueding E, Anscher S, Dolan P. Anticarcinogenic and other protective effects of dithiolthiones. In: *Basic Life Sciences.* Vol 39. New York, NY: Plenum Press; 1986;483–489.

64. Stich HF, Rosin MP. Naturally occurring phenolics as antimutagenic and anticarcinogenic agents. *Adv Exp Med.* 1984; 177:1–29.

65. Adlercreutz H. Western diet and western diseases: some hormonal and biochemical mechanisms and associations. *Scand J Clin Lab Invest.* 1990;50(suppl 201):3–23.

66. Messina M, Barnes S. The role of soy products in reducing risk of cancer. *J Natl Cancer Inst.* 1991;83:541–546.

67. Ness AR, Powles JW. Fruit and vegetables, and cardiovascular disease: a review. *Int J Epidemiol.* 1997;26(1):1–13.

68. Trowell H. Ischemic heart disease and dietary fiber. *Am J Clin Nutr.* 1972;25(9):926–932.

69. Morris JN, Marr JW, Clayton DG. Diet and heart: a postscript. *Br Med J.* 1977;2(6098):1307–1314.

70. Marr JW, Morris JN. Dietary intake and the risk of coronary heart disease in Japanese men living in Hawaii. [letter] *Am J Clin Nutr.* 1981 Jun; 34(6):1156–1157.

71. Kromhout D, Bosschieter EB, de Lezenne Coulander C. Dietary fibre and 10-year mortality from coronary heart disease, cancer,

and all causes. The Zutphen study. *Lancet.* 1982;2(8297):518–522.

72. Gordon T, Kagan A, Garcia-Palmieri M, Kannel WB, Zukel WJ, Tillotson J, Sorlie P, Hjortland M. Diet and its relation to coronary heart disease and death in three populations. *Circulation.* 1981;63(3):500–515.

73. Khaw KT, Barrett-Connor E. Dietary fiber and reduced ischemic heart disease mortality rates in men and women: a 12-year prospective study. *Am J Epidemiol.* 1987;126(6):1093–1102.

74. Kushi LH, Lew RA, Stare FJ, Ellison CR, el Lozy M, Bourke G, Daly L, Graham I, Hickey N, Mulcahy R, Kevaney J. Diet and 20-year mortality from coronary heart disease. The Ireland-Boston Diet-Heart Study. *N Engl J Med.* 1985;312(13):811–818.

75. Fehily AM, Yarnell JW, Sweetnam PM, Elwood PC. Diet and incident ischaemic heart disease: the Caerphilly Study. *Br J Nutr.* 1993;69(2):303–314.

76. Humble CG, Malarcher AM, Tyroler HA. Dietary fiber and coronary heart disease in middle-aged hypercholesterolemic men. *Am J Prev Med.* 1993;9(4):197–202.

77. Rimm EB, Ascherio A, Giovannucci E, Spiegelman D, Stampfer MJ, Willett WC. Vegetable, fruit, and cereal fiber intake and risk of coronary heart disease among men. *JAMA.* 1996;275(6):447–451.

78. Pietinen P, Rimm EB, Korhonen P, et al. Intake of dietary fiber and risk of coronary heart disease in a cohort of Finnish men. The Alpha-Tocopherol, Beta-Carotene Cancer Prevention Study. *Circulation.* 1996;94(11): 2720–2727

79. Kushi LH, Meyer KA, Folsom AR, Jacobs DR Jr, Wallace RB. Dietary fat and fiber and death from coronary heart disease in women. [Abstract] In: *Abstracts of the 38th Annual Conference on Cardiovascular Disease Epidemiology and Prevention.* Dallas, Tex: American Heart Association; 1998;3.

80. Ripsin CM, Keenan JM, Jacobs DR Jr, Elmer PJ, Welch RR, Van Horn L, Liu K, Turnbull WH, Thye FW, Kestin M, et al. Oat products and lipid lowering. A meta-analysis. *JAMA.* 1992;267(24):3317–3325. [Published correction appears in *JAMA.* 1992;2;268(21):3074]

81. Food and Drug Administration. T97-5. FDA allows whole oat foods to make health claim on reducing the risk of heart disease. Available at: http://www.fda.gov/bbs/topics/ANSWERS/ANS00782.html. Accessed January 21, 1997.

82. Swain JF, Rouse IL, Curley CB, Sacks FM. Comparison of the effects of oat bran and low-fiber wheat on serum lipoprotein levels and blood pressure. *N Engl J Med.* 1990;322:147–52.

83. Kestin M, Moss R, Clifton PM, Nestel PJ. Comparative effects of three cereal brans on plasma lipids, blood pressure, and glucose metabolism in mildly hypercholesterolemic men. *Am J Clin Nutr.* 1990;52:661–666.

84. Anderson JW, Story L, Sieling B, Chen WJL, Petro MS, Story J. Hypocholesterolemic effects of oat bran or bean intake for hypercholesterolemic men. *Am J Clin Nutr.* 1984;40:1146–1155.

85. Mathur KS, Khan MA, Sharma RD. Hypocholesterolemic effect of bengal gram. *Br Med J.* 1968; 1:30–31.

86. Bell LP, Hectorne K, Reynolds H, Balm TK, Hunninghake DB. Cholesterol-lowering effects of psyllium hydrophilic mucilloid: adjunct therapy to a prudent diet for patients with mild to moderate hypercholesterolemia. *JAMA.* 1989;261:3419–3423.

87. Aro A, Uusitupa M, Voutilainen E, Korhonen T. Effects of guar gum in male subjects with hypercholesterolemia. *Am J Clin Nutr.* 1984;39:911–916.

88. Zavoral JH, Hannan P, Fields DJ, Hanson MN, Frantz ID, Kuba K, Elmer P, Jacobs DR Jr. The hypolipidemic effect of locust bean gum food products in familial hypocholesterolemic adults and children. *Am J Clin Nutr.* 1983;38:285–294.

89. Kay RM, Truswell AS. Effect of citrus pectin on blood lipids and fecal steroid excretion in man. *Am J Clin Nutr.* 1977;30:171–175.

90. The Lipid Research Clinics Coronary Primary Prevention Trial results. I. Reduction in incidence of coronary heart disease. *JAMA.* 1984;251(3):351–364.

91. The Lipid Research Clinics Coronary Primary Prevention Trial results. II. The relationship of reduction in incidence of coronary heart disease to cholesterol lowering. *JAMA.* 1984;251(3):365–374.

92. Rossner S, Andersson IL, Ryttig K. Effects of a dietary fibre supplement to a weight reduction programme on blood pressure: a randomised, double-blind, placebo-controlled trial. *Acta Med Scand.* 1988;223:353–357.

93. Fehily AM, Milbank JE, Yarnell JW, Hayes TM, Kubiki AJ, Eastham RD. Dietary determinants of lipoproteins, total cholesterol, viscosity, fibrinogen, and blood pressure. *Am J Clin Nutr.* 1982;36(5):890–896.

94. Fehily AM, Burr ML, Butland BK, Eastham RD. A randomized

controlled trial to investigate the effect of a high fibre diet on blood pressure and plasma fibrinogen. *J Epidemiol Community Health*. 1986;40:334–337.

95. Margetts BM, Beilin LJ, Vandongen R, Armstrong B. A randomized controlled trial of the effects of dietary fibre on blood pressure. *Clin Sci.* 1987;72:343–350.

96. Anderson JW, O'Neal DS, Riddell-Mason S, Floore TL, Dillon DW, Oeltgen PR. Postprandial serum glucose, insulin, and lipoprotein responses to high- and low-fiber diets. *Metabolism*. 1995; 44(7):848–854.

97. Tappy L, Gugolz E, Wursch P. Effects of breakfast cereals containing various amounts of beta-glucan fibers on plasma glucose and insulin responses in NIDDM subjects. *Diabetes Care*. 1996;19(8):831–834.

98. Marshall JA, Bessesen DH, Hamman RF. High saturated fat and low starch and fibre are associated with hyperinsulinaemia in a non-diabetic population: the San Luis Valley Diabetes Study. *Diabetologia*. 1997; 40(4):430–438.

99. Salmeron J, Manson JE, Stampfer MJ, Colditz GA, Wing AL, Willett WC. Dietary fiber, glycemic load, and risk of non-insulin-dependent diabetes mellitus in women. *JAMA*. 1997;277(6):472–477.

100. Salmeron J, Ascherio A, Rimm EB, et al. Dietary fiber, glycemic load, and risk of NIDDM in men. *Diabetes Care*. 1997;20(4):545–550.

101. Steinberg D, Witztum JL. Lipoproteins and atherogenesis: current concepts. *JAMA*. 1990;264:3047–3052.

102. Aviram M. Modified forms of low density lipoprotein and atherosclerosis. *Atherosclerosis*. 1993;98:1–9.

103. Gey KF, Puska P. Inverse correlation between plasma vitamin E and mortality from ischemic heart disease in cross-cultural epidemiology. *Am J Clin Nutr*. 1991;53:326S–334S.

104. Simon JA, Schreiber GB, Crawford PB, Frederick MM, Sabry ZI. Dietary vitamin C and serum lipids in black and white girls. *Epidemiology*. 1993;4:537–542.

105. Jacques PF, Sulsky SI, Perrone GA, Schaefer EJ. Ascorbic acid and plasma lipids. *Epidemiology*. 1994;5:19–26.

106. Reaven PD, Khouw A, Beltz WF, Parthasarathy S, Witztum JL. Effect of dietary antioxidant combinations in humans. *Arterioscler Thromb*. 1993; 13:590–600.

107. Knekt P, Reunanen A, Jarvinen R, Seppanen R, Heliovaara M, Aromaa A. Antioxidant vitamin intake and coronary mortality in

a longitudinal population study. *Am J Epidemiol.* 1994;139(12): 1180–1189.

108. Stampfer MJ, Hennekens CH, Manson JE, Colditz GA, Rosner B, Willett WC. Vitamin E consumption and the risk of coronary disease in women. *N Engl J Med.* 1993;328:1444–1449.

109. Rimm EB, Stampfer MJ, Ascherio A, Giovannucci E, Colditz GA, Willett WC. Vitamin E consumption and the risk of coronary heart disease in men. *N Engl J Med.* 1993;328:1450–1456.

110. Kushi LH, Folsom AR, Prineas RJ, Mink PJ, Wu Y, Bostick RM. Dietary antioxidant vitamins and death from coronary heart disease in postmenopausal women. *N Engl J Med.* 1996;334(18):1156–1162.

111. Losonczy KG, Harris TB, Havlik RJ. Vitamin E and vitamin C supplement use and risk of all-cause and coronary heart disease mortality in older persons: the Established Populations for Epidemiologic Studies of the Elderly. *Am J Clin Nutr.* 1996;64(2):190–196.

112. Meyer F, Bairati I, Dagenais GR. Lower ischemic heart disease incidence and mortality among vitamin supplement users. *Can J Cardiol.* 1996;12(10):930–934.

113. Hertog MGL, Feskens EJM, Hollman PCH, Katan MB, Kromhout D. Dietary antioxidant flavonoids and risk of coronary heart disease: the Zutphen Elderly Study. *Lancet.* 1993;342:1007–1011.

114. Hertog MGL, Hollman PCH, Katan MB, Kromhout D. Estimation of daily intake of potentially anticarcinogenic flavonoids and their determinants in adults in the Netherlands. *Nutr Cancer.* 1993;20:21–29.

115. Knekt P, Jarvinen R, Reunanen A, Maatela J. Flavonoid intake and coronary mortality in Finland: a cohort study. *Br Med J.* 1996; 312(7029):478–481.

116. Rimm EB, Katan MB, Ascherio A, Stampfer MJ, Willett WC. Relation between intake of flavonoids and risk for coronary heart disease in male health professionals. *Ann Intern Med.* 1996;125(5):384–389.

117. Hegsted DM, Ausman LM, Johnson JA, Dallal GE. Dietary fat and serum lipids: an evaluation of the experimental data. *Am J Clin Nutr* 1993;57(6):875–883. [Published correction appears in *Am J Clin Nutr* 1993;58(2):245]

118. Clarke R, Frost C, Collins R, Appleby P, Peto R. Dietary lipids and blood cholesterol: quantitative meta-analysis of metabolic ward studies. *Br Med J.* 1997; 314(7074):112–117.

119. Mensink RP, Katan MB. Effect of monounsaturated fatty acids

versus complex carbohydrates on high-density lipoproteins in healthy men and women. *Lancet.* 1987;17;1(8525):122–125.

120. Willett WC, Sacks F, Trichopoulou A, et al. Mediterranean diet pyramid: a cultural model for healthy eating. *Am J Clin Nutr.* 1995;61(6 suppl): 1402S–1406S.

121. Mensink RP, Katan MB. Effect of dietary trans fatty acids on high-density and low-density lipoprotein cholesterol levels in healthy subjects. *N Engl J Med.* 1990;323 (7):439–445.

122. Zock PL, Katan MB. Trans fatty acids, lipoproteins, and coronary risk. *Can J Physiol Pharmacol.* 1997;75(3):211–216.

123. Kushi LH, Kottke TE. Dietary fat and coronary heart disease: evidence of a causal relation. In: Goldbloom RB, Lawrence RS, eds. *Preventing Disease: Beyond the Rhetoric.* New York: Springer-Verlag; 1990:385–400.

124. Shekelle RB, Shryock AM, Paul O, Lepper M, Stamler J, Liu S, Raynor WJ Jr. Diet, serum cholesterol, and death from coronary heart disease. The Western Electric study. *N Engl J Med.* 1981;304(2):65–70.

125. Anderson JT, Jacobs DR Jr, Foster N, Hall Y, Moss D, Mojonnier L, Blackburn H. Scoring systems for evaluating dietary pattern effect on serum cholesterol. *Prev Med.* 1979 Sep; 8(5):525-537.

126. McGee D, Reed D, Stemmerman G, et al. The relationship of dietary fat and cholesterol to mortality in 10 years: the Honolulu Heart Program. *Int J Epidemiol.* 1985;14(1):97–105.

127. Shekelle RB, Stamler J. Dietary cholesterol and ischaemic heart disease. *Lancet.* 1989;1(8648): 1177–1179.

128. Kromhout D, Bosschieter EB, de Lezenne Coulander C. The inverse relation between fish consumption and 20-year mortality from coronary heart disease. *N Engl J Med.* 1985; 312(19):1205–1209.

129. Ascherio A, Rimm EB, Giovannucci EL, Spiegelman D, Stampfer M, Willett WC. Dietary fat and risk of coronary heart disease in men: cohort follow up study in the United States. *Br Med J.* 1996;313(7049):84–90.

130. Hu FB, Stampfer MJ, Manson JE, et al. Dietary fat intake and the risk of coronary heart disease in women. *N Engl J Med.* 1997; 337(21):1491–1499.

131. Pietinen P, Ascherio A, Korhonen P, et al. Intake of fatty acids and risk of coronary heart disease in a cohort of Finnish men. The Alpha-Tocopherol, Beta-Carotene Cancer Prevention Study. *Am J Epidemiol.* 1997;145(10):876–887.

132. Willett WC, Ascherio A. Trans
fatty acids: are the effects only
marginal? *Am J Public Health.*
1994;84(5):722–724.

133. Sacks FM, Donner A, Castelli
WP, et al. Effect of ingestion of
meat on plasma cholesterol of
vegetarians. *JAMA.*
1981;246(6):640–644.

134. Phillips RL, Lemon FR, Beeson
WL, Kuzma JW. Coronary heart
disease mortality among Seventh-Day Adventists with
differing dietary habits: a preliminary report. *Am J Clin Nutr.*
1978;(10 suppl):S191–S198.

135. Snowdon DA, Phillips RL, Fraser
GE. Meat consumption and fatal
ischemic heart disease. *Prev
Med.* 1984;13(5):490–500.

136. Chang-Claude J, Frentzel-Beyme
R, Eilber U. Mortality pattern of
German vegetarians after 11
years of follow-up. *Epidemiology.* 1992;3(5):395–401.

137. Thorogood M, Mann J, Appleby
P, McPherson K. Risk of death
from cancer and ischaemic heart
disease in meat and non-meat
eaters. *Br Med J.* 1994;308
(6945):1667–1670

138. Sullivan JL. Iron and the sex
difference in heart disease risk.
Lancet. 1981;1:1293–1294.

139. Salonen JT, Nyssonen K, Korpela
H, Tuomilehto J, Seppanen R,
Salonen R. High stored iron
levels are associated with excess
risk of myocardial infarction in
eastern Finnish men. *Circulation.* 1992;86:803–811.

140. Magnusson MK, Sigfusson N,
Sigvaldson H, Johannesson GM,
Magnusson S, Thorgeirsson G.
Low iron-binding capacity as a
risk factor for myocardial
infarction. *Circulation.* 1994;
89:102–108.

141. Morrison HI, Semenciw RM, Mao
Y, Wigle DT. Serum iron and risk
of fatal acute myocardial infarction. *Epidemiology.* 1994;5:243–
246.

142. Sempos CT, Looker AC, Gillum
RF, Makuc DM. Body iron stores
and the risk of coronary heart
disease. *N Engl J Med.* 1994;
330:1119–1124.

143. Ascherio A, Willett WC, Rimm
EB, Giovannucci EL, Stampfer
MJ. Dietary iron intake and risk
of coronary heart disease among
men. *Circulation.* 1994;89:969–
974.

144. Ueland PM, Refsum H, Brattstrom
L. Plasma homocyst(e)ine and
cardiovascular disease. In: Francis
RBJ, ed. *Atherosclerotic Cardio-
vascular Disease Hemostasis, and
Endothelial Function.* New York,
NY: Marcel Dekker, Inc.; 1992:
183–236.

145. Stampfer MJ, Malinow MR,
Willett WC, et al. A prospective
study of plasma homocyst(e)ine
and risk of myocardial infarction
in US physicians. *JAMA.* 1992;
268:877–881.

146. Selhub J, Jacques PF, Wilson PWF, Rush D, Rosenberg IH. Vitamin status and intake as primary determinants of homocysteinemia in an elderly population. *JAMA*. 1993;270: 2693–2698.

147. Freedman LS, Clifford C, Messina M. Analysis of dietary fat, calories, body weight, and the development of mammary tumors in rats and mice: a review. *Cancer Res*. 1990;50 (18):5710–5719.

148. Carroll KK. Experimental studies on dietary fat and cancer in relation to epidemiological data. *Prog Clin Biol Res*. 1986;222:231–248.

149. Armstrong B, Doll R. Environmental factors and cancer incidence and mortality in different countries, with special reference to dietary practices. *Int J Cancer*. 1975;15:617–631.

150. Prentice RL, Sheppard L. Dietary fat and cancer: consistency of the epidemiologic data, and disease prevention that may follow from a practical reduction in fat consumption. *Cancer Causes Control* 1990;1(1):81–97. [Published correction appears in *Cancer Causes Control*. 1990; 1(3):253]

151. Hunter DJ, Willett WC. Nutrition and breast cancer. *Cancer Causes Control*. 1996;7(1):56–68.

152. Hunter DJ, Spiegelman D, Adami HO, et al. Cohort studies of fat intake and the risk of breast cancer—a pooled analysis. *N Engl J Med*. 1996;334(6):356–361.

153. Prentice RL. Measurement error and results from analytic epidemiology: dietary fat and breast cancer. *J Natl Cancer Inst*. 1996;88(23):1738–1747.

154. Greenwald P, Sherwood K, McDonald SS. Fat, caloric intake, and obesity: lifestyle risk factors for breast cancer. *J Am Diet Assoc*. 1997;97(7 suppl):S24–S30.

155. Kolonel LN. Nutrition and prostate cancer. *Cancer Causes Control*. 1996;7(1):83–94.

156. Hill HA, Austin H. Nutrition and endometrial cancer. *Cancer Causes Control*. 1996;7(1):19–32.

157. Hirayama T. A large-scale cohort study on the relationship between diet and selected cancers of digestive organs. In: Bruce WR, Correa P, Lipkin M, et al., eds. *Gastrointestinal Cancer: Endogenous Factors. Banbury Report 7*. Cold Spring Harbor, NY: Cold Spring Harbor Laboratory; 1981:409–426.

158. Kune S, Kune GM, Watson F. Case-control study of dietary etiologic factors: the Melbourne Colorectal Cancer Study. *Nutr Cancer*. 1987;9:21–42.

159. Willett WC, Stampfer MJ, Colditz GA, Rosner BA, Speizer FE. Relation of meat, fat, and fiber intake to the risk of colon cancer in a prospective study among

women. *N Engl J Med.* 1990;323:1664–1672.

160. Giovannucci E, Rimm EB, Stampfer MJ, Colditz GA, Ascherio A, Willett WC. Intake of fat, meat, and fiber in relation to risk of colon cancer in men. *Cancer Res.* 1994;5:2390–2397.

161. Goldbohm RA, van den Brandt PA, van 't Veer P, et al. A prospective cohort study on the relation between meat consumption and the risk of colon cancer. *Cancer Res.* 1994;54(3): 718–723.

162. Severson RK, Nomura AMY, Grove JS, Stemmerman GN. A prospective study of demographics, diet, and prostate cancer among men of Japanese ancestry in Hawaii. *Cancer Res.* 1989;49: 1857–1860.

163. Hsing AW, McLaughlin JK, Schuman LM, et al. Diet, tobacco use, and fatal prostate cancer: results from the Lutheran Brotherhood Cohort Study. *Cancer Res.* 1990;50:6836–6840.

164. Hirayama T. Epidemiology of prostate cancer with special reference to the role of diet. *Natl Cancer Inst Monogr.* 1979;53: 149–155.

165. Le Marchand L, Kolonel LN, Wilkens LR, Myers BC, Hirohata T. Animal fat consumption and prostate cancer: a prospective study in Hawaii. *Epidemiology.* 1994; 5:276–282.

166. Giovannucci E, Rimm EB, Colditz GA, Stampfer MJ, Ascherio A, Chute CC, Willett WC. A prospective study of dietary fat and risk of prostate cancer. *J Natl Cancer Inst.* 1993;85:1571–1579.

167. Snowdon DA, Phillips RL, Choi W. Diet, obesity, and risk of fatal prostate cancer. *Am J Epidemiol.* 1984; 120:244–250.

168. Phillips RL, Snowdon DA. Association of meat and coffee use with cancers of the large bowel, breast, and prostate among Seventh-day Adventists: preliminary results. *Cancer Res.* 1983;43:2403s–2408s.

169. Mills PK, Beeson WL, Phillips RL, Fraser GE. Cohort study of diet, lifestyle, and prostate cancer in Adventist men. *Cancer.* 1989; 64:598–604.

170. Demirer T, Icli F, Uzunalimoglu O, Kucuk O. Diet and stomach cancer incidence: a case-control study in Turkey. *Cancer.* 1990; 65:2344–2348.

171. Lee HH, Wu HY, Chuang YC, et al. Epidemiologic characteristics and multiple risk factors of stomach cancer in Taiwan. *Anticancer Res.* 1990;10:875–882.

172. Hirayama T. Epidemiology of breast cancer with special reference to the role of diet. *Prev Med.* 1978;7:173–195.

173. Toniolo P, Riboli E, Shore RE, Pasternak BS. Consumption of

meat, animal products, protein, and fat and risk of breast cancer: a prospective cohort study in New York. *Epidemiology.* 1994;5:391–397.

174. Gaard M, Tretli S, Loken EB. Dietary fat and the risk of breast cancer: a prospective study of 25,892 Norwegian women. *Int J Cancer.* 1995;63(1):13–17.

175. Friedman E, Isaksson P, Rafter J, Marian B, Winawer S, Newmark H. Fecal diglycerides as selective endogenous mitogens for premalignant and malignant human colonic epithelial cells. *Cancer Res.* 1989;49:544–554.

176. Committee on Nitrite and Alternative Curing Agents in Foods, Assembly of Life Sciences, National Academy of Sciences. *The Health Effects of Nitrate, Nitrite, and N-Nitroso Compounds.* Washington, DC: National Academy Press; 1981.

177. Sugimura T. Carcinogenicity of mutagenic heterocyclic amines formed during the cooking process. *Mutation Res.* 1985; 150:33–41.

178. Furihata C, Matsushima T. Mutagens and carcinogens in foods. *Ann Rev Nutr.* 1986;6:67–94.

179. Steineck G, Gerhardsson de Verdier M, Overvik E. The epidemiological evidence concerning intake of mutagenic activity from the fried surface and the risk of cancer cannot justify preventive measures. *Eur J Cancer Prev.* 1993;2:293–300.

180. Babbs CF. Free radicals and the etiology of colon cancer. *Free Rad Biol Med.* 1990;8:191–200.

181. Interagency Board for Nutrition Monitoring and Related Research. *Nutrition Monitoring in the United States. Chartbook I: Selected Findings from the National Nutrition Monitoring and Related Research Program.* Ervin B, Reed D, eds. Hyattsville, Md: Public Health Service; 1993.

182. Putnam JJ, Allshouse JE. Food consumption, prices, and expenditures, 1996: Annual data, 1970–94. Washington, DC; Food and Consumer Economics Division, Economic Research Service, US Department of Agriculture; 1996. Statistical Bulletin 928.

183. Labarthe DR. Dietary imbalance. In: *Epidemiology and Prevention of Cardiovascular Diseases: A Global Challenge.* Gaithersburg, Md: Aspen Publishers; 1998:133–165.

184. Kushi LH, Folsom AR, Jacobs DR Jr, Luepker RV, Elmer PJ, Blackburn H. Educational attainment and nutrient consumption patterns: the Minnesota Heart Survey. *J Am Diet Assoc.* 1988;88:1230–1236.

185. Shimakawa T, Sorlie P, Carpenter MA, et al. Dietary intake patterns

and sociodemographic factors in the atherosclerosis risk in communities study. ARIC Study Investigators. *Prev Med.* 1994; 23(6):769–780.

186. Zephier EM, Ballew C, Mokdad A, et al. Intake of nutrients related to cardiovascular disease risk among three groups of American Indians: the Strong Heart Dietary Study. *Prev Med.* 1997;26(4):508–515.

187. Bureau of Health Professions, Health Resources and Services Administration, Public Health Service, US Department of Health and Human Services. *Health Status of Minorities and Low-Income Groups.* 3rd ed. Washington, DC: US Government Printing Office; 1991.

188. US Department of Health and Human Services. *Healthy People 2000: National Health Promotion and Disease Prevention Objectives.* Washington, DC: US Government Printing Office; 1990. DHHS publication (PHS) 91-50213.

189. Brewster L, Jacobson MF. *The Changing American Diet.* Washington, DC: Center for Science in the Public Interest; 1978.

190. Jacobs DR Jr, Meyer KA, Kushi LH, Folsom AR. Whole grain intake is associated with reduced total and cause-specific death rates in older women: The Iowa Women's Health Study. *Am J Publ Health.* (In press).

191. Sellers TA, Kushi LH, Potter JD. Can dietary intake patterns account for the familial aggregation of disease? Evidence from adult siblings living apart. *Genetic Epidemiol.* 1991;8:105–112.

192. Story M, Faulkner P. The prime-time diet: A content analysis of eating behavior and food messages in television program content and commercials. *Am J Public Health.* 1990;80:738–740.

193. US Department of Agriculture, Food and Consumer Service. National School Lunch Program and School Breakfast Program: School Meal Initiatives for Healthy Children. Final Rule. 7 CFR Parts 210 and 220. *Federal Register.* 1995;60(113):31187–31222. Available at: http://schoolmeals.nal.usda.gov:8001/regs/regs.html.

194. Caspersen CJ. Physical activity epidemiology: concepts, methods, and applications to exercise science. *Exerc Sport Sci Rev.* 1989;17:423–473.

195. Doll R, Peto R. The causes of cancer: quantitative estimates of avoidable risks of cancer in the United States today. *J Natl Cancer Inst.* 1981;66:1192–1308.

196. Wynder E, Gori GB. Contribution of the environment to cancer incidence: An epidemiologic

exercise. J Natl Cancer Inst 1977; 58:825-832.

197. US Department of Agriculture, Human Nutrition Information Service. *The Food Guide Pyramid.* Washington, DC: US Department of Agriculture; 1992. Home and Garden Bulletin 252.

198. US Department of Health and Human Services, Public Health Service. *Healthy People 2000: Midcourse Review and 1995 Revisions.* Washington, DC: US Department of Health and Human Services; 1995.

199. Manoff RK. *Social Marketing: The New Imperative for Public Health.* New York, NY: Praeger Publishers; 1985.

200. Balch, GI. Nutrition education for adults: a review of research. Prepared for: Alexandria, Va: US Department of Agriculture, Food and Consumer Service, Office of Analysis and Evaluation; 1994.

201. Glanz K, Lankenau B, Foerster S, Temple S, Mullis R, Schmid T. Environmental and policy approaches to cardiovascular disease prevention through nutrition: opportunities for state and local action. *Health Educ Q.* 1995;22(4):512–527.

202. McAlister A. Behavioral journalism: Beyond the marketing model for health communication. *Am J Health Promotion.* 1995; 9(6):417–420.

203. Center for Nutrition Policy and Promotion, US Department of Agriculture. *A Catalog of National Nutrition Education Promotion Projects.* Washington, DC: US Department of Agriculture; 1997.

204. Wootan, M. A comparison of mass media versus community-based programs to promote low-fat milk consumption. Paper presented at: CDC National Conference on Chronic Disease Prevention and Control; December 1997; Washington, DC.

205. Goodman RM, Wheeler FC, Lee PR. Evaluation of the Heart to Heart Project: Lessons from a community-based chronic disease prevention program. *Am J Health Promotion.* 1995; 9(6):443–455.

206. Susser M. Editorial: the tribulations of trials—intervention in communities. *Am J Public Health.* 1995;85(2):156–158.

207. Stone EJ, Pearson TA, Fortmann SP, McKinlay JB. Community-based prevention trials: challenges and directions for public health practice, policy and research. *Ann Epidemiol.* 1997;7(suppl 7):S113–S120.

208. US Department of Health and Human Services. *Physical Activity and Health: A Report of the Surgeon General.* Atlanta, Ga: US Department of Health and Human Services, Centers for

Disease Control and Prevention, National Center for Chronic Disease Prevention and Health Promotion; 1996.

209. Blair SN, Horton E, Leon AS, et al. Physical activity, nutrition and chronic disease. *Med Sci Sports Exerc.* 1996;28(3):335–349.

210. Lytle L, Achterberg C. Changing the diet of America's children: What works and why? *J Nutr Educ.* 1995;27(5):250–260.

211. Taras HL, Gage M. Advertised foods on children's television. *Arch Pediatric & Adolescent Med.* 1995;149:649–652.

212. Foerster SB, Gregson J, Beall DL, et al. The California Children's 5 a Day—Power Play! Campaign: Evaluation of a Large-Scale Social Marketing Initiative. *Fam Commun Health.* 1998;21(1):46–64.

213. American Society for Clinical Nutrition/American Institute of Nutrition. Position paper on trans fatty acids. *Am J Clin Nutr.* 1996;63:663–670.

214. Buring JE, Hennekens CH. Antioxidant vitamins and cardiovascular disease. *Nutr Rev.* 1997;55(1):S53–S60.

215. Byers T. Hardened fats, hardened arteries? *N Engl J Med.* 1997;337(21):1444–1445.

216. Gillman MW, Cupples LA, Millen BE, Ellison RC, Wolf PA. Inverse association of dietary fat with development of ischemic stroke in men. *JAMA.* 1997;278(24):2145–2150.

217. National Academy of Sciences, Institute of Medicine. *Dietary Reference Intakes for Calcium, Phosphorus, Magnesium, Vitamin D, and Fluoride.* Washington, DC: National Academy Press; 1997.

SUGGESTED READING

Balch, GI. *Nutrition education for adults: a review of research.* Prepared for: US Department of Agriculture, Food and Consumer Service, Office of Analysis and Evaluation, Alexandria, Va, 1994.

Center for Nutrition Policy and Promotion, US Department of Agriculture. *A Catalog of National Nutrition Education Promotion Projects.* Washington, DC: US Department of Agriculture; 1997.

Meisler JG, St Jeor S. Summary and recommendations from the American Health Foundation's Expert Panel on Healthy Weight. *Am J Clin Nutr.* 1996;63(3 suppl):474S–477S.

US Department of Health and Human Services. *Physical Activity and Health: A Report of the Surgeon General.* Atlanta, GA: US Department of Health and Human Services, Centers for Disease Control and Prevention, National Center for Chronic

Disease Prevention and Health Promotion; 1996.

Wheelock V, ed. *Implementing Dietary Guidelines for Healthy Eating*. London, England: Chapman & Hall; 1997.

World Cancer Research Fund/ American Institute for Cancer Research. *Food, Nutrition and the Prevention of Cancer: A Global Perspective*. Washington, DC: American Institute for Cancer Research; 1997.

RESOURCES

American Cancer Society, Inc.
1599 Clifton Road, NE
Atlanta, GA 30329-4251
(800) ACS-2345
http://www.cancer.org

American Dietetic Association
216 West Jackson Boulevard
Chicago, IL 60606-6995
(312) 899-0040
http://www.eatright.org

American Heart Association
7272 Greenville Avenue
Dallas, TX 75231-4596
(214) 373-6300
http://www.amhrt.org

Center for Food Safety & Applied Nutrition
Food and Drug Administration
200 C Street SW
Washington, DC 20204
http://vm.cfsan.fda.gov/list.html

Center for Nutrition Policy and Promotion
U.S. Department of Agriculture
1120 20th Street NW
Suite 200, North Lobby
Washington, DC 20036
http://www.usda.gov/fcs/cnpp.htm

Center for Science in the Public Interest
1875 Connecticut Avenue, NW, Suite 300
Washington, DC 20009
Telephone: (202) 332-9110
Fax: (202) 265-4954
http://www.cspinet.org

Food and Nutrition Service
U.S. Department of Agriculture
3101 Park Center Drive
Alexandria, VA 22302-1594
http://www.usda.gov/fcs/fcs.htm

National Center for Chronic Disease Prevention and Health Promotion
Centers for Disease Control and Prevention, Mail Stop K-46
4770 Buford Highway, NE
Atlanta, GA 30341-3717
Telephone: (770) 488-5820
Fax: (770)488-5473
http://www.cdc.gov/nccdphp/

9

HIGH BLOOD PRESSURE

ICD-9 401-405

High blood pressure refers to levels of systolic and/or diastolic blood pressure associated with increased risks of morbidity or mortality. The gradients of risk for sequelae such as acute myocardial infarction or stroke are continuous and without any apparent thresholds.[1, 2] The precise numerical criteria defining high blood pressure are therefore arbitrary.

The prevalence of high blood pressure in the United States increases markedly with age, from approximately 4% at ages 18 through 24 to nearly 65% at ages 80 and older.[3] This increasing prevalence reflects the fact that, for most people in the United States, blood pressure increases over each decade of age. Not all populations in the world experience such an increase, however, which indicates that this shift is not a necessary concomitant of aging.

For blood pressure classification of adults 18 years of age or older, the 1997 Joint National Committee on Prevention, Detection, Evaluation, and Treatment of High Blood Pressure (JNC-VI)[2] defined hypertension based on the level of systolic and diastolic blood pressure (Table 9.1). People in the high-normal category are at risk for developing higher levels of blood pressure as they grow older.[4] In a recent trial, researchers demonstrated that certain lifestyle changes reduced blood pressure levels in people in the normal and high-normal range.[5] The terms mild, moderate, and severe have been carried over from the early investigation of the effect of treatment on reducing blood pressure. However, the current guidelines no longer recommend using these terms, because they inappropriately understate the risks and importance of intervention for most people who are so classified.

Isolated systolic hypertension is especially common in older people and has specific pathophysiologic concomitants. In recent trials, such as the Systolic Hypertension in the Elderly Program (SHEP), investigators have demonstrated the efficacy

Darwin R. Labarthe, MD, PhD
Edward J. Roccella, PhD, MPH

Table 9.1—Classification of Blood Pressure for Adults Aged 18 Years and Older[a]

Category	Systolic (mm Hg)		Diastolic (mm Hg)	Follow-up Recommended[b]
Optimal[c]	<120	and	<80	—
Normal	<130	and	<85	Recheck in 2 years
High-normal	130-139	or	85-89	Recheck in 1 year[d]
Hypertension[e]				
Stage 1	140-159	or	90-99	Confirm within 2 months[d]
Stage 2	160-179	or	100-109	Evaluate or refer to source of care within 1 month
Stage 3	180-209	or	≥110	Evaluate or refer to source of care immediately or within 1 week depending on clinical situation

[a]Not taking hypertensive drugs and not acutely ill. When systolic and diastolic pressure fall into different categories, the higher category should be selected to classify the individual's blood pressure status. For instance, 160/92 should be classified as Stage 2, and 174/120 should be classified as Stage 3. Isolated systolic hypertension (ISH) is defined as SBP ≥140 mm Hg and DBP <90 mm Hg and staged appropriately (eg, 170/85 is defined as Stage 2 ISH).

[b]Modify the scheduling of follow-up according to reliable information about past blood pressure measurements, other cardiovascular risk factors, or target organ disease.

[c]Optimal blood pressure with respect to cardiovascular disease risk is SBP <120 and DBP <80. However, unusually low readings should be evaluated for clinical significance.

[d]Provide advice about lifestyle modifications.

[e]Based on the average of 2 or more readings taken at each of 2 or more visits after an initial screeening.

Source: Joint National Committee on Prevention, Detection, Evaluation, and Treatment of High Blood Pressure.[2]

and safety of treating this condition,[6] which has been associated with a two- to fivefold increase in death from all causes and from cardiovascular disease in particular. Further aspects of measurement and classification are addressed in Suggested Readings on page 285.

SIGNIFICANCE

High blood pressure contributes substantially to the risks of coronary heart disease, thromboembolic stroke, and other complications of advanced atherosclerosis as well as to damage of the heart, brain, kidneys, and other organs.[1] Its impact on disability is therefore only partially reflected in data on hypertension, which alone disabled some 3 million Americans from 1990 through 1992. If the numbers of people disabled by heart disease and cerebrovascular disease are added, the total is greater than 9 million.[7]

Recently, as many as 50 million Americans either had high blood pressure, which is defined as systolic blood pressure of 140 mm Hg or greater and/or diastolic blood pressure of 90 mm Hg or greater, or were taking antihypertensive medication.[2] This estimate is derived from a random sample of American adults (NHANES III), in addition to extrapolations from large data sets on the young applied to the 1990 census population.

This represents a decrease in the number of people with hypertension from the 60 million reported more than a decade ago (NHANES II). In both surveys, the estimates are high because they reflect only a single occasion of measurement.[8] The number of people who would have high blood pressure readings on repeated occasions and who would therefore be potential candidates for interventions, may actually be one-third or more below this estimate, because many people exhibit lower levels of blood pressure on repeated measurements. Thus, risk, and the indication for individual treatment,

should be estimated on the basis of the average of several measurements. Nonetheless, an elevated blood pressure reading on one occasion may be a harbinger of repeated sustained elevations in the future.

Over the past 3 decades, researchers have discovered the benefits of reversing high blood pressure through both nonpharmacologic[5, 9, 10] and pharmacologic[11, 12] interventions as well as the potential for the primary prevention of high blood pressure. These approaches present a major public health opportunity and challenge for the next century.

PATHOPHYSIOLOGY

Most people with hypertension have essential hypertension—that is, it has no identifiable cause. Relatively few people have secondary hypertension, or hypertension resulting from a specific defect, such as hypertension caused by renal disease or endocrine abnormalities.

The pathophysiologic cause of most essential hypertension is unknown. However, just as pneumonia is caused by a variety of infectious agents that may present similar clinical pictures, so too essential hypertension probably has a number of distinct causes.[13] The factors involved include age, heredity, race, sex, smoking habits, dietary patterns, serum cholesterol, glucose intolerance, weight, and renin activity. The primary difficulty in uncovering the specific mechanism(s) responsible for hypertension in most people is that blood pressure is regulated by a variety of interrelated peripheral and/or central adrenergic, renal, hormonal, and vascular systems.

High blood pressure that is sustained over several years is accompanied by pathological changes in blood vessels and target organs, especially the kidneys, heart, eyes, and brain. These changes can be direct effects of pressure, consequences of injury to the blood vessel walls, or caused by accelerated development of atherosclerotic plaques. Despite these changes, treatment of established high blood pressure can substantially reduce a person's risk of developing complications. However, the risks have not been reduced as effectively for those who have already developed organ damage as for those still free of such damage.

DESCRIPTIVE EPIDEMIOLOGY

High-Risk Groups

The incidence of high blood pressure when studied among adults in 13 communities in the United States in the mid-1970s was 6.8% per year for Black men, 5.5% for Black women, 2.6% for White men, and 2.6% for White women.[14] In cross-sectional surveys, about twice as many Blacks as Whites and Mexican Americans in the United States are found to have high blood pressure,[15] regardless of the specific blood pressure criteria used. Blacks develop high blood pressure at an earlier age than Whites and experience it more severely.[2] An inverse relation between blood pressure levels and occupational and socio-economic status has long been recognized in the United States.[2] Blood pressure differences by race or ethnicity also have been found to reflect socioeconomic differences, but higher blood pressure levels in Blacks persist even after controlling for socioeconomic variables.[16]

Internationally, investigators have identified an inverse relation between education and blood pressure levels. A recent report from the INTERSALT Study,[17] conducted in 32 countries, suggests that about half of this inverse association was accounted for by five factors: urinary sodium excretion, potassium excretion, body mass index (weight divided by a squared term of height), alcohol intake, and smoking. These investigators caution against making too facile a distinction between unmodifiable and modifiable risk factors.

Consistently, the strongest predictor of future high blood pressure has been the level of blood pressure at initial observation. Hence, the high-normal group identified previously is of great prognostic importance.

Geographic Distribution

Around the world, the prevalence of high blood pressure varies widely. Some populations exhibit no increase in mean blood pressure levels with age, and high blood pressure is virtually absent in these populations. Within the United States, few reliable data are available for assessing regional variation. An exception is that the southeastern states have long been identified as the "Stroke Belt," reflecting a higher prevalence of severe or uncontrolled high blood pressure, especially among Blacks, than is found in the rest of the country.[3] Population distributions according to race and socioeconomic status tend to identify areas of especially high risk, such as low-income urban areas.

Time Trends

Data are available for the United States from national probability samples over the period 1960 to 1962 to 1988 to 1991. They indicate that the distribution of high blood pressure has shifted to lower values—at the center or median as well as the upper extreme or 90th percentile of the distribution—over these 30 years.[18] The prevalence of high blood pressure has varied between 21% (1971 to 1974) and 14% (1988 to 1991) among persons aged 18 to 74 years in the civilian, noninstitutionalized population.

Major changes have occurred in the control status of those affected, however. The percentage of people who are aware that they have high blood pressure has increased from 53% to 89%; the proportion of those people receiving active treatment has increased from 35% to 79%; and the proportion of people with adequately controlled blood pressure levels (ie, blood pressure, with medication, is below 160/95 mm Hg) has increased from 16% to 64%.[8] The latter two trends indicate the major nationwide impact that control efforts can have.

RISK FACTORS

Magnitude of Risk Factors

Measuring a person's risk for developing high blood pressure depends greatly on the criteria for classification, the number of occasions on which measurements are taken, and other circumstances of the investigation. Only a small proportion (perhaps fewer than 5%) of people with high blood pressure are found to have a specific pathophysiologic cause for this condition. For high blood pressure in general, a variety of environmental factors and predisposing genetic components have been investigated.

Although the initial level of blood pressure is the strongest predictor of the level of subsequent measurements, it has been shown in extended follow-up studies that weight gain in the interval between measurements is another strong predictor of increasing blood pressure among adults. People with a family history of high blood pressure also have an increased risk.

Modifiable risk factors include obesity, high alcohol intake, a diet high in sodium and low in potassium, and physical inactivity. In cross-sectional analyses of INTERSALT Study data, the contribution of sodium and potassium intake (estimated by urinary excretion), body mass index, and alcohol intake were assessed for their contributions to blood pressure differences between populations (Table 9.2).[17] For each variable and certain derived indices, regression analyses were used to estimate the predicted difference in average population values of systolic blood pressure for a given reduction in the level of each factor. These analyses provide a quantitative index of risk in which the contributions of each factor or index can be compared.

Population-Attributable Risk

The quantitative contributions of specific factors to the risk of developing specific blood pressure levels are rarely presented in the same way as conventional attributable risks, but such data would be useful. Again, the INTERSALT Study results provide some insight. The projected effect of combined lifestyle changes would be

Table 9.2—Predicted Difference in Population Average Systolic Blood Pressure with Given Differences in Lifestyle Variables

Lifestyle Variable	Present Level[a]	Improved Level	Predicted Difference
Na	170 mmol[a]	70 mmol	-2.17 (mm Hg)
K	55 mmol[a]	70 mmol	-0.67
Na/K	3.09[a]	1.00	-3.36
BMI	25.0 k/m^2 [a]	23.0 k/m^2	-1.55
High alcohol	≥300 mL/week[b]	1-299 mL/week	-2.81
Improved levels of both Na/K and BMI	—	—	-4.91
Expected difference if heavy drinkers also reduced alcohol	—	—	-5.33

[a]Approximate median level found in INTERSALT.
[b]Reported by about 15% of respondents.
Na, sodium; K, potassium; Na/K, sodium/potassium ratio; BMI, body mass index.
Note. Adapted from Stamler et al.[17]

to reduce the population average value for systolic blood pressure by about 5 mm Hg. This difference could reduce coronary heart disease deaths by 9%, stroke deaths by 14%, and all causes of death by 7% (these estimates were made by using a multivariate risk score developed on the basis of data from several longitudinal studies in the United States and the United Kingdom).[17] (The attributable risks for the contributions of blood pressure to cardiovascular events are discussed in Chapter 11.)

PREVENTION AND CONTROL MEASURES

Prevention

Primary prevention of high blood pressure was the focus of a 1992 National High Blood Pressure Education Program report.[3] The report emphasized that despite the clear benefit of detecting and treating hypertension, this approach alone will not prevent all of the high blood pressure-related cardiovascular disease in the community. First, blood pressure-related vascular complications can occur before the onset of established hypertension, because the blood pressure-cardiovascular disease risk relationship is continuous and progressive, even within the "normal" range of blood pressure. Second, it is difficult to ensure that all people with hypertension are detected and treated ad-

equately. Finally, many hypertensive treatment regimens are expensive, especially those including new drugs, and almost all carry the potential for some adverse effects.

The report recommended that primary prevention of hypertension be accomplished through interventions with the general population (population strategy), with the objective of achieving a downward shift in the distribution of blood pressure. This approach can be complemented by special attempts to lower blood pressure among populations that are most likely to develop hypertension (targeted strategy). These population groups include African Americans, people with high-normal blood pressure, people with a family history of hypertension, and individuals with one or more lifestyle factors that contribute to age-related increases in blood pressure.

As discussed earlier, the lifestyle factors that have been shown to be risk factors for hypertension include a high sodium intake, excessive caloric intake, physical inactivity, excessive alcohol consumption, and deficient intake of potassium. These lifestyle factors have formed the basis for intervention strategies that have shown promise in the prevention of high blood pressure.[11] For example, recent research has shown that physical activity has an independent capacity to lower blood pressure.[10] Reports on these and other lifestyle interventions have shown that previously controlled hypertension can be maintained without medication and that the progression to undesirable high blood pressure levels can be averted.

The evidence is less convincing for stress management, for altering macronutrient consumption, and for supplementing the diet with calcium, magnesium, fish oils, or fiber. Present data are insufficient to make a final judgment on the potential role of these factors in the primary prevention of hypertension.

Screening and Early Detection

Recommendations for detection, evaluation, and treatment of high blood pressure are given in a series of reports by the Joint National Committee. These reports have been updated and released every 4 years by the National High Blood Pressure Education Program (NHBPEP), which is administered by the National Heart, Lung, and Blood Institute. The reports address various aspects of high blood pressure control in considerable detail and with extensive reference to recent research. Whereas screening of whole populations to identify unrecognized cases of high blood pressure was a strong recommendation in the early years of the NHBPEP, the emphasis now is on maintaining treatment and control among those already identified.

Screening remains important for certain underserved and high-risk populations, however. Current screening recommendations are shown in Table 9.1.

The Working Group on Hypertension Control in Children and Adolescents, a working committee of the NHBPEP, reflects the recognition that primary prevention is most effective when it begins during childhood. The first and second reports from this task force, released in 1977 and 1987 (and updated in 1996), addressed concerns about blood pressure measurement and the identification of children at risk between birth and age 18.[19-21] Criteria for referral and evaluation are based on percentile ranks of blood pressure readings derived from the pooled data of several cross-sectional surveys of blood pressure. Table 9.3 shows 95th percentiles that are considered elevated. Given the known relation between relative ranks of blood pressure and relative growth in children, those children who are high in percentile ranks for blood pressure but also rank high for height are considered to have normal blood pressure.

Treatment, Rehabilitation, and Recovery

The JNC-VI report appreciated the importance of risk stratification and treatment (Table 9.4). Suggested treatment plans are based on the

Table 9.3—Ninety-fifth Percentiles of Blood Pressure by Selected Ages, by the 50th and 75th Height Percentiles

Age, y	Girls' SBP/DBP		Boys' SBP/DBP	
	50th Percentile for Height	75th Percentile for Height	50th Percentile for Height	75th Percentile for Height
1	104/58	105/59	102/57	104/58
6	111/73	112/73	114/74	115/75
12	123/80	124/81	123/81	125/82
17	129/84	130/85	136/87	138/88

Source: Adapted from a report by the National High Blood Pressure Education Program Working Group on Hypertension Control in Children and Adolescents.[21]
SBP, systolic blood pressure; DBP, diastolic blood pressure.

level of blood pressure, plus consideration of the presence or absence of cardiovascular risk factors. As a result, some hypertensive individuals (blood pressure $\geq$140/90) may be placed on lifestyle modification of up to 1 year in an attempt to control blood pressure. Others who have high-normal blood pressures of 130 to 139 systolic blood pressure (SBP) or 85 to 89 diastolic blood pressure (DBP) with target organ damage or clinical cardiovascular disease should be placed on drug therapy. The treatment program should include the leading options among available drugs. These drugs should be used in stepwise fashion to increase dosage and potency until blood pressure is under control (Figure 9.1).

Drug therapy should begin at less than full dose. If high blood pressure control is not achieved, clinicians may increase dose of the drug of second class or substitute another class of agent. Long-acting combination therapy is also suggested as a way to improve adherence to medical regimens. Reduced intensity of therapy is to be considered after at least 1 year of successful blood pressure control. A number of special circumstances and precautions are also noted, such as those concerning children, older people, and other special groups at risk.

The rationale for such intervention is based on a large body of experience in clinical trials of antihypertensive therapy. These trials have persuasively demonstrated major reductions in morbidity and mortality with effective treatment, especially when introduced before target organ damage is evident.[22]

Table 9.4—Risk Stratification and Treatment

Blood Pressure Stages (mm Hg)	Risk Group A (No Risk Factors) No TOD/CCD[a]	Risk Group B (At Least 1 Risk Factor, Not Including Diabetes; No TOD/CCD)	Risk Group C (TOD/CCD and/or Diabetes, With or Without Other Risk Factors)
High-normal (130-139/85-89)	Lifestyle modification	Lifestyle modification	Drug therapy[b]
Stage 1 (140-159/90-99)	Lifestyle modification (up to 12 months)	Lifestyle modification[c] (up to 6 months)	Drug therapy
Stages 2 and 3 ($\geq$160/$\geq$100)	Drug therapy	Drug therapy	Drug therapy

[a]TOD/CCD indicates target organ disease/clinical cardiovascular disease.

[b]For those with heart failure, renal insufficiency, or diabetes.

[c]For patients with multiple risk factors, clinicians should consider drugs as initial therapy plus lifestyle modifications.

Note. For example, a patient with diabetes and a blood pressure of 142/94 mm Hg plus left ventricular hypertrophy should be classified as having stage 1 hypertension with target organ disease (left ventricular hypertrophy) and with another major risk factor (diabetes). This patient would be categorized as "Stage 1, Risk Group C," and recommended for immediate initiation of pharmacologic treatment. Lifestyle modification should be adjunctive therapy for all patients recommended for pharmacologic therapy.

Source. Joint National Committee on Prevention, Detection, Evaluation, and Treatment of High Blood Pressure.[2]

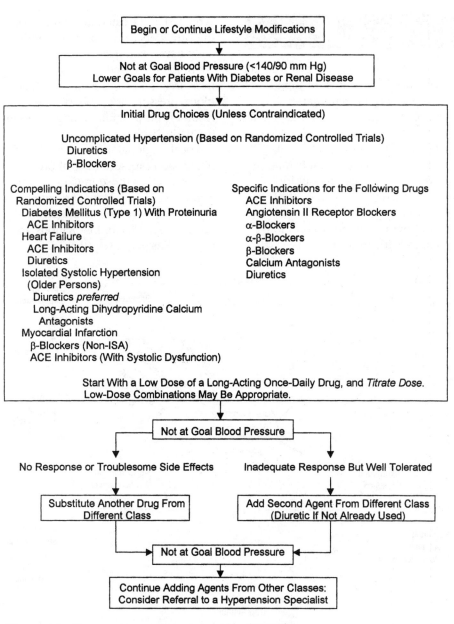

Figure 9.1—Hypertension treatment algorithm (JNC VI).

McClellan and Wilber reviewed 20 public health programs for high blood pressure detection and control: eight in urban settings, eight in rural settings, and four in selected worksites.[23] From the profiles of these programs, the investigators derived a "composite model for community hypertension control" (Figure 9.2).

This model's emphasis on motivating individuals at risk to be screened and treated and on preparing providers to respond appropriately have been major aspects of the NHBPEP. Increased public awareness, treatment, and control of high blood pressure are probably the result of this program, inaugurated in the early 1970s.

Local, regional, and statewide high blood pressure control programs, such as those in Connecticut, Kentucky, Maine, Maryland, and Wisconsin, have demonstrated diverse strengths and limitations and, in some instances (eg, the Two-

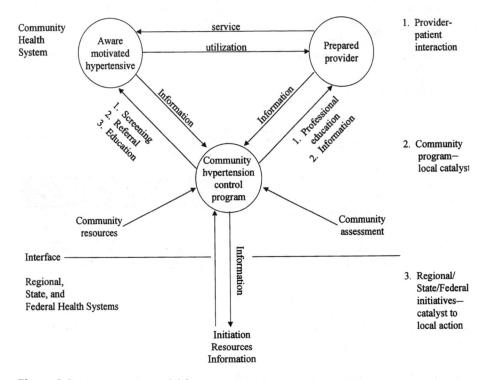

Figure 9.2—A composite model for community hypertension control.

County Program in Kentucky), have been shown to reduce mortality significantly.[24]

Another important aspect of high blood pressure is its joint occurrence with other major risk factors for cardiovascular disease. This well-documented circumstance points to the value of addressing several risk factors together in one program. Thus, high blood pressure programs should take into account the extent of additional risk related to age, sex, smoking habits, lipid profile, diabetes, physical inactivity, and other contributing factors. These risks can be identified at entry to the program or as they emerge over time, possibly as side effects of pharmacologic treatment. The experiences of several community-based cardiovascular risk reduction programs that address multiple factors can be informative to practitioners and policymakers striving to prevent cardiovascular diseases.[25]

Finally, the Working Group on Primary Prevention of Hypertension recommended a national campaign for the primary prevention of high blood pressure.[3] To accomplish this goal, the campaign, at a minimum, would include the following components: (1) public education on the role of lifestyle in the etiology of hypertension; (2) education programs for the food industry (manufacturers and retailers) and food service institutions (restaurants, schools, hospitals, etc.) to encourage them to provide the public with healthier foods; and (3) an education and support program for health care professionals. Such a comprehensive program will support healthy lifestyle changes among the general public.

The health objectives for the United States presented in Healthy People 2000 include increased measurement and awareness of blood pressure levels among adults generally, and in worksites employing 50 or more persons.[26] At least 90% of persons aged 18 years or older should have had blood pressure measured within the past 2 years and know whether the result was normal or high, an increase from 61% in 1985. Worksites which offer blood pressure control programs should increase from 16.5% in 1985 to at least 50%. These objectives are currently being updated for the year 2010.

AREAS OF FUTURE RESEARCH AND DEMONSTRATION

Much has been learned in the past 3 decades that now permits effective high blood pressure control for millions of people in the United States. However, not all people at risk are reached by such programs, and many important challenges remain. Further research is needed to achieve the prevention and control of high blood pressure.

To address research priorities in this field, the National Heart, Lung, and Blood Institute charged a task force to prepare a report on high blood pressure research aimed at achieving the greatest potential benefit to Americans through the 1990s.[27] From a public health point of view, the leading questions were those relating to population-based research. The priority areas were characterized broadly as follows:

• Continued evaluation of the cost-effectiveness of community-based hypertension control programs, with the aim of achieving complete control of high blood pressure in entire communities, and especially among high-risk, underserved, and other special populations.

• Assessment of the benefits of primary prevention programs, both in terms of changes in the population distribution of blood pressure and in the frequency of effective blood pressure control.

• Research focused on the development of strategies for incorporating prevention activities into primary care practice and the changing health care delivery system(s).

• Research on the determinants of high blood pressure at the population level, the individual risks of complications of high blood pressure, and the mechanisms of action of such factors.

• Research on the factors influencing the control of high blood pres-

sure in Blacks and other racial minorities.

These priorities represent the major strategies needed at the population level to ensure this nation's continuing progress toward the primary prevention and community control of high blood pressure. They identify groups in special need of intervention and call for progress toward understanding the determinants of high blood pressure.

REFERENCES

1. Kannel WB, Stokes J III. Hypertension as a cardiovascular risk factor. In: Bulpitt CJ, ed. *Handbook of Hypertension, Vol. 6: Epidemiology of Hypertension.* New York, NY: Elsevier Science Publishers; 1985:15–34.

2. Joint National Committee on Prevention, Detection, Evaluation, and Treatment of High Blood Pressure. The sixth report of the Joint National Committee on Detection, Evaluation, and Treatment of High Blood Pressure (JNC VI). *Arch Intern Med.* 1997;157:2413–2446.

3. National High Blood Pressure Education Program. Working group report on primary prevention of hypertension. National Heart, Lung, and Blood Institute, NIH. *Arch Intern Med.* 1993;153: 186–208.

4. Leitschuh M, Cupples LA, Kannel W, Gagnon D, Chobanian A. High-normal blood pressure progression to hypertension in the Framingham Heart Study. *Hypertension.* 1991;17:22–27.

5. The Trials of Hypertension Prevention Collaborative Research Group. The effects of nonpharmacologic interventions on blood pressure of persons with high normal levels. Results of the trials of hypertension prevention, phase I. *JAMA.* 1992;267:1213–1220.

6. SHEP Cooperative Research Group. Prevention of stroke by antihypertensive drug treatment in older persons with isolated systolic hypertension. Final results of the Systolic Hypertension in the Elderly Program (SHEP). *JAMA* 265:3255–3264, 1991.

7. National Heart, Lung, and Blood Institute. *Fact Book Fiscal Year 1995.* Washington, DC: US Dept of Health and Human Services, Public Health Service, National Institutes of Health; 1995.

8. Roccella EJ, Horan MJ. The National High Blood Pressure Education Program: measuring progress and assessing its impact. *Health Psych.* 1988; 7(suppl):297–303.

9. Horan MJ, Roccella EJ. Non-pharmacologic treatment of hypertension: does it work? *Eur Heart J.* 1987;8(suppl):77–86.

10. Arroll B, Beaglehole R. Does physical activity lower blood pressure: a critical review of the clinical trials. *J Clin Epidemiol.* 1992;45:439–447.

11. MacMahon SW, Cutler JA, Furberg CD, Payne GH. The effects of drug treatment for hypertension on morbidity and mortality from cardiovascular disease: a review of randomized controlled trials. *Prog Cardiovasc Dis.* 1986;29(suppl 1):99–118.

12. Collins R, Peto R, MacMahon S, et al. Blood pressure, stroke, and coronary heart disease. Part 2, short-term reductions in blood pressure: overview of randomised drug trials in their epidemiological context. *Lancet.* 1990;335:827–838.

13. William GH, Braunwald E. Hypertensive vascular disease. In: Braunwald E, Isselbacher KJ, Petersdorf RG, Wilson JD, Martin JB, Fauci AS, eds. *Principles of Internal Medicine.* 11th ed. New York, NY: McGraw-Hill Inc; 1987:1024–1037.

14. Apostolides AY, Cutter G, Daugherty SA, et al. Three year incidence of hypertension in thirteen US communities. *Prev Med.* 1982;11:487–499.

15. Burt VL, Whelton P, Roccella EJ, et al. Prevalence of hypertension in the US adult population. Results from the Third National Health and Nutrition Examina-

tion Survey, 1988–1991. *Hypertension* 1995;25:305—313.

16. Hypertension Detection and Follow-up Program Cooperative Group. Five-year findings of the Hypertension Detection and Follow-up Program. II. Mortality by race, sex, and age. *JAMA.* 1979;242:2572–2577.

17. Stamler J, Rose G, Stamler S, Elliott P, Dyer A, Marmot M. INTERSALT Study findings. Public health and medical care implications. *Hypertension.* 1989;14:570–577.

18. Burt VL, Cutler JA, Higgins M, et al. Trends in the prevalence, awareness, treatment, and control of hypertension in the adult US population. Data from the Health Examination Surveys, 1960 to 1991. *Hypertension* 26:60–69, 1995.

19. Report of the Task Force on Blood Pressure Control in Children. *Pediatrics.* 1977;59: 797–820.

20. Report of the Second Task Force on Blood Pressure Control in Children. *Pediatrics.* 1987;79:1–25.

21. National High Blood Pressure Education Program Working Group on Hypertension Control in Children and Adolescents. Update on the 1987 Task Force Report on High Blood Pressure in Children and Adolescents: a Working Group report from the National High Blood Pressure Education Program. *Pediatrics.* 1996;98:649–658.

22. Cutler JA, MacMahon SW, Furberg CD. Controlled clinical trials of drug treatment for hypertension: a review. *Hypertension.* 1989;13(suppl. I):I-36–I-44.

23. McClellan W, Wilber JA. A decade's experience with hypertension control programs in the United States: the empirical basis for a model of community control programs. In: Rosenfeld JB, Silverberg DS, Viskiper R, eds. *Hypertension Control in the Community.* London: John Libbey; 1985:1–16.

24. Kotchen JM, McKean HE, Jackson-Thayer S, Moore RW, Straus R, Kotchen TA. Impact of a rural high blood pressure control program on hypertension control and cardiovascular disease mortality. *JAMA.* 1986; 255:2177–2182.

25. Pearson TA, Boekeloo BA, Graziano S. Community based cardiovascular risk reduction programs. *Maryland Med J.* 1988;37:836–839.

26. Public Health Service, U.S. Department of Health and Human Services. *Healthy People 2000. National Health Promotion and Disease Prevention Objectives. Full Report, with Commentary.* Washington, DC:

US Govt Printing Office; 1991. DHHS publication (PHS) 91-50212.

27. National Heart, Lung, and Blood Institute. *Report of the Task Force on Research in Hypertension.* Washington, DC: US Dept of Health and Human Services, Public Health Service; 1991.

SUGGESTED READING

Joint National Committee on Prevention, Detection, Evaluation, and Treatment of High Blood Pressure. The sixth report of the Joint National Committee on Detection, Evaluation, and Treatment of High Blood Pressure (JNC VI). *Arch Intern Med.* 1997;157:2413–2446.

Lawrence M, Neil A, Mant D, Fowler G, eds. *Prevention of Cardiovascular Disease. An Evidence-Based Approach.* New York: Oxford University Press Inc; 1996.

McClellan W, Wilber JA. A decade's experience with hypertension control programs in the United States: the empirical basis for a model of community control programs. In: Rosenfeld JB, Silverberg DS, Viskiper R, eds. *Hypertension Control in the Community.* London: John Libbey; 1985:1–16.

National Heart, Lung, and Blood Institute. Report of the Task Force on Research in Hypertension. Washington, DC: US Dept of Health and Human Services, Public Health Service; 1991.

National High Blood Pressure Education Program. Working group report on primary prevention of hypertension. National Heart, Lung, and Blood Institute, NIH. *Arch Intern Med.* 1993;153:186–208.

The Trials of Hypertension Prevention Collaborative Research Group. The effects of nonpharmacologic interventions on blood pressure of persons with high normal levels. Results of the trials of hypertension prevention, phase I. *JAMA.* 1992;267:1213–1220.

RESOURCES

American Heart Association
7272 Greenville Avenue
Dallas, TX 75231-4596
(214) 373-6300

National Heart, Lung, and Blood Institute Information Center
PO Box 30105
Bethesda, MD 20824-0105
(301) 951-3260

10

CHOLESTEROL

Multiple longitudinal studies have demonstrated that the risk of coronary heart disease (CHD) increases as the level of serum cholesterol increases.[1, 2] The relationship between total serum cholesterol and the risk of CHD appears to be continuous and graded. [1-3] That is, there appeared to be no "threshold" level at which total cholesterol becomes a risk factor for CHD.[3] "High blood cholesterol" or hypercholesterolemia are terms used to describe a level of cholesterol in the blood that is associated with an increase in the risk of atherosclerosis and cardiovascular disease, particularly CHD.

On the basis of data from the Third Health and Nutrition Examination Survey, 31% of US adults have borderline high (200 to 239 mg/dL) cholesterol levels and 20% have high (more than 240 mg/dL) levels.[4] In addition, 16% of men and women have low-density lipoprotein (LDL)

levels in the high-risk range (LDL > 160 mg/dL). Thus, a large portion of Americans are at risk for CHD because of hypercholesterolemia. However, the prevalence of those with high blood cholesterol fell from prior reports,[4] indicating the effectiveness of public health measures to reduce high blood cholesterol.

The public health burden from high blood cholesterol results from both the health and economic consequences of cardiovascular disease. High blood cholesterol is thought to account for approximately 30% of CHD and up to 20% of strokes in the United States (see Chapter 11 on cardiovascular diseases). In addition, considerable health care resources are required for the screening and treatment of persons with high blood cholesterol.

PATHOPHYSIOLOGY

Elevated levels of serum cholesterol play an important role in the development of atherosclerosis— a disease in which cholesterol accumulates in the walls of arteries and

Patrick E. McBride, MD, MPH
Robert F. Anda, MD, MS

contributes to the development of plaques that can inhibit blood flow or acutely rupture leading to acute CHD events or death.[5, 6] "Fatty streaks" are the earliest atherosclerotic lesions that can be easily recognized and are the result of the accumulation of lipid and lipid-containing monocytes (that have penetrated beneath the endothelium) in the innermost arterial wall. These lesions are flat or only slightly elevated and do not significantly narrow the involved artery.[7] It has been known for several decades that fatty streaks begin in early childhood and that the extent of fatty streaks in early life is related to levels of serum cholesterol and other risk factors.[8] Fibrous plaques are raised lesions resulting from the accumulation of lipids, lipid-containing cells, and the proliferation of connective tissue in the arterial wall. It remains unclear whether fibrous plaques arise from fatty streaks, but it appears that many do. These lesions generally appear in the second decade of life and are associated with serum lipoprotein concentrations.[5, 9, 10]

Fibrous plaques can become progressive and become complicated by calcification, hemorrhaging, and ulceration. Platelet aggregation and thrombus formation can occur and become incorporated into these complicated plaques. Ultimately, occlusion of the artery by the plaque or thrombus (clot) formation as a result of inflammation and rupture of the plaque can result in infarction and organ damage.[6] When one or more of the coronary arteries is seriously narrowed or when thrombosis occurs at the site of an advanced plaque, the supply of blood to the heart can be critically lowered and manifest as angina pectoris or myocardial infarction. Recent evidence indicates that lesions that are 40% to 50% stenotic related to the diameter of the artery lumen, which are highly lipid-rich lesions, are the most likely to rupture and to precipitate acute myocardial infarction and other CVD clinical syndromes.[11] These partially occluding lesions are also more likely to respond to lipid-lowering therapy by changing their morphology, structure, and function to become more stable, suggesting further evidence for the benefits of cholesterol screening and therapy.[11]

Because cholesterol is insoluble in water, it is transported in the blood after being surrounded by plasma proteins called apoproteins. The combination of lipid and apoprotein are called lipoprotein particles, which are essentially "oil droplets" composed of cholesterol esters and triglycerides and are made water soluble by the hydrophilic composition of the surface layer protein of the particle.[12]

There are four major classes of lipoprotein particles. Most cholesterol is carried by LDL. The other three lipoproteins are very low density lipoprotein (VLDL) which carries mostly triglycerides, intermediate density lipoprotein (IDL), and high density lipoprotein (HDL).[12]

LDL cholesterol is delivered to cells (primarily in the liver) by a process that involves the attachment of circulating LDL to LDL receptors, which are located on the surface of the cell. The cholesterol is used by the cell for the synthesis of plasma membranes, bile acids, and steroid hormones or is stored by the cell. Because the receptor has a high affinity for LDL particles and the receptor can cycle multiple times in and out of the cell, large amounts of cholesterol can be delivered to body tissues.[12]

Damage to the endothelial lining of arteries and lipid infiltration appear to be involved in the genesis of atherosclerosis.[6, 13] The lipids contained in atherosclerotic lesions are thought to be primarily derived from LDL.[13] When LDL receptor function is diminished in response to regulatory signals (such as a high saturated fat diet) or as a result of genetic defects, cholesterol levels in the plasma rise and can contribute to the development of atherosclerosis.[12, 13] Oxidized LDL and VLDL have high affinity for the LDL receptor and are involved in the formation of foam cells and the initiation and progression of atherosclerotic lesions.[13]

The relationship between cholesterol and the risk of CHD has been refined by understanding the contribution of specific lipoproteins to the risk of CHD.[13] High levels of the major carrier of cholesterol, LDL, have been consistently associated with an increased risk for CHD.[14] More recently, elevated VLDL (or triglycerides) has also been shown to be associated with increased risk of CHD.[15, 16] In contrast, higher levels of HDL cholesterol are associated with reduced risk for CHD.[14]

DESCRIPTIVE EPIDEMIOLOGY

High-Risk Groups

The proportion at risk of high blood cholesterol increases substantially with age and is slightly higher among men and Caucasians and those with a family history of premature CHD.[4]

Geographic Distribution

The mean level of total cholesterol varies widely between populations. In the 1950s, the Seven Countries Study found a correlation between the proportion of men (in each country) with serum cholesterol more than 250 mg/dL and CHD mortality.[17] In the Ni-Hon-San Study, three cohorts of Japanese men living in southern Japan, Hawaii, and San Francisco, both CHD incidence and serum cholesterol levels were higher in San Francisco than Hawaii, and higher in Hawaii than Japan, which suggests a cultural contribution to increased risk.[17]

Time Trends

Data from the National Health and Nutrition Examination Surveys indicate that the mean cholesterol level of the adults in the United States has been declining since 1980. Between the 1960 to 1962 and the 1988 to 1991 surveys the age-adjusted mean serum cholesterol values decreased by 12 to 17 mg/dL. For men, this represented a decrease from 217 to 205 mg/dL and for women, a decrease from 222 to 205 mg/dL.[18] However, the declines among Black men and women and White men with less than 9 years of education were substantially less.

RISK FACTORS

Dietary Fatty Acids

The most important modifiable risk factor for high blood cholesterol is dietary fat intake, especially saturated fat. The fact that some populations whose diets are substantially lower in fat than the US diet also have substantially lower levels of total cholesterol suggests that diet plays a major role in the high prevalence of high blood cholesterol in the United States. This idea is supported by migration studies such as the Ni-Hon-San Study.[17] However, diet in the United States is relatively uniform (high in total and saturated fat); yet, there is substantial variability in plasma cholesterol levels. Thus, genetic factors—such as those that control the activity of LDL receptors—play an important role in determining cholesterol levels.[19] Nonetheless, because of the high saturated fat intake in the United States, diet is probably an important factor in the occurrence of high blood cholesterol for a large number of US adults.[20, 21]

Most of the fat in human diets is in the form of fatty acids, with "medium chain" fatty acids (chain lengths of 12, 14, 16, or 18 carbons) being the most common. These fatty acids are divided into three groups: saturated (completely saturated with hydrogen and have no double bonds), monounsaturated (one double bond), and polyunsaturated (two or more double bonds). Intake of saturated fatty acids raises total serum cholesterol levels and may increase LDL cholesterol levels by decreasing the activity of LDL receptors.[20] Therefore, current guidelines for cholesterol reduction focus primarily on the amount of saturated fat in the diet.

Polyunsaturated fatty acids are of two types based on the location of the double bond: omega-6 and omega-3. Omega-6 saturated fatty acids are common in plant oils (corn, safflower, soybean, sunflower oils). Clinical and animal studies provide evidence that, when substituted for saturated fatty acids in the diet, omega-6 polyunsaturated fatty acids result in lowering of total and LDL cholesterol, but usually some lowering of HDL cholesterol as well. Omega-3 polyunsaturated fatty acids are common in marine fish and some plant oils; these fatty acids also lower LDL cholesterol and reduce CHD risk.[22]

Monounsaturated fatty acids are especially abundant in olive oil and canola oil.[19–21] Clinical studies indicate that substitution of monounsaturated for saturated fatty acids reduces serum total and LDL cholesterol without reducing HDL cholesterol.

Because of the high correlation between intake of saturated fatty acids and cholesterol, it is difficult to distinguish the independent effect of dietary cholesterol and saturated fat on atherogenesis. However, reviews of the association of dietary intake of cholesterol with the risk of CHD concluded that dietary cholesterol is atherogenic in humans.[21, 23]

Dietary Fiber and Antioxidants

Increased intake of dietary soluble fiber (such as oat bran) has been shown to reduce serum cholesterol.[24] The mechanism by which soluble fiber reduces serum cholesterol is not clear. It is not known whether the reduction of serum cholesterol by increasing dietary fiber is due to a concomitant reduction of dietary fat or to an intrinsic cholesterol lowering property of soluble fiber.[24]

The role of intake of fruits, vegetables, and other sources of micronutrients, including antioxidants, is becoming increasingly important related to reduced incidence of CHD.[21] A number of antioxidants appear to protect lipoproteins from becoming atherogenic via oxidation.[12, 25] Epidemiologic studies indicate an association of reduced CHD with increased intake of fruits and vegetables.[25] Whether the amounts found in diets rich in antioxidants are adequate or supplemental antioxidants for those at high risk are required remains open to debate, though clinical trials suggest that supplemental doses of antioxidants, such as alpha-tocopherol (vitamin E) will be necessary for a treatment effect.[25,26] Clinical trials of alpha-tocopherol that used high doses (400 to 800 IU daily) showed significant benefits, while low-dose trials (50 IU daily) did not.[25] Other antioxidant supplements are under investigation but to date have not demonstrated significant benefits in clinical trials.

Genetic Disorders

Familial hypercholesterolemia (FH) is a genetic disorder that involves the functioning of LDL receptors. About one in every 500 persons are heterozygous for FH; the number of LDL receptors is reduced by about half in these persons, resulting in LDL cholesterol levels that are about twice normal. Homozygous FH is substantially less common, but results in cholesterol levels that are about four times normal. In these persons, premature atherosclerosis and CHD are common.[26] Many other genetically determined abnormalities involving cholesterol metabolism have been described.[26] The most common of these is called familial-combined hyperlipidemia or combined dyslipidemia. Persons with this disorder have multiple abnormalities of lipoproteins, including high LDL, high triglyceride, and low HDL.[21, 26] It has been demonstrated that the lipoproteins in persons with this disorder are more prone to oxidation and are more atherogenic than normal lipoproteins.[21] Low HDL, high lipoprotein(a), and other lipid disorders are commonly noted in persons with CHD.[27]

Other Factors Influencing Cholesterol Levels

Obesity is associated with an increase in LDL-cholesterol levels, a decrease in HDL cholesterol levels, and an increase in the fasting triglyceride levels,[28] and body mass index is positively correlated with total cholesterol levels.[29] Physical inactivity[30] and smoking[31] are associated with lower levels of HDL cholesterol. Although alcohol use is associated with higher levels of HDL cholesterol it is not recommended as a means for raising HDL cholesterol due to other deleterioius effects.[22]

PREVENTION AND CONTROL MEASURES

The reduction of risk for CHD by the use of cholesterol-lowering medications has been demonstrated in randomized trials.[32] Older primary prevention studies examined the potential to reduce CHD events but were not powered to study effects on total mortality. For example, the Lipid Research Clinics Coronary Primary Prevention Trial reduced the incidence of cardiac events by 19% in persons receiving cholestryamine compared to those receiving placebo[33, 34] and the Helsinki Heart Study reported a 34% reduction in the incidence of nonfatal myocardial infarction and cardiac death in the men who received gemfibrozil.[35] A limitation of the primary prevention trials of cholesterol lowering agents is that they were limited to White, middle aged men with very high total cholesterol levels due to the necessity to study very high risk groups for primary prevention. More recently, numerous randomized clinical trials, including primary and secondary prevention trials, have demonstrated that cholesterol treatment for high-risk individuals (including men, women and the elderly) is safe and reduces cardiovascular events and total mortality.[35-42] The benefits of cholesterol treatment are particularly clear in patients with known CHD as this is a high-risk group and multiple studies have shown that cholesterol treatment stabilizes atherosclerotic plaques.[40-42] The results of randomized trials using cholesterol lowering medications have been extensively reviewed elsewhere.[36]

The National Cholesterol Education Program (NCEP) was launched in 1987 to develop national health policy and specific recommendations to reduce the risk of CHD by lowering cholesterol levels in the United States. The NCEP guidelines include a population approach to cholesterol reduction, recommendations for identifying and treating adults at high risk of CHD due to cholesterol disorders, an approach for screening and cholesterol reduction in children and adolescents, and laboratory guidelines among other initiatives.[43-45] Most other national health organizations have endorsed the NCEP guidelines with some exceptions.

The NCEP guidelines provide for both a "population" and a "high-risk" strategy for cholesterol reduction in the United States.[43, 44] The population strategy assumes that widespread changes in lifestyle will result in substantial reductions in the CHD burden. At the same time, the high-risk approach addresses the needs of persons with cholesterol abnormalities (especially those with other CHD risk factors) or preexisting CHD who have a greatly increased risk for a future CHD event and would benefit most from cholesterol reduction. Despite the apparent differences in the two strategies for cholesterol reduction, they should not be viewed as mutually exclusive. In fact, universal screening of adults is a part of both the population and high-risk approaches.[43, 44] Current guidelines for public screening call for referral of persons with elevated cholesterol levels to their health care provider where the high-risk guidelines would then be applied.

The Population Approach

The NCEP Report of the Expert Panel on Population Strategies for Blood Cholesterol Reduction[44] (Population Panel) provides a rationale and guidelines for widespread cholesterol reduction in the United States. The panel concluded that "...changing eating patterns will influence blood cholesterol levels and that eating patterns can be changed, while preserving the nutritional adequacy, variety, and affordability of good tasting food. The panel regards reduction of dietary saturated fats from both animal and vegetable sources as being of greatest importance."

The panel concluded that the eating patterns of Americans can change through a combination of public education and actions by the sectors of society that influence the availability, purchase, preparation, and consumption of foods. The diet recommended by the NCEP for healthy Americans is listed in Table 10.1. These dietary guidelines are considered appropriate for the general population, including healthy women and persons 65 years of age and older. The guidelines also apply to healthy children as they join in the eating patterns of other members of the family (after 2 years of age). To achieve the recommended nutrient intakes, the panel recommended the consumption of foods that contain lower amounts of saturated fatty acids, total fat, and cholesterol. This type of diet should include the choice of a variety of foods to ensure recommended intake of carbohydrates, protein, and other nutrients. Desirable weight should be maintained.

Table 10.1—Diet Recommended for Healthy Americans by the National Cholesterol Education Program

---

- Less than 10% of total calories from saturated fatty acids.
- An average of 30% of total calories or less from all fat.
- Dietary energy levels needed to reach or maintain a desirable body weight.
- Less than 300 mg/dL of cholesterol per day.

Universal Screening of Adults

The NCEP'S Adult Treatment Panel[43] (ATP II) recommended that all adults have their blood cholesterol measured at least once every 5 years. The Population Panel recommended that public screening should be used to supplement screening in the health care setting only under conditions that ensure adherence to high quality standards.[44, 45] These standards include assuring the performance and standardization of cholesterol analyzers, appropriate training and supervision of staff, and providing reliable information about cholesterol levels and dietary practices to lower cholesterol to the screenee. The classification of total cholesterol into three groups—desirable, borderline-high, and high—and the recommended follow-up and referral pattern are shown in Table 10.2. It should be emphasized that public screening is not a substitute for health care and should not be used for monitoring the cholesterol levels of individuals under treatment.

Adult Treatment Panel Guidelines

The NCEP's Expert Panel on Detection, Evaluation, and Treatment of High Blood Cholesterol in Adults[43] (Adult Treatment Panel II [ATP II]) outlined the patient-based high-risk approach to identify individuals who would benefit from intensive intervention efforts. ATP II recommended

Table 10.2—The National Cholesterol Education Program Categories of Total Cholesterol and the Referral Recommendations for Public Screenings

Category (level)	Referral Recommendation
Desirable (total cholesterol <200 mg/dL)	Repeat blood cholesterol measurement within 5 years.
Borderline-high (total cholesterol 200–239 mg/dL)	Refer to physician if patient has a history of CHD[a] or if two or more CHD risk factors are detected by interview. Otherwise, repeat cholesterol measurement within 1 year.
High (total cholesterol ≥240 mg/dL)	Refer patient to physician for follow-up lipoprotein analysis.

[a]CHD indicates coronary heart disease.

that serum total cholesterol and HDL cholesterol be measured in all adults (20 years of age and over) at least once every 5 years and that the measurement may be done in the nonfasting state. The initial phase of case finding is based on total cholesterol and the presence of risk factors for CHD. The cutpoint for high cholesterol (more than 240 mg/dL) corresponds to approximately the 75th percentile of cholesterol levels of the US adult population.

The initial classification of risk then uses a combination of total cholesterol, HDL cholesterol and CHD risk factors to determine the need for follow-up and further evaluation. Because the assessment of LDL cholesterol provides a better measure of risk for CHD than total cholesterol, and other lipoproteins predict future risk and help define therapy, persons at highest risk (known atherosclerosis, family history of premature CHD, or cholesterol disorder, or patients with multiple risk factors) are recommended to undergo a full lipoprotein analysis.

The subsequent classification of patients and therapy is based upon the level of LDL cholesterol calculated from lipoprotein analysis, the lipid disorder identified, and the presence of CHD risk factors. Persons whose risk places them in need of treatment are then recommended dietary therapy. The recommended diets are presented in two "steps." The "Step-One" diet calls for the reduction of the major sources of saturated fatty acids and cholesterol in the diet. Step-One recommends less than 30% of total daily calories be derived from fat, less than 10% be derived from saturated fat, and a total of less than 300 mg of daily

287

cholesterol. This "diet" is consistent with national nutritional recommendations for all Americans. For patients who do not respond adequately to the Step-One diet, the Step-Two diet calls for reducing the intake of saturated fatty acids to less than 7% of total daily calories and cholesterol to less than 200 mg/day. If, after 3 to 6 months of dietary therapy, the goal cholesterol reduction is not achieved, medication may be considered. The specific, detailed guideline report is available elsewhere.[43]

Guidelines for Children and Adolescents

Guideline development for children and adolescents was based on several major factors. First, studies indicate that the process of atherosclerosis begins in childhood and that this process is related to elevated levels of blood cholesterol.[5–8] Second, cholesterol levels in children "track" over time and adolescents with high cholesterol levels are more likely to have high levels as adults.[47] Third, high blood cholesterol aggregates in families as a result of shared environments and genetic factors and children and adolescents with elevated total or LDL cholesterol frequently come from families with a high incidence of CHD.[48, 49] Finally, US children and adolescents have higher blood cholesterol levels and higher intakes of saturated fatty acids

and cholesterol than their counterparts in many other countries.[49] Therefore, the NCEP's Expert Panel on Blood Cholesterol Levels in Children and Adolescents[49] recommended both a population approach and an individualized approach that includes selective screening of children and adolescents. It should be noted, however, that screening children and young adults for high blood cholesterol is controversial.[50, 51]

As with adults, the *population approach* is intended to reduce the average levels of blood cholesterol of children and adolescents through populationwide changes in eating patterns of children over the age of 2 years. The diet is the same as recommended for adults. Because the fast growth of infants and children up to the age of 2 years requires a diet with a higher percentage of calories from fat, the recommendations are not intended for this age range. Toddlers 2 and 3 years of age may safely make the transition to the recommended eating pattern as they begin to eat with the family.

The *individualized approach* is designed to identify and treat children who are at greatest risk of having high blood cholesterol levels as adults and an increased risk of CHD. To accomplish this, selective screening of children and adolescents who have a family history of premature cardiovascular disease or at least one parent with high blood cholesterol is recommended. This screening should be done in the context of regular and continuing health care.

The screening protocol varies according to the reason for screening. For young people screened because of hypercholesterolemia in a parent, the initial test should be total cholesterol. For those tested because of a documented history of premature cardiovascular disease in a parent or grandparent or those with a complex cholesterol disorder in a parent, the initial test should be a lipoprotein analysis because of the high proportion of lipoprotein abnormalities in these children.

As with adults, dietary therapy with the Step-One or Step-Two diet (if necessary) is recommended. Medication therapy should only be considered for children more than 10 to 12 years old if the goal LDL cholesterol is not achieved after evaluating for secondary clinical causes, at least 6 months of dietary therapy, and other needed lifestyle changes.

EXAMPLES OF PUBLIC HEALTH INTERVENTIONS

The major public health intervention to reduce cholesterol levels is the application of NCEP guidelines in the community. In addition, community intervention projects such as the Pawtucket Heart Health Program, the Minnesota Heart Health Program, and the Stanford Five City Project have addressed cardiovascular disease risk factors, including high blood cholesterol (see Chapter 11 on cardiovascular disease).

AREAS OF FUTURE RESEARCH AND DEMONSTRATION

While clinical trials of cholesterol lowering medications have shown that the risk of CHD is lowered by cholesterol reduction, the estimated public health benefit in terms of total event and mortality reduction appears to vary substantially by age, cholesterol level, and presence of other CHD risk factors.[2, 26, 52] Secondary prevention trials have included women and the elderly and have documented benefits for these patients with cholesterol therapy.[36] Further information is needed on the benefits of cholesterol reduction as primary prevention among women, young men, the elderly, and other subgroups, related to mortality and quality of life.

The "optimal" diet in terms of dietary fat composition is being debated.[52] For example, there is interest in the role of diets such as the so-called "Mediterranean" diet, which is high in total fat (30% to 40% of calories) but is associated with low rates of CHD; in this type of diet, the majority of fat intake is from olive oil. Because the adoption of a low fat diet can reduce HDL-cholesterol as well as LDL cholesterol, the potential benefits in terms of risk of CHD may be attenuated. Theoretically, the ideal dietary changes would lower LDL cholesterol while HDL cholesterol is increased or unchanged. Whether diets rich in antioxidants or other micronutrients can offer protection from higher intakes of fats, and which dietary or supplemental antioxidants is the best combination, is also unknown. Studies should test whether antioxidants are enough to protect against CHD despite hyperlipidemia.

It is now known that there is a variety of each type of lipoprotein particle in human serum. Some patients will have inherited disorders that predict the presence of smaller, more dense and atherogenic lipoproteins.[52] The variety of cholesterol disorders, with heterogeneous lipoproteins, needs careful evaluation for absolute predictive risk levels and the success with treatment for these disorders.[52, 53] Other factors, such as dietary intake and the presence of abnormal metabolism, contribute to the oxidation and atherogenicity of lipoproteins. Effective treatment of these disorders needs research.[52] Genetic testing and gene therapy will be important areas of research and development to develop enhanced treatment strategies for high-risk individuals.[53]

Studies on motivating behavior change, both for population and individual levels, are key to further reducing CHD. Much is known about preventing disease; yet, American physicians and the public continue to fail to apply known guidelines into practice. Methods to support improved adherence to lifestyle changes and medical guidelines are sorely needed. Healthcare systems must be reorganized to ensure the delivery of proven preventive strategies and medical therapies.

REFERENCES

1. Kannel WB, Castelli WP, Gordon T, et al. Serum cholesterol, lipoproteins, and the risk of coronary heart disease. *Ann Intern Med*. 1971;74:1–12.
2. Ockene IS, Ockene JK (eds). *Prevention of Coronary Heart Disease*. Boston, Mass: Little Brown & Co, 1992.
3. Stamler J, Wentworth D, Neaton JD, for the MRFIT Research Group. Is the relationship between serum cholesterol and risk of premature death from coronary heart disease continuous and graded? Findings in 356,222 primary screenees of the Multiple Risk Factor Intervention Trial (MRFIT). *JAMA*. 1986;256: 2823–2828.
4. Sempos CT, Cleeman JI, Carroll MD, et al. Prevalence of high

blood cholesterol among US adults: An update based on guidelines from the Second Report of the National Cholesterol Education Program Adult Treatment Panel. *JAMA*. 1993; 269:3009–3014.

5. McGill HC Jr, McMahan CA, Malcom GT, Oalmann MC, Strong JP, for the PDAY Research Group. Effects of serum lipoproteins and smoking on atherosclerosis in young men and women. *Arterioscler Thromb Vasc Biol*. 1997;17:95–107.

6. Fuster V, Badimon L, Badimon JJ, Cheseboro JH. The pathogenesis of coronary artery disease and the acute coronary syndromes (first of two parts). *N Engl J Med*. 1992;326:242–250.

7. Berenson GS, Srinivasan SR, Freedman DS, Radhakrishnamurthy, Dalferes ER. Review: atherosclerosis and its evolution in childhood. *Am J Med Sci*. 1987;294:429–440.

8. Newman WP, Freedman DS, Voors AW, et al. Relation of serum lipoprotein levels and systolic blood pressure to early atherosclerosis. The Bogalusa Heart Study. *N Engl J Med*. 1986;314:138–144.

9. Klag MJ, Ford DE, Mead LA, et al. Serum cholesterol in young men and subsequent cardiovascular disease. *N Engl J Med*. 1993;328:313–318.

10. Solberg LA, Strong JP. Risk factors and atherosclerotic lesions: a review of autopsy studies. *Arteriosclerosis*. 1983; 3:187–198.

11. Little W, Downes T, Applegate R. The underlying coronary lesion in myocardial infarction: implications for coronary arteriography. *Clin Cardiol*. 1991;14:868–874.

12. Brown MS, Goldstein JL. A receptor mediated pathway for cholesterol homeostasis. *Science*. 1986;232:34–47.

13. Steinberg D, Witztum JL. Lipoproteins and atherogenesis. Current concepts. *JAMA*. 1990; 264:3047–3052.

14. Gordon DJ, Rifkind BM. High-density lipoprotein—the clinical implications of recent studies. *N Engl J Med*. 1989;321:1311–1316.

15. Hodis HN, Mack WJ. Triglyceride-rich lipoproteins and the progression of coronary artery disease. *Curr Opin Lipidol*. 1995;6:209–214.

16. Stampfer MJ, Krauss RM, Ma J, et al. A prospective study of triglyceride level, low-density lipoprotein diameter, and risk of myocardial infarction. *JAMA*. 1996;276:882–888.

17. Worth RM, Kato H, Rhoads GG, et al. Epidemiologic studies of CHD and stroke in Japanese men living in Japan, Hawaii, and California: Mortality. *Am J Epidemiol*. 1975;102:481.

18. Johnson CL, Rifkind BM, Sempos CT, et al. Declining serum total cholesterol levels among US adults: The National Health and Nutrition Examination surveys. *JAMA.* 1993;269:3002–3008.

19. Denke MA. Review of human studies evaluating individual dietary responsiveness in patients with hypercholesterolemia. *Am J Clin Nutr.* 1995;62: 471S–477S.

20. Grundy SM, Denke MA. Dietary influences on serum lipids and lipoproteins. *J Lipid Res.* 1990;31: 1149–1172.

21. Krauss RM, Deckelbaum RJ, Fisher EN, et al. Dietary guidelines for healthy American adults: a statement for physicians and health professionals by the Nutrition Committee, American Heart Association. *Circulation.* 1996;94:1795–1800.

22. Stone NJ. Fish consumption, fish oil, lipids, and coronary heart disease. *Circulation.* 1996;94: 2337–2340.

23. Stamler J, Shekelle RB. Dietary cholesterol and human coronary heart disease: the epidemiologic evidence. *Arch Pathology Lab Med.* 1988;113:1032–1040.

24. Ripsin CM, Keenan JM, Jacobs DR, et al. Oat products and lipid lowering: a meta-analysis. *JAMA.* 1992;267:3317–3325.

25. Diaz MN, Frei B, Vita JA, Keaney JF Jr. Antioxidants and athero-sclerotic heart disease. *N Engl J Med.* 1997;337:408–416

26. Stone NJ, Blum CB, Winslow E. *Management of Lipids in Clinical Practice.* Caddo, Okla: Professional Communications, Inc; 1997.

27. Genest J Jr, McNamara JR, Ordovas JM, et al. Lipoprotein cholesterol, apolipoprotein A-I and B and lipoprotein (a) abnormalities in men and premature coronary artery disease. *J Am Coll Cardiol* 1992;19:792-802.

28. Baumgartner RN, Roche AF, Chumlea C, et al. Fatness and fat patterns: Associations with plasma lipids and blood pressures in adults, 18 to 57 years of age. *Am J Epidemiol.* 1987;126: 614–629.

29. Higgins M, Kannel WB, Garrison RJ, et al. Hazards of obesity: The Framingham experience. *Acta Medica Scand.* 1987;723(suppl): 23–26.

30. Haskell W, Taylor H, Wood P, et al. Strenuous physical activity, treadmill exercise test performance and plasma high-density lipoprotein cholesterol: The Lipid Research Clinics Program Prevalence Study. *Circulation.* 1980;62(suppl IV):53–61.

31. Criqui M, Wallace R, Heiss G, et al. Cigarette smoking and plasma high-density lipoprotein cholesterol: The Lipid Research Clinics

Program Prevalence Study. *Circulation.* 1980;62(suppl IV):70–76.

32. Holme I. An analysis of randomized trials evaluating the effect of cholesterol reduction on total mortality and coronary heart disease incidence. *Circulation.* 1990;82:1916–1924.

33. The Lipid Research Clinics Coronary Primary Prevention Trial Results. I. Reduction in incidence of coronary heart disease. *JAMA.* 1984;251:351–364.

34. The Lipid Research Clinics Coronary Primary Prevention Trial Results. II. The relationship of the reduction in incidence of coronary heart disease to cholesterol lowering. *JAMA.* 1984;251:365–374.

35. Frick MH, Elo O, Haapa K, et al. Helsinki Heart Study: primary prevention trial with gemfibrozil in middle aged men with dyslipidemia. Safety of treatment, changes in risk factors, and incidence of coronary heart disease. *N Engl J Med.* 1987; 317:1237–1245.

36. Superko HR, Krauss RM. Coronary artery disease regression: convincing evidence for the benefit of aggressive lipoprotein management. *Circulation* 1994;90:1056–1069.

37. Sheperd J, Cobbe SM, Ford I, et al. Prevention of coronary heart disease with pravastatin in men with hypercholesterolemia. *N Engl J Med* 1995;333:1301–1307.

38. Kane JP, Malloy MJ, Ports TA, et al. Regression of coronary atherosclerosis during treatment of familial hypercholesterolemia with combined drug regimens. *JAMA.* 1990:264:3007–3012.

39. Salonen R, Nyyssonen K, Pokkala E, et al. Kuoppio Atherosclerosis Prevention Study (KAPS): A population-based primary prevention trial of the effects of LDL lowering on atherosclerotic progression in femoral and carotid arteries. *Circulation.* 1995;92:1758–1764.

40. Scandanavian Simvastatin Survival Group. Randomised trial of cholesterol lowering in 4,444 patients with coronary heart disease: The Scandanavian Simvastatin Survival Study (4S). *Lancet.* 1994;344:1383–1389.

41. Furberg CD, Adams HP, Applegate WB, et al for the Asymptomatic Carotid Artery Progression Study (ACAPS) Research Group. Effect of lovastatin on early carotid atherosclerosis and cardiovascular events. *Circulation.* 1994;90:1679–1687.

42. Sacks FM, Pfeffer MA, Moye LA, et al, for the Cholesterol and Recurrent Events Trial Investigators. The effects of pravastatin on coronary events after myocardial infarction in patients with

average cholesterol levels. *N Engl J Med*. 1996;335:1001–1009.

43. Expert Panel on Detection, Evaluation, and Treatment, of High Blood Cholesterol in Adults. Second Report of the National Cholesterol Education Program (NCEP) Expert Panel on detection, evaluation, and treatment of high blood cholesterol in adults (Adult Treatment Panel II). *Circulation*. 1994;89: 1329–1445.

44. National Institutes of Health. *Report of the Expert Panel on Population Strategies for Blood Cholesterol Reduction*. Washington, DC: Dept of Health and Human Services, Public Health Service; November 1990. NIH publication 90-3046.

45. National Institutes of Health. *Recommendations Regarding Public Screening for Measuring Blood Cholesterol*. Washington, DC: Dept of Health and Human Services. Public Health Service; June 1989.NIH publication 89-3045.

46. National Institutes of Health. *Recommendations for Improving Blood Cholesterol Measurement*. Washington, DC: Dept of Health and Human Services, Public Health Service; February 1990. NIH publication 90-2964.

47. Freedman DS, Chear Cl, Srinivasan SR, Webber LS, Berenson GS. Tracking of serum lipids and lipoproteins in children over an 8-year period: The Bogalusa Heart Study. *Prev Med*. 1985;14:203–216.

48. Lauer RM, Lee J, Clarke WR. Factors affecting the relationship between childhood and adult cholesterol levels. The Muscatine Study. *Pediatrics*. 1988;82:309–318.

49. National Institutes of Health. *Report of the Expert Panel on Blood Cholesterol Levels in Children and Adolescents*. Washington, DC: Dept of Health and Human Services, Public Health Service; November 1990. NIH publication 91-2732.

50. Newman TB, Browner WS, Hulley SB. The case against childhood cholesterol screening. *JAMA*. 1990;3039–3043.

51. Cleeman JI, Grundy SM. National Cholesterol Education Program recommendations for cholesterol testing in young adults: a science based approach. *Circulation*. 1997;95:1646–1650.

52. Grundy SM. Small LDL, atherogenic dyslipidemia, and the metabolic syndrome. *Circulation*. 1997;95:1–4.

53. Grundy SM. Cholesterol and coronary heart disease: the 21st century. *Arch Intern Med*. 1997;157:1177–1184.

SUGGESTED READING

Denke MA. Cholesterol-lowering diets: a review of the evidence. *Arch Intern Med.* 1995;155:17–26.

Grundy SM. Cholesterol and coronary heart disease: the 21st century. *Arch Intern Med.* 1997: 1177–1184.

Miller M, Vogel R. *The Practice of Coronary Disease Prevention.* Baltimore, Md: William & Wilkins; 1996.

National Institutes of Health. *Report of the Expert Panel on Blood Cholesterol Levels in Children and Adolescents.* Washington, DC: Dept of Health and Human Services, Public Health Service; November 1990. NIH publication 91-2732.

National Institutes of Health. *Report of the Expert Panel on Population Strategies for Blood Cholesterol Reduction.* Washington, DC: Dept of Health and Human Services, Public Health Service; NIH publication 90-3046.

Report of the Expert Panel on Detection, Evaluation, and Treatment, of High Blood Cholesterol in Adults. National Cholesterol Education Program: second report of the Expert Panel on Detection, Evaluation, and Treatment of High Blood Cholesterol in Adults (Adult Treatment Panel II). *Circulation.* 1994;89: 1329–1445.

Stone NJ, Blum CB, Winslow E. *Management of Lipids in Clinical Practice.* Caddo, Okla: Professional Communications Inc; 1997.

RESOURCE

National Cholesterol Education Program
National Heart, Lung, and Blood Institute
National Institutes of Health
Building 31, Room 4A-21
Bethesda, MD 20892
(301) 496-0554

11

CARDIOVASCULAR DISEASE

ICD-9 390-448

ardiovascular disease (CVD) refers to a wide variety of heart and blood vessel diseases, including coronary heart disease, hypertension, stroke, and rheumatic heart disease. In the United States today, CVD is of paramount public health importance because of its widespread nature and the potential for intervention. Over 57 million Americans have one or more type of CVD.[1] CVD is the leading cause of death and disability in the United States. More than 951 000 Americans died of CVD in 1995, accounting for nearly 41% of all US deaths in that year.[2]

SIGNIFICANCE

Death rates for CVD vary markedly by age, race, and sex.[1] Mortality from CVD is highest among older adults, but, despite much higher CVD rates in older age groups, more than 148 000 Americans under the age of 65 died from CVD in 1995.[2] Although the age-adjusted CVD

Craig J. Newschaffer, PhD
Carol A. Brownson, MSPH
Linda J. Dusenbury, MS, RN

mortality rate for US men in 1995 was 55% higher than for women, CVD is still the leading cause of death in women, and, in fact, more female (60 400) than male (56 700) lives were claimed by CVD in that year. In 1995, the age-adjusted death rates were 326 per 100 000 for Black men, 218 for White men, 210 for Black women, and 125 for White women.[2] Hispanic women have higher age-adjusted death rates for ischemic heart disease than non-Hispanic women but lower stroke mortality rates than non-Hispanic women. Hispanic men have lower mortality rates than non-Hispanic men for both heart disease and stroke. Asian Americans appear to be at lower risk of CVD mortality than Whites, but for Asian Americans, as for Hispanic Americans, African Americans and Whites, CVD causes are the leading contributor to mortality.[3]

Mortality captures only a portion of the health burden imposed by CVD. CVD was responsible for almost 6 million hospitalizations in 1994 and is a leading cause of disability as an estimated 8 million Americans attributed disability to

CVD in 1992.[1] The economic costs of CVD reached an estimated $259 billion in direct and indirect costs in 1997, according to the Centers for Disease Control and Prevention.[4]

CVD mortality rates remain higher in the United States than in many other industrialized nations. When compared with 35 industrialized nations in 1994, the United States ranked 16th (ie, 19 nations were lower) in CVD mortality among both men and women aged 35 through 74. The US mortality rates were roughly midway between the extremely high rates observed in the Russian Federation and Eastern Europe and the low rates observed in Japan, France, Spain, and Switzerland.[1] In the United States, CVD mortality has declined steadily from its peak. Over the last 15 years alone, US age-adjusted mortality rates for the major causes of CVD mortality have dropped approximately 30% (Figure 11.1).[2]

PATHOPHYSIOLOGY

Atherosclerosis, the underlying disease process of the major forms

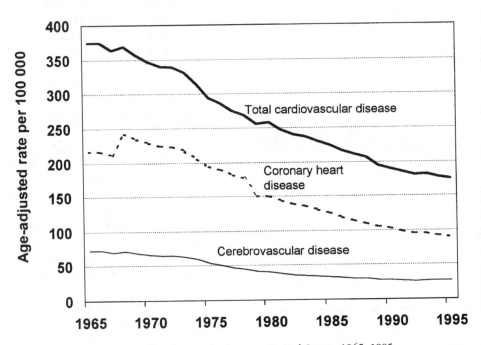

Figure 11.1—Cardiovascular disease death rates, United States, 1965–1995.

of CVD, is a slowly progressive condition in which the inner layers of the artery walls become thick, irregular, and rigid. The process is complex, with contributing factors including deposition of fat and cholesterol, migration and proliferation of smooth muscle cells, and formation of raised fibrous lesions. With the progression of atherosclerosis, the arteries narrow, the blood flow is decreased, and there is greater likelihood that the built-up material, or plaque, will disrupt, creating a traveling blood clot (or embolism). (See also Chapter 10 on cholesterol).

CVD is usually manifested clinically in middle age or later, but atherosclerosis begins in childhood. Atherosclerosis is associated with several modifiable risk factors including those well known as risk factors for CVD: high blood cholesterol, high blood pressure, cigarette smoking, physical inactivity, diabetes, and obesity.[5] The advent of noninvasive means of evaluating atherosclerosis has fostered the epidemiologic study of asymptomatic CVD. Control of modifiable risk factors, at both the population and individual levels, remains the key to primary and secondary prevention of CVD.

Stroke and coronary heart disease, the two forms of CVD making the greatest direct contribution to mortality, share the underlying mechanism

of atherosclerosis, but they are not influenced equally by the many known CVD risk factors. Coronary heart disease is rarely found in populations without elevated cholesterol. In contrast, stroke is a disease most strongly associated with high blood pressure with less contribution coming from cholesterol and other risk factors. This chapter provides a detailed discussion of the two major forms of CVD, coronary heart disease and stroke.

CORONARY HEART DISEASE
ICD-9 410-414, 429.2

SIGNIFICANCE

Coronary heart disease (CHD) is the leading cause of death in the United States today, accounting for nearly 480 000 deaths in 1995. CHD represents over half (51%) of the cardiovascular disease deaths and over one-fifth (21%) of the deaths from all causes.[2] Each year there are more than 1.5 million new or recurrent heart attacks. The American Heart Association estimates that over 13 million Americans alive today have a history of CHD. Over 2 million hospital admissions each year involve diagnoses of CHD, and the costs associated with medical care, lost earnings, and lost productivity due to CHD were estimated at $90.9 billion for 1997.[1]

PATHOPHYSIOLOGY

Coronary heart disease, also called ischemic heart disease or coronary artery disease, is a term used to identify several disorders that reduce the blood supply to the heart muscle. This impairment of circulation to the heart is most frequently the result of narrowing of the coronary arteries by atherosclerosis. The onset, and much of the progression, of atherosclerosis is subclinical (ie, without symptoms) with the most common emergent clinical manifestations of coronary atherosclerosis being angina pectoris (chest pain), myocardial infarction (heart attack), and sudden death. Historically, CHD epidemiology has been dependent on studies of these clinical manifestations as endpoints. However, the incorporation of new technologies into epidemiologic investigations, such as the B-mode ultrasound of the carotid arteries used in the Atherosclerosis Risk Factors in Communities (ARIC) studies, is allowing for new insights about risk factors for early-stage CHD. Those implicated through these studies thus far include traditional CHD risk factors as well as genetic changes at the cellular level, infectious agents, micronutrients, and hemostatic factors.[6-10]

DESCRIPTIVE EPIDEMIOLOGY

High-Risk Groups

Throughout life, men have much higher CHD mortality rates than women. Overall, the age-adjusted death rate for CHD in the United States is more than twice as high for men as it is for women. Yet, in women, CHD is still the single greatest mortality risk, with the age-adjusted mortality rate three times greater than that for breast cancer.[2]

CHD risk increases with age independent of known CHD risk factors. Approximately 55% of all heart attacks occur in people aged 65 or older and 85% of the people who die of heart attacks are over age 65.[1] CHD is the leading cause of death for men and women over 65 years of age and the second leading cause of disability in older men and women.[11] For men, major increases in CHD begin in the 35- to 44-year age group. For women, the marked increase is delayed until after menopause. Subclinical CHD is more prevalent in older than in younger individuals and has been shown to be associated with the same risk factors linked to clinical disease at younger ages, thereby suggesting that risk factor modification in older individuals may still be a very cost-effective public health strategy.[11]

For men and women combined, CHD death rates are higher among

Blacks than Whites until advanced age, at which point they are higher among Whites. Black men experience a slightly higher death rate from CHD than White men. In 1995, the age-adjusted death rate for White men was 124 per 100 000 compared with 133 per 100 000 for Black men. It is the difference in female death rates that accounts for the bulk of the discrepancy in CHD mortality between Blacks and Whites. With a rate of 81.6 CHD deaths per 100 000 in 1995, Black women die at 1.35 times the rate of White women.[2]

Although national data on CHD mortality among Americans of Hispanic origin are limited, existing data suggest that their age-adjusted CHD death rates are comparable to those of non-Hispanics among women and slightly (just 6%) lower among men. Americans of Asian and Pacific Island origin have age-adjusted CHD mortality rates approximately half that of White Americans.[3]

A family history of premature CHD increases the risk of CHD. The clustering of CHD in families is not fully understood but is believed to be a combination of genetics and higher levels of risk factors within these families (eg, similar dietary patterns).

CHD incidence and mortality rates are higher among people of lower socioeconomic status than among those in the middle or upper classes.[12] The greatest declines in CHD mortality over time among White men and women in the United States have been among those with the highest levels of income and education and among workers in white-collar jobs.[13,14] Not surprisingly, the gradient of CHD mortality associated with socioeconomic status is similar to the gradient of risk factors; for example, cigarette smoking, obesity, and high blood pressure are more common among people with lower income and education levels.[12] However, neighborhood socioeconomic status effects may persist above those related to differing distributions of individual level risk factors. Complex interaction between individual- and neighborhood-level socioeconomic status on CHD risk factors in African American men has been documented. For example, lower individual socioeconomic status in higher average socioeconomic neighborhoods correlated with certain adverse CHD risk factor profiles as did higher socioeconomic status in more deprived neighborhoods.[15]

Geographic Distribution

In the United States, CHD death rates are highest in New York, Michigan, and most Ohio and Mississippi River states while lowest in most southwestern states. In 1993, the age-adjusted death rates varied from a high of 135.9 per 100 000 in New York to a low of 54.2 per 100 000 in New Mexico.[1] The CHD death rate for the United States is approximately midway between those of other industrialized countries. A World Health Organization study of CHD deaths rates from 1985 showed extremely high rates in the United Kingdom, Ireland, and some of the Nordic and eastern European countries. Low rates were noted in certain southern European countries, France, and Japan. In the countries studied, the highest CHD death rate was as much as 10 times the lowest rate.[16]

Time Trends

CHD has been the leading cause of death in the United States for most of this century, with death rates from CHD peaking in 1963. Since 1968, the decline in CHD mortality has been consistent and nearly uniform across race and sex groups. The decline is steeper in younger than in older age groups.[17] By 1995, the age-adjusted mortality rate for CHD was 90 per 100 000, representing a decline of about 63% since 1968 (see Figure 11.1)[2, 17] In recent years, the rate of decline in CHD deaths has slowed somewhat among Black men and women and White women but not among White men.[18] The decline in CHD mortality is not fully under-stood, but changes in lifestyle, reductions in risk factor prevalence, and improvements in medical care and treatment of CHD are thought to have contributed.[19] A statistical model drawing on data from a variety of sources in the published medical literature estimated that about one-quarter of the decline in CHD mortality from 1980 to 1990 can be attributed to primary prevention with the majority attributable to treatment and risk factor reduction among those diagnosed with CHD.[20] Population follow-up in the Twin Cities area found that CHD risk factor profiles improved from the mid-1980s through the mid-1990s. Further, in-hospital CHD mortality during this period declined dramatically. Approximately 25% of the decrease in 28-day hospital CHD mortality was estimated to be attributable to increased use of thrombolytic (or "clot bursting") therapy for myocardial infarction patients.[21]

RISK FACTORS

Coronary risk factors can be classified as either modifiable or nonmodifiable. Among modifiable risk factors, the major independent risk factors for CHD are high blood pressure, elevated blood cholesterol, cigarette smoking, and physical inactivity. Other modifiable risk factors include diabetes, obesity, elevated blood homocysteine, dietary factors, and environmental tobacco smoke. Alcohol use and stress may also contribute to CHD risk. Nonmodifiable risk factors are discussed under the previous heading of high-risk groups. Note, however, that not all high-risk groups are defined by nonmodifiable factors. Improved socioeconomic status, for example, while not typically a direct goal of medical or public health intervention, certainly is a legitimate objective for social and economic policy.

Magnitude of Risk Factors

High blood pressure, or hypertension, is a strong independent risk factor for morbidity and mortality from CHD.[22] Hypertension is a condition in which blood pressure is persistently elevated above levels that are considered desirable: systolic blood pressure ≥140 mm Hg and/or diastolic blood pressure ≥90 mm Hg.[23] Using that conventional

Table 11.1—Modifiable Risk Factors for Coronary Heart Disease, United States

Magnitude	Risk Factor	Best Estimate (%) of Population Attributable Risk (Range)
Strong (relative risk >4)	None	—
Moderate (relative risk 2–4)	High blood pressure (≥140/90 mm Hg)	25 (20–29)
	Cigarette smoking	22 (17–25)
	Elevated cholesterol (≥200 mg/dL)	43 (39–47)
	Diabetes (fasting glucose ≥140 mg/dL)	8 (1–15)
Weak (relative risk <2)	Obesity[a]	17 (7–32)
	Physical inactivity	35 (23–46)
	Environmental tobacco smoke exposure	18 (8–23)
Possible	Psychological factors	—
	Alcohol use[b]	
	Elevated plasma homocysteine	—
	Infectious agents	—

[a]Based on body mass index >27.8 kg/m^2 for men and >27.3 kg/m^2 for women.
[b]Moderate to heavy alcohol use may increase risk, whereas light use may reduce risk.
Note. Data compiled from references 30–32, 58, and 75–78.

definition, and including people who are taking antihypertensive medication, the American Heart Association estimates that high blood pressure afflicts nearly one-fourth of the adult population.[1] People with elevated blood pressure are 2 to 4 times as susceptible to CHD as are people with normal blood pressure (Table 11.1).[12] However, it is important to note that risk of CHD generally increases as levels of systolic or diastolic blood pressure rise whether or not one is looking at a population group above or below a particular hypertension cutpoint. Therefore, blood pressure reduction by individuals labeled "normotensive" by conventional definitions can also be beneficial. Studies suggest that a prolonged reduction of only 5 to 6 mm Hg in diastolic blood pressure results in a 20% to 25% reduction in CHD.[24] Although drug therapy to reduce high blood pressure has resulted in lower overall rates of cardiovascular disease deaths, major studies of drug treatment for high blood pressure have failed to demonstrate a reduction in CHD deaths, possibly as a result of the untoward effects of antihypertensive therapy on other risk factors.[25] (High blood pressure is discussed in greater detail in Chapter 9.).

Cigarette smoking is a major cause of CHD among both men and women. Smokers have twice the risk of heart attack as nonsmokers.

Smoking is also the major risk factor for sudden death from heart attack, with smokers having 2 to 4 times the risk of nonsmokers. The risk increases with the number of cigarettes smoked.[26]

An estimated 23% of women and 27% of men in the United States smoke cigarettes.[27] Overall, cigarette smokers have CHD death rates 70% higher than those of nonsmokers, with heavy smokers (ie, two or more packs per day) dying from CHD at a rate 2 to 3 times that of nonsmokers. Studies have shown, however, that people who stop smoking experience a rapid and substantial reduction in CHD mortality. For people who have smoked a pack or less per day, within 10 years of quitting, death rates from CHD drop to the level of people who have never smoked.[26]

In addition, growing evidence suggests that exposure to environmental tobacco smoke (also called passive smoking or secondhand smoke) increases the risk of CHD.[28,29] Follow-up of a very large group of never-smoking US women showed that those with regular exposure to passive smoke at home or at work had a 90% increased risk of developing CHD compared to those unexposed.[30] Furthermore, arteriography of nonsmoking women with CHD found the actual number of stenotic arteries to be correlated with the amount of passive smoke exposure from husbands[31] and, in a population-based sample, environmental tobacco smoke exposure increased the risk of atherosclerosis progression (measured by ultrasound) approximately 20%.[32] The emerging association of environmental tobacco smoke exposure and the number one cause of death is elevating the importance of this critical public health issue to new heights.

Cholesterol is the blood lipid most strongly associated with CHD. The risk of CHD increases steadily as blood cholesterol levels in a population increase. Blood cholesterol levels below 200 mg/dL in middle-aged adults seem to confer low risk for CHD.[33] At levels of 240 mg/dL and over, the risk approximately doubles.[34] More than half of all adults have total cholesterol levels of 200 mg/dL or greater, and about one in four has blood cholesterol levels of 240 mg/dL or greater.[35, 36] Most excess CHD occurs among people with levels of 220 to 310 mg/dL.[33] For people with cholesterol levels in the 250 to 300 mg/dL range, each 1% reduction in cholesterol level results in about a 2% reduction in CHD morbidity and mortality.[35]

Cholesterol is transported in the blood by low-density lipoproteins (LDL), very–low density lipoproteins (VLDL), and high-density lipoproteins (HDL); 60% to 70% of the total serum cholesterol is contained in the LDL.[37] High levels of LDL are a leading factor in the progression of atherosclerosis and in the subsequent development of CHD.[33,37] Even those particles categorized as LDL differ greatly in size and density, and recent work has shown that development of a greater frequency of smaller LDL particles precedes the onset of clinical CHD by several years.[38] The VLDL, which are composed primarily of triglyceride, comprise 10% to 15% of the total serum cholesterol. Evidence supporting the association between elevated blood triglyceride and CHD has been mounting in recent years.[39]

The level of HDL is inversely related to CHD; the lower the level of HDL, the higher the risk of CHD, particularly at levels below 35 mg/dL.[37,40] The ratio of total cholesterol to HDL is also used as a predictor of CHD. The optimal ratio for low CHD risk is considered to be less than 3.5.[41] HDL level correlates inversely with LDL size and triglyceride level, and this coupled with the complex metabolic interrelationships of these particles makes it more difficult to separate the independent contributions of various lipids to CHD. It is quite possible that all play a role; one hypothesis is that LDL may be more important in early-stage atherogenesis, while low HDL and triglyceride elevation develops closer to the clinical onset of CHD.[42] (For more information on cholesterol, refer to Chapter 10.)

Another plasma constituent, homocysteine, is receiving increased attention as a potentially modifiable risk factor for acute CHD events. Plasma homocysteine levels have been found to be positively associated with risk of CHD events[43,44] and, although homocysteine level tends to correlate with a poor CHD risk factor profile,[45] there is evidence that there is an independent effect.[46] Molecular epidemiology studies, however, have not been clear-cut. About half the individuals with certain inborn metabolic errors leading to extremely high homocysteine levels have strokes before the age of 30.[47] Yet, those with other genetic defects associated with moderately high homocysteine levels, about equal to "high" levels in the general population, have not been shown to be at increased risk for CHD events.[48] Nonetheless, since dietary intake of folic acid, vitamin B12 and, perhaps, B6 correlate with lower homocysteine levels in normal populations[49] and since pharmacologic doses of folic acid have been shown to lower homocysteine levels,[50] there is intense interest in completing our understanding of the potential role of homocysteine in CHD.

Although the underlying mechanisms relating diabetes and CHD are still not well understood, diabetes mellitus is generally considered a major CHD risk factor. Diabetes affects about 6% of the adult population in America.[51] It has been diagnosed in more than 10 million persons, and an additional 5 million are suspected to have undiagnosed diabetes.[52] CHD is the most common cause of morbidity and mortality among people with diabetes and individuals with diabetes experience CHD rates 2 to 4 times higher than those without the disease.[51] CHD risk among people with diabetes is higher for women than men, in part because of a greater prevalence of obesity among women.[51] In general, the manifestations and outcomes of coronary events are more severe and more lethal among people with diabetes than among others of the same age.[53] (Refer to Chapter 14 for additional information on the epidemiology and control of diabetes.)

Obesity has widely been defined as a body weight greater than 120% of desirable weight for height.[54] Another measure of overweight commonly used in the United States is body mass index, which is a ratio of weight to height (kg/m^2). A body mass index greater than 27.8 in men or 27.3 in women indicates overweight.[55] By either criterion the prevalence of overweight in the United States has risen dramatically since the early 1970s. Twenty-five years ago one in four Americans were overweight. Today a striking one in three Americans are overweight.[56, 57] Poverty is related to obesity in women, and obesity is more common among minority populations, especially women.[58]

Death due to CHD is associated with obesity at the upper range of body weight; that is, a relative weight of 140% or greater or a body mass index greater than or equal to 30.[41,53] In men and women under age 50, relative weight of 130% or greater is associated with twofold increases in the risk of developing CHD.[59] Obesity is associated other CHD risk factors. For example, the prevalence of high blood pressure and diabetes is 3 times higher among overweight people than among those of normal body weight.[54] Obesity is also associated with higher levels of total blood cholesterol as well as LDL and lower levels of HDL.[53, 57] The indirect CHD risk from obesity mediated by these other risk factors is substantive and, at higher levels of overweight, increased obesity risk has been shown even after adjusting for these factors.[59] At moderate levels, the indirect effects no doubt persist, but direct effects are less certain. Although the health effects of long-term weight loss have proven difficult to study, there is some evidence of reduced cardiovascular mortality among overweight individuals with obesity-related problems like hypertension who intentionally lose weight.[60]

Recent studies suggest that the distribution of fat deposits on the body may also affect CHD risk.

Upper body or abdominal fat ("central obesity" "apple shape") appears to increase risk more than lower body fat (pear shape). Men and women in the upper quintile of subscapular skin fold as well as men with a waist-to-hip ratio greater than 1.0 and women with a ratio greater than 0.8 experience increased CHD risk.[53,54,61] The tendency toward abdominal disposition of body fat seems to increase CHD risk across all levels of BMI.[62]

Physical inactivity is increasingly recognized as a major risk factor for CHD. More than 60% of US adults do not engage in the recommended amount of physical activity with one-quarter being completely sedentary.[63] Physical activity decreases body weight, decreases blood pressure, and improves insulin sensitivity.[63] (Refer to Chapter 7 for additional information on the epidemiology and control of physical inactivity.) Mounting evidence suggests that small amounts of physical activity can also have a significant impact on heart disease mortality.[64,65] The greatest benefits appear to occur with the move from a completely sedentary life-style to very modest levels of activity.

Moderate to heavy alcohol consumption is known to raise blood pressure levels and to increase CHD mortality. However, in most studies, including several recent investigations,[66–68] light regular drinking (two or fewer drinks per day) has been associated with modest reductions in CHD risk. The principal pathway for this protection appears to be through increased HDL cholesterol.[69] The relationship to other risk factors and the social consequences of alcohol use, however, preclude any public health recommendation for alcohol use (see Chapter 6).

Psychological factors and stress also have been studied in relation to the development of CHD.[70, 71] Perhaps the most widely studied is the Type A behavior pattern, characterized by excessive competitiveness, hostility, impatience, fast speech, and quick motor movements.[72] Considerable

attention has been devoted to the exploration of specific psychological factors, including anger, job stress, anxiety, and social support. Causal connections between these specific psychological risk factors and CHD have yet to be clearly established, but evidence supporting a causal role for anger, both as an event trigger and a long-term risk factor, and social support, particularly important in extending survival among those with disease, is mounting.[71,73]

Lastly, risk factors for heart disease tend to cluster; that is, individuals with CHD are likely to have more than one risk factor. The greater the level of any single risk factor, the

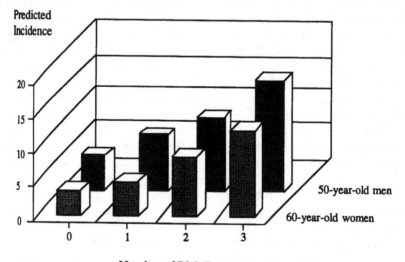

Number of Risk Factors

Figure 11.2—Predicted coronary heart disease incidence (8-year risk per 1000) by number of risk factors, Framingham, Massachusetts.[74] Risk factors defined as cholesterol 200–239 md/dL; systolic blood pressure ≥140 mm Hg; current cigarette smoking.

greater the chance of developing CHD. Moreover, the likelihood of developing CHD increases markedly when risk factors manifest simultaneously. There is at least an additive contribution to CHD risk for the major risk factors of high blood pressure, smoking, and high cholesterol, as evident in the findings of the Framingham study (Figure 11.2).[74-79]

Population-Attributable Risk

CHD is a multifactorial disease, and precisely quantifying the contribution of each risk factor to overall heart disease is difficult. We can, however, roughly gauge the importance of risk factors by estimating population-attributable risk, which is the percentage of CHD that could be prevented by eliminating a particular risk factor in the population. There are several things that need to be remembered when considering population-attributable risks, the two most important being that (1) when there are many factors contributing to a disease, as is the case with CHD, these percentages will sum to more than 100%; and (2) when risk factors are continuous, like blood pressure or cholesterol level, the population-attributable risk estimated depends greatly on the cut-point chosen to designate who is at high risk. Table 11.1 shows the proportion of CHD mortality that can be attributed to the risk factors discussed above.

PREVENTION AND CONTROL MEASURES

Prevention

Because of the multiple risk factors involved in coronary heart disease, modest changes in one or more risk factors can have a large public health impact. Primary prevention of CHD involves controlling the major preventable risk factors: hypertension, high blood cholesterol, tobacco use, diet and physical inactivity (see Chapters 5, 7, 8, 9, and 10). Other effective methods of prevention include diabetes control, weight management, and limitations in alcohol consumption.

The multifactorial nature of CHD etiology calls for multiple intervention strategies. In addition to the early detection and control of risk factors in adults, prevention approaches may include early and systematic health education regarding the importance of lifestyle behaviors in young people, such as cigarette smoking, diet, and physical activity. Other prevention interventions can include policy-related or environmental changes such as improved food choices in schools, improved food labeling in grocery stores, elimination of cigarette vending machines, and provision of smoke-free environments. (The multifaceted approach to risk reduction is discussed in Chapter 4 on intervention strategies.)

When considering prevention strategies, it is also important to recognize that CHD is affected by the social and economic characteristics of a community, including levels of income and education and occupations. Positive changes in public health are, therefore, often the result of general social and economic development policies, rather than public health policies per se.[13]

Screening and Early Detection

The principal methods of early detection for CHD include screening for high blood pressure (see Chapter 9) and for elevated serum cholesterol (see Chapter 10) and assessing behavioral factors such as tobacco use, dietary fat intake, and physical activity level.

Routine screening for diabetes among the general adult population is not recommended.[54] The American Diabetes Association recommends screening only people at risk for having or developing diabetes, pregnant women, and people with possible complications or symptoms of diabetes. The preferred test is a fasting plasma glucose test.[80]

Screening electrocardiograms are not recommended for the general population but may be appropriate for individuals at increased risk of CHD. This group includes men over 40 with two or more CHD risk factors, high-risk sedentary men planning to begin an exercise program, and people who would endanger the safety of others if they were to experience sudden cardiac events.[54]

Treatment, Rehabilitation, and Recovery

Advances in the treatment of CHD have contributed substantially to major reductions in mortality over the past 3 decades. Hospital coronary care units, coronary artery bypass graft surgery, percutaneous transluminal coronary angioplasty (also called balloon angioplasty), coronary stenting, thrombolytic therapy, new lipid-lowering medications, and out-of-hospital emergency response teams have revolutionized the treatment of CHD. Treatment can involve medical therapy, interventional cardiology, or, most typically, some combination of these. The total number of interventional cardiology procedures performed in the United States have been increasing through the early 1990s, driven largely by increases in coronary stenting, a moderately invasive approach to opening clogged coronary arteries that is more resistant to reclosing than other equally invasive procedures.[81] Finally, cardiac rehabilitation— prevention of CHD complications through diet, exercise, weight control, and smoking cessation--has reduced mortality and improved functional capacity and quality of life among patients with clinical CHD.[82]

EXAMPLES OF PUBLIC HEALTH INTERVENTIONS

Two major primary prevention strategies have been used in attempts to reduce cardiovascular mortality rates: the high-risk and the community-based (or population-based) approaches. The high-risk approach aims to identify high-risk individuals through population screening and to refer them for treatment. The Oslo Heart Study,[83] the Multiple Risk Factor Intervention Trial,[84] the European Collaborative Trial of Multifactorial Prevention of Coronary Heart Disease,[85] and the Lipid Research Clinics Coronary Primary Prevention Trial,[86] are examples of this approach.

The community-based approach aims to reduce cardiovascular disease by changing behaviors and/or policies in whole populations. This is a relatively new concept that is based on the principles of community organization. The idea is to involve communities in the development and implementation of programs or interventions.

The oldest community-based cardiovascular disease prevention program is the North Karelia (Finland) Project, which began in 1972 and provided a broad range of risk factor interventions. Those targeted at individuals and groups included smoking cessation programs, nutrition education aimed at housewives, and the use of natural helper networks. At the community level, interventions were directed at the media and at food producers and distributors. Physicians and community nurses played a key role in providing both clinical services and health education. Combined, these efforts resulted in reduced heart disease morbidity and mortality in North Karelia.[87]

Subsequently, the National Heart, Lung, and Blood Institute (NHLBI) funded four sites for major research and demonstration field trials: the Stanford (California) Three Community Study, the Stanford Five-City Project, the Minnesota Heart Health Program, and the Pawtucket (Rhode Island) Heart Health Program. The Three Community Study, funded in 1971, investigated the influence of a large-scale media intervention on health behavior. Evaluation showed the use of media to be effective and the addition of face-to-face intervention even more powerful in producing behavior changes.[88, 89]

In the Five-City Project, funded from 1978 through 1992, two treatment and two control cities were compared for changes in knowledge and changes in risk factors. The 5-year intervention was based on social learning theory, a communication-behavior change model, community organization principles, and social marketing methods. The treatment cities received 26 hours of exposure to general education and specific risk factor campaigns, resulting in increased knowledge and a reduction of CHD risk factors.[90]

In 1980, the Minnesota Heart Health Program was initiated by the University of Minnesota. The program combined community organization, cardiovascular disease risk factor screening and counseling, smoking cessation contests, physical activity promotion, mass media campaigns, and other interventions to reduce heart disease risk factors in three communities in Minnesota and North Dakota.[91]

The Pawtucket Heart Health Program, funded for 11 years beginning in 1980, was based on community psychology principles. A cornerstone of this program's approach was the use of volunteers. The intervention strategy involved mobilizing the community and involving them in all aspects of the program.[92, 93]

Largely because of a strong favorable but unanticipated secular trend in CHD risk factors in control communities, these interventions tended to have less power to demonstrate overall effectiveness at the community level than originally anticipated. However, within each intervention program individual components frequently were shown to be successful in analyses of intermediate or process outcomes as well as in analyses of principal endpoints that were limited to

subpopulations most likely to be exposed to the component (eg, school children participating in school-based components of community interventions).[94] A recent review of 50 published analyses of particular components from the above-mentioned major community-based CVD intervention program all showed positive findings on CVD risk factors.[94] While there is no doubt a greater chance that studies demonstrating effectiveness get published than those that do not, it seems reasonable to conclude that the major community-based interventions have provided valuable lessons on effective mechanisms for population-based CVD prevention and control.

From the Stanford projects, the utility of channel-specific interventions (eg, worksite exercise challenges etc.) to maximize reach and change behavior became evident.[95] In addition, interventionists learned that they needed to work within the formal political and institutional structure and the informal opinion leadership network. In some instances, community members need to be mobilized to modify the formal rules and regulations of a community to implement and maintain changes in risk factors.[96] In Minnesota, it was apparent that changes in different outcomes (eg, knowledge, behavior changes) necessitated different targeted strategies. For example, awareness was most influenced by general community events—fun walks, health fairs etc. for older persons and women. Similar to the experience of the Stanford study, specific settings such as work sites yielded better behavior change results than general community settings.[95] The most cost-effective efforts were those done in existing community channels: schools, work sites, etc. where participants spend considerable time. The need to institutionalize these competitions and programs with limited resources and staff time from service providers was an ongoing issue.[95] Finally, Pawtucket investigators found it useful and important not only to establish formal, continuing relationships with community organizations already providing CVD risk reduction services but also to establish and maintain positive working relationships with community organizations that did not ordinarily view themselves as having a role in CVD risk reductions (eg, places of worship). Leaders in these sites needed to buy in and be actively involved in planning and implementation for greatest participation to be realized.[95]

Since the NHLBI demonstrations, smaller-scale efforts have been undertaken at other sites. One is the New York State Healthy Heart Program, an effort based on community wide strategies for influencing risk behaviors developed and tested in the major NHLBI studies. The challenge has been to apply these strategies on a limited budget for hard-to-affect populations. The eight programs in high-risk communities are sponsored and coordinated by the New York State Department of Health through its Mary Lasker Heart and Hypertension Institute.[97]

Also employing some of the methods and lessons learned from the early NHLBI projects, the Centers for Disease Control and Prevention joined with states and other agencies to fund other community-based intervention programs, including the South Carolina Cardiovascular Disease Prevention Project,[98] the Bootheel Heart Health Project,[99] the Bemidji (Minnesota) Cardiovascular Disease Prevention Project, a collaborative project with the Indian Health Service,[100] and several projects using their Planned Approach to Community Health.[101]

In sum, there were numerous insights gained from these pioneering community CVD prevention interventions, relating to the following: using mass media effectively, building on existing settings/institutions, creating strategies for making a healthy heart lifestyle "doable"; developing approaches to support environmental as well as legislative and policy changes; and establishing and maintaining community coalitions. One of the most important common threads in the truly exemplary prevention and control programs was their reliance on multiple channels and multiple levels. This strategy appears to be critical in effecting lasting change. A model exemplifying this approach is the Multi-level Approach to Community Health (MATCH) model.[102] Under the model, the four specific channels suggested are work sites, schools, health care, and community sites. Interventions can be directed to the individual, organizational, or policy level in any of these sites. Table 11.2 gives an example of an organizational-level MATCH intervention in the "school" channel. Other, multi-level models that appear to be successful include the Spectrum of Prevention, used successfully in California for its tobacco control program, and the social ecology approach being used in other countries, such as Australia.

Public health leaders are now approaching consensus on high yield strategies to help change social/community norms regarding other critical CHD risk factors, including physical activity and nutrition. As these strategies are tested and refined, various experts are recommending that they be implemented through the population-based approach like MATCH.[103–107] However, as these are begun, individual and organizational practice efforts should also be launched as complements to changing community norms. Specific counseling and skill building approaches delivered by influential leaders including physicians, nurse practitioners, physician assistants, and other health care

Table 11.2 — Example of an Organizational-level MATCH Intervention in the "School" Channel: "Organizational Change for School Lunch Modifications for Cardiovascular Health."

Intervention objectives:	*Policy:* Adopt "Go for Health" program, establish and distribute policy supporting lower fat and sodium diets for children authorizing changes in school food service menus, food purchasing, and food preparation practices.
Targets of intervention:	*Policy makers:* School superintendent, food service director, school principals.
	Staff: School food service workers, cafeteria managers.
Intervention approaches:	*Policy:* Consulting to policy makers.
	Practice: Training of staff

Note. Adapted from Simons-Morton DG et al.[103]

providers can assist and motivate individuals to change their behavior.

AREAS OF FUTURE RESEARCH AND DEMONSTRATION

Epidemiologic research on CHD will likely focus on emerging, yet not completely understood, modifiable factors, like plasma homocysteine, as well as known, but complex, risk factors like serum cholesterol. Studies focusing on subclinical endpoints will be important in revealing undiscovered risk factors potentially significant in primary prevention. For example, further exploration of the importance of infection and inflammation in increasing the risk of atherosclerosis may prove fruitful. Population-based studies devising novel means of using information on known risk factors, like a recently proposed algorithm to improve decision rules for medical treatment of hypercholesterolemia,[108] may also be crucial to advancing secondary prevention strategies.

There is also growing interest and recognition of the importance of conducting more research and demonstration efforts involving policy and environmental approaches to reduce CHD risk factors. Partnerships with nontraditional partners will be essential for success. Population-based prevention research should focus on CHD re-search in special populations such as women, children, older adults, and racial and ethnic minorities, addressing the applicability of current knowledge to these populations and designing population-specific interventions. Finally, despite the huge potential for public health benefits, CHD control efforts have been modest at many state and local health department levels. Both levels need to have an infusion of resources and expertise to build capacity and expand activities in CHD control.

CEREBROVASCULAR DISEASE
ICD-9 430-438

SIGNIFICANCE

Cerebrovascular disease is the third leading cause of death in the United States, accounting for 157 991 deaths in 1995. It represents over one-sixth of all cardiovascular disease deaths and 7% of deaths from all causes.[2] The most severe clinical manifestation of CVD is stroke, with transient ischemic attacks (TIA) comprising a generally less-severe clinically apparent manifestation of CVD. In addition, subclinical or "silent" stroke is quite prevalent. Stroke is also a major cause of morbidity, with an estimated 500 000 Americans suffering strokes each year. Nearly 4 million Americans are survivors of stroke, and many are disabled as a result. In 1992, over 1 million Americans age 15 and older had disabilities resulting from stroke.[1] Stroke-associated societal costs, including costs of medical care and lost productivity, were estimated to exceed $40 billion in 1997 alone.[1]

PATHOPHYSIOLOGY

Stroke includes a group of diseases that affect the arteries of the central nervous system. Stroke results when an artery in the brain is either ruptured or clogged by a blood clot (thrombus), a wandering clot (embolus), or atherosclerotic plaque. Nerve cells in the affected part of the brain die within minutes, often resulting in neurologic impairment.

Cerebral thrombosis and cerebral embolism, referred to as ischemic stroke, account for 70% to 80% of strokes in the United States.[34] The most common stroke is cerebral thrombosis, which is caused when a blood clot forms and blocks blood flow in the cerebral artery. This is generally the result of atherosclerosis in the cerebral vessels. Cerebral embolism occurs when a clot breaks loose from another part of the body, often the heart, and lodges in a cerebral artery. TIAs are distinguished from ischemic stroke by the short-term nature of their symptoms. Over 75% of TIAs are believed to last less than 5 minutes, but, by

definition, they can last up to an hour. These attacks are "transient" because the blockage of the affected cerebral artery is only temporary, with the thrombus or embolus quickly dislodging, allowing restored blood flow.[34] Typically, a TIA does not result in lasting nuerologic impairment.

Cerebral hemorrhage is the other principal cause of stroke. It is the result of a ruptured blood vessel that bleeds into the brain tissue (intracerebral hemorrhage) or into the space between the brain and the skull (subarachnoid hemorrhage). Cerebral hemorrhage accounts for about 17% of all strokes.[34]

DESCRIPTIVE EPIDEMIOLOGY

High-Risk Groups

The incidence of stroke is strongly related to age. Only about 28% of stroke victims are under age 65. After age 55, the rate of stroke incidence doubles in each successive decade.[1] Stroke mortality also increases sharply with age. In 1995, the stroke death rate ranged from 46 per 100 000 in 55- to 64-year-olds to 1637 per 100 000 in people 85 years old and older.[2]

Differences in stroke mortality between Blacks and Whites in the United States are marked. Overall age-adjusted rates are over 80% higher among Blacks than Whites.[2] The ratios are greatest for men under

65 years of age and women under 45 years of age where the death rate among similar aged Blacks is over 3 times that of Whites.[2] Men in general have about a 17% higher age-adjusted stroke mortality rate than women.[2] This difference is slightly greater under age 65.

In the United States, men of Hispanic origin have a 10% lower rate of stroke death and women of Hispanic origin a 5% lower rate of stroke death than their White counterparts.[3] The stroke death rates among Asian Americans and Pacific Islanders as well as among Native Americans and Alaska Natives appear to be comparable to, or somewhat lower than, those for White Americans.[3]

Individuals with diabetes are also at higher risk of stroke. The occurrence of stroke is 2 to 6 times higher among people with diabetes than among those without it, and the risk is higher for women than for men.[109] Diabetes is associated with increased prevalence of other stroke risk factors, nonetheless, diabetes alone, independent of other risk factors, has been estimated to increase the incidence of stroke somewhere between 2 and 3 times.[110]

The risk of stroke is greatly increased among people who previously have had a stroke or a TIA. Approximately one-third of people who have had one or more TIA will later have a stroke. People who have had TIAs are nearly 10 times more likely to have a stroke than are people of the same age and sex who have not had TIA. However, only about 10% of all strokes are preceded by TIAs.[34]

Asymptomatic carotid bruit doubles the risk of TIAs and stroke. A carotid bruit—the abnormal sound of blood flowing through a partially blocked carotid artery—is a general marker for advanced atherosclerosis, the underlying risk factor. It develops more often in people with diabetes or hypertension.[74] In addition, about 15% of strokes occur in people with atrial fibrillation, the most common cause of cerebral embolism.

The risk for stroke is higher for people with a family history of stroke. Positive paternal family history is associated with a doubling of stroke risk, while maternal family history increases stroke risk about 40%. The effect of family history appears to be about the same in Blacks and Whites.[111] Finally, the postpartum period is a time of significant relative increase in stroke risk for women, although the absolute risk in this group is still quite modest.[112]

Geographic Distribution

In the United States, stroke rates are highest in a group of states clustered in the Southeast: Alabama, Arkansas, Georgia, Indiana, Kentucky, Louisiana, Mississippi, North

Death Rates Per
100,000 Population

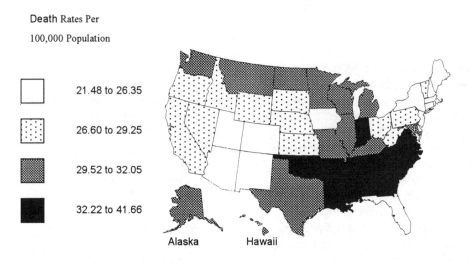

☐	21.48 to 26.35
▦	26.60 to 29.25
▨	29.52 to 32.05
■	32.22 to 41.66

Alaska   Hawaii

Figure 11.3—Stroke death rates by state, United States, 1993.[1]

Carolina, South Carolina, Tennessee, and Virginia (Figure 11.3). In 1993, age-adjusted stroke mortality ranged from a high of 41 per 100 000 in South Carolina to a low of 22 per 100 000 in New Mexico.[1] Regional differences in stroke rates are more pronounced in Whites than in Blacks; however, Blacks residing in nonmetropoliton areas irrespective of region have far greater stroke risk, even after adjusting for known stroke risk factors, than Blacks residing in metropolitan areas.[113] Countries with the highest rate of stroke in 1985 were Bulgaria, Hungary, and the former Soviet Union. Those with very low rates were Canada, Iceland, and Switzerland.[16] In a more recent international incidence comparison of rates from 1984 or later in 11 western nations, overall and subtype specific age- and sex-standardized incidence was fairly

similar across most nations (somewhere between 300 and 500 per 100 000 per year) with significantly lower rates reported in France and significantly higher rates in Russia.[114]

Time Trends

The decline in stroke mortality has been striking. Since 1950, mortality rates in the United States have dropped over 65%.[115] The trend has been uniformly downward for both sexes and all race groups, with steeper declines for younger adults and people of other than White race. In more recent years, between 1979 and 1995, there has been a 20% decline in the stroke mortality rate. The rate of decline during the 1980s varied by region, with rates dropping fastest in the South.[116] Additionally, a slowing of the rate of decline was seen toward the end of that decade.[117] In the first half of the 1990s, mortality rates have actually increased slightly.[2,118] The underlying causes for the historical decline in stroke mortality have not been well established, but the decline has been attributed in part to the control of hypertension, secondary prevention of stroke among TIA patients, and, to a lesser extent, the decline in smoking.[119] Similarly, the reasons behind the recent plateauing and upturn are not yet completely understood.

RISK FACTORS

The list of risk factors for stroke is extensive. Modifiable factors include hypertension, cigarette smoking, obesity, and total cholesterol level. In addition, physical inactivity and alcohol consumption are controllable factors that may contribute directly or indirectly to stroke risk.

Magnitude of Risk Factors

Hypertension is the major risk factor for stroke and the only one consistently found to be related to all types of stroke (Table 11.3).[119] Both isolated systolic hypertension and elevations in diastolic blood pressure powerfully predispose to stroke. The risk of stroke increases exponentially as the diastolic blood pressure increases throughout the range from 70 to 110 mm Hg. An increase of 7.5 mm Hg in diastolic blood pressure doubles the risk of stroke.[23] Among adults 55 through 64 years of age in the Framingham study, the risk of cerebral infarction was 10- to 20-fold

Table 11.3—Modifiable Risk Factors for Stroke, United States

Magnitude	Risk Factor	Best Estimate (%) of Population Attributable Risk (Range)
Strong (relative risk >4)	High blood pressure (systolic $\geq$140 mm Hg)	26 (20–50)
Moderate (relative risk 2-4)	Cigarette smoking	12 (11–25)
	Diabetes	3 (0–7)
	Elevated cholesterol ($\geq$220 mg/dL)	10 (0–20)
	Obesity[a]	20 (15–25)
Possible	Physical inactivity	—
	Alcohol use	—
	Very low cholesterol (<160mg/dl)[b]	—

[a]Based on body mass index >27.8 kg/m^2 for men and >27.3 kg/m^2 for women.
[b]May increase risk of hemorrhagic stroke.
Note: Data compiled from references 110, 130–32.

higher for people with hypertension than for those without it.[120] The combined results of clinical trials and epidemiologic studies suggest that small reductions of elevated diastolic blood pressure (eg, reductions of as little as 5 mmHg) are associated with at least significant (40% to 45%) reductions in the incidence of both fatal and nonfatal strokes.[25, 121, 122] Although somewhat less studied, there is now evidence that reduction in mean systolic pressure among individuals with isolated systolic hypertension also leads to real declines in stroke incidence.[110] Finally, it is also important to note that blood pressure is also associated with risk of recurrent stroke among individuals with a history of cerebrovascular disease.[123]

Current smokers are at over twice the risk of stroke as never smokers.[124-127] The smoking-associated relative risk does, however, differ by age with the association strongest for people under age 55 and diminishing to little or none after age 75.[124] Smoking cessation reduces the risk of both ischemic stroke and subarachnoid hemorrhage. The risk declines quickly, within the first 5 years relative risks approach those of people who have never smoked.[110,127]

The relationship between stroke risk and serum cholesterol is unclear. A combined analysis of prospective observational studies found no association between baseline total cholesterol and subsequent stroke risk.[128] The theory has been proposed, however, that the association with total cholesterol is masked because it is dependent on stroke subtype. Low cholesterol has been shown in some studies to increase the risk of hemorrhagic stroke, while high cholesterol has been associated with increased risk of ischemic stroke. In the aforementioned meta-analysis, there was no significantly increased stroke risk associated with low cholesterol even in the Asian subpopulation, which has generally low cholesterol levels and high proportions of hemorrhagic strokes. Other meta-analyses (synthesized results of clinical trials of cholesterol-lowering drugs) have reported treatment-associated increases in the risk of fatal stroke. While more research is needed on cholesterol and specific stroke subtypes, because people at risk of stroke are also at a high risk of developing CHD, avoidance of high serum cholesterol most likely offers substantial net cardiovascular benefit.

Obesity is associated with increased risk of fatal and nonfatal stroke with relative risk in the range of 1.5 to 2.0.[110] After adjustment for other cardiovascular disease risk factors, which of course cluster with obesity, there is some evidence of an independent risk increase linked to being overweight. Moreover, being overweight during young adulthood, weight gain in adulthood, higher waist-to-hip ratio, and larger subscapular skinfold thickness have also been associated with stroke risk in a number of research studies. Not surprisingly, a few studies have also reported that increased physical activity also protects against stroke risk.[110]

During the time period when oral contraceptives contained high estrogen levels, there were convincing reports of associations between their use and thrombotic stroke. Studies of the low-dose oral contraceptives prescribed today have yielded mixed results. Recent investigations do not provide much evidence for a positive association with stroke risk, except among women with other stroke risk factors where oral contraceptive use remains contraindicated.[129]

Population-Attributable Risk

An estimated 26% of stroke deaths in the United States are attributed to elevated blood pressure (Table 11.2).[130–134] The overall attributable risk estimate for incident stroke associated with smoking is 12%.[110] However, the smoking attributable risk varies greatly by age and sex, with about half the fatal strokes among both men and women under the age of 65 attributed to smoking. After age 65, smoking accounts for 24% of the fatal strokes among men and 6% among women.[124] The

population-attributable risk for stroke associated with obesity has been estimated between 15% and 25%.[110] Finally, the attributable risk for elevated cholesterol (ie, $\geq$ 220 mg/ dL) ranges from 0% to 20%[130, 131] while diabetes accounts for a relatively small proportion, 2% to 5%, of stroke deaths.[110] The same issues in interpreting population-attributable risks raised in the previous discussion of CHD apply here as well.

PREVENTION AND CONTROL MEASURES

Prevention

The best method for reducing the burden of stroke in the population appears to be control of modifiable risk factors for stroke. Treatment of high blood pressure is the most efficacious method of primary prevention of a first stroke, although it is somewhat less effective in preventing recurrent stroke.[119] Data have shown that the 10% of the population at highest risk for stroke have a set of four modifiable risk factors: hypertension, cigarette smoking, elevated cholesterol, and abnormal glucose tolerance.[34] As many as half of all strokes could be prevented if these people were to be identified and treated.[131]

Secondary Prevention

There are no definitive tests for early detection of stroke. All adults should be routinely screened for hypertension and elevated serum cholesterol. Clinicians should also investigate their patients' dietary patterns, smoking behavior, and level of physical activity. The effectiveness of screening for carotid bruits is unproved. Clinical trials of carotid endarectomy, a once popular surgical procedure used to clear clogged arteries in the neck that had also been proposed as an early intervention in individuals with asymptomatic carotid atherosclerosis, have reached generally negative conclusions. Noninvasive ultrasound or magnetic resonance angiography technology has been proposed as a means of improving screening by increasing the proportion of screen positive individuals with more severe disease—the group most likely to benefit from treatment.[122] However, the extent to which these additional diagnostic modalities change risk-benefit equations for early intervention remains to be seen.

Treatment, Rehabilitation, and Recovery

Over the past decade, dramatic advances in technology have led to a much improved understanding of the pathophysiology of stroke. Advanced imaging techniques such as computerized axial tomography (CAT) scanning, magnetic resonance imaging (MRI), and radionuclide angiography (nuclear brain scan)

have greatly aided treatment decision making. Another group of tests, which includes electroencephalogram (EEG), measures electrical activity in the brain. Another category includes a variety of tests such as ultrasound for measuring blood flow. Clinicians can now individualize stroke treatment according to the characteristics of disease in each person.[133] Reducing risk factors, altering blood coagulability, and performing surgery are the cornerstones of stroke treatment. Among individuals with a history of TIAs or minor stroke, antiplatelet therapy (aspirin or other medications) clearly reduces the risk of future stroke, but it has not been shown to be effective in the primary prevention of stroke among either a general population or among groups of asymptomatic individuals.[134]

Acute anticoagulation therapy (with agents like tissue plasminogen activator) is now standard treatment for ischemic strokes. Because studies have shown that the time between stroke onset and initiation of drug therapy is critical to conferring therapeutic benefit, attention has now focused on development of effective means of ascertaining event onset time and standard approaches for rapid management of stroke patients.[129] Because stroke is a major cause of disability, rehabilitation, including physical therapy, speech therapy, and occupational therapy, is essential to maximize the return of functional capacity.

EXAMPLES OF PUBLIC HEALTH INTERVENTIONS

Only a few public health interventions have specifically targeted stroke. (Interventions targeted at risk factors common to both CHD and stroke are discussed in the CHD section and in Chapters 5, 8, 9, and 10 on tobacco use, diet and nutrition, high blood pressure, and cholesterol.) In 1990, a large-scale stroke intervention was initiated by NHLBI. Called the Stroke Belt Initiative, this program targeted the 11 high-risk states in an attempt to reduce their disproportionately high stroke mortality. These states are using a variety of community-based and mass media approaches to reach populations at highest risk for stroke, particularly Blacks.[135] For example, the Alabama Department of Health partnered with churches, hospitals, blood donation centers, the Red Cross and others in 12 counties across the state to locate medically indigent uncontrolled hypertensives and bring them into hypertension control programs. In addition, the hypertension control services being offered by health departments in 60 Alabama counties were reviewed to assure that they met quality of care standards.

AREAS OF FUTURE RESEARCH AND DEMONSTRATION

In spite of the fact that it is the third leading cause of death, there are a surprising number of unanswered questions in stroke epidemiology, prevention, and control. A number of potentially modifiable risk factors, including cholesterol, body weight, and physical activity should be explored further. The factors behind the attenuation of the decline in stroke mortality rates in the United States are deserving of further inquiry. Continued study of diagnostic, treatment, and rehabilitation technologies all can make new inroads in reducing the morbidity burden associated with stroke. Further refinement of approaches used by health systems to foster rapid diagnosis of and early drug therapy for incident stroke also hold promise for improving overall treatment effectiveness. Finally, more community-based research on stroke risk factor modification approaches should be undertaken to develop more effective methods of primary prevention.

REFERENCES

1. American Heart Association. *1997 Heart and Stroke Statistical Update.* Dallas, Tex: National Center; 1996. AHA Publication 55-0524.

2. Anderson RN, Kochonck KD, Murphy SL. A Report of Final Mortality Statistics, 1995. *Month Vital Stat Rep.* 1997;45(11)(suppl 2) Hyattsville, Md: National Center for Health Statistics; 1997. DHHS publication 97-1120.

3. Centers for Disease Control and Prevention. *Chronic Disease in Minority Populations.* Atlanta, Ga; 1992.

4. Centers for Disease Control and Prevention. *Preventing Cardiovascular Disease: Addressing the Nation's Leading Killer - At a Glance 1997.* Atlanta, Ga; 1997.

5. Labarthe DR, Eissa M, Varas C. Childhood precursors of high blood pressure and elevated cholesterol. *Ann Rev Public Health.* 1991;12:519–541.

6. Folsom AR, Eckfeldt JH, Weitzman S, et al. Relation of carotid artery wall thickness to diabetes mellitus, fasting glucose and insulin, body size, and physical activity. The Atherosclerosis Risk in Communities Study Investigators. *Stroke.* 1994;25:66–73.

7. deAndrade M, Thandi I, Brown S, et al. Relationship of the apolipoprotein E polymorphism with carotid artery atherosclerosis. *Am J Hum Genet.* 1995;56:1379–1390.

8. Nieto FJ, Adam E, Sorlie P, et al. Cohort study of cytomegalovirus infection as a risk factor for carotid intimal-medial thickening, a measure of subclinical atherosclerosis. *Circulation.* 1996;94:922–927.

9. Ma J, Folsom AR, Melnick SL, et al. Associations of serum and dietary magnesium with cardiovascular disease, hypertension, diabetes, insulin, and carotid arterial wall thickness: the atherosclerosis risk in communities study. *J Clin Epidemiol.* 1995;48:927–940.

10. Folsom AR, Wu KK, Shahar E, et al. Association of hemostatic variables with prevalent cardiovascular disease and asymptomatic carotid artery atherosclerosis. The Atherosclerosis Risk in Communities Study Investigators. *Arterioscler Thromb.* 1993;12:1829–1836.

11. Corti MC, Guralnik JM, Bicato C. Coronary heart disease risk factors in older persons. *Aging Clin Exp Res.* 1996;9:75–79.

12. Jenkins CD. Epidemiology of cardiovascular diseases. *J Consult Clin Psychol.* 1988;56:324–332.

13. Wing S, Casper M, Riggan W, et al. Socioenvironmental characteristics associated with the onset of decline of ischemic heart disease mortality in the United States. *Am J Public Health.* 1988;78:923–926.

14. Wing S, Barnett E, Casper M, et al. Geographic and socioeconomic variation in the onset of

decline of coronary heart disease mortality in white women. *Am J Public Health*. 1992;82:204–209.

15. Diezroux AV, Nieto FJ, Muntanal C, et al. Neighborhood environments and coronary heart disease. *ADE* 1997;146:48—63.

16. Uemura K, Pisa Z. Trends in cardiovascular disease mortality in industrialized countries since 1950. *World Health Stat Q*. 1988;41:156–168.

17. Higgins MW, Luepker RV, eds. Appendix: Mortality from coronary heart disease and related causes of death in the United States, 1950–85. In: *Trends in Coronary Heart Disease Mortality: The Influence of Medical Care*. New York, NY: Oxford University Press Inc; 1988:279–297.

18. Sempos C, Cooper R, Kovar MG, McMillen M. Divergence of the recent trends in coronary mortality for the four major race-sex groups in the United States. *Am J Public Health*. 1988;78: 1422–1427.

19. Goldman L, Cook EF. Reasons for the decline in coronary heart disease mortality: medical interventions versus life-style changes. In: Higgins MW, Luepker RV, eds. *Trends in Coronary Heart Disease Mortality: The Influence of Medical Care*. New York, NY: Oxford University Press Inc; 1988:67–75.

20. Hunink MMG, Goldman L, Tosteson ANA, et al. The recent decline in mortality from coronary heart disease, 1980-1990: The effect of secular trends in risk factors and treatment. *JAMA*. 1997;277:535-42.

21. McGovern PG, Pankow JS, James S, et al. Recent trends in acute coronary heart disease— mortality, morbidity, medical care, and risk factors. *New Engl J Med*. 1996;334:884–890.

22. Hennekens CH, Satterfield S, Hebert PR. Treatment of elevated blood pressure to prevent coronary heart disease. In: Higgins MW, Luepker RV, eds. *Trends in Coronary Heart Disease Mortality: The Influence of Medical Care*. New York, NY: Oxford University Press Inc; 1988:103–108.

23. US Dept of Health and Human Services. *The 1988 Report of the Joint National Committee on Detection, Evaluation, and Treatment of High Blood Pressure*. Bethesda, Md: National Institutes of Health; 1988. NIH publication 88-1088.

24. MacMahon S, Peto R, Cutler J, et al. Blood pressure, stroke, and coronary heart disease. Part 1, prolonged differences in blood pressure: prospective observational studies corrected for the regression dilution bias. *Lancet*. 1990;335:765–774.

25. Collins R, Peto R, MacMahon S, et al. Blood pressure, stroke, and coronary heart disease. Part 2, short-term reductions in blood pressure: overview of randomised drug trials in their epidemiological context. *Lancet.* 1990;335:827–838.

26. US Dept of Health and Human Services. *The Health Consequences of Smoking: Cardiovascular Disease. A Report of the Surgeon General.* Rockville, Md: Public Health Service, Office on Smoking and Health; 1984. DHHS publication PHS 84-50204.

27. Centers for Disease Control. Cigarette smoking among adults—United States, 1995. *MMWR.* 1997;46:1217–1220.

28. Glantz SA, Parmley WW. Passive smoking and heart disease: epidemiology, physiology, and biochemistry. *Circulation.* 1991;83:1–12.

29. Steenland K. Passive smoking and the risk of heart disease. *JAMA.* 1992;267:94–99.

30. Kawachi I, Colditz GA, Speizer FE, et al. A prospective study of passive smoking and coronary heart disease. *Circulation.* 1997;95:2374–2379.

31. He Y, Lam TH, Li LS, et al. The number of stenotic coronary arteries and passive smoking exposure from husbands in lifelong non-smoking women in Xi'an, China. *Atherosclerosis.* 1996;127:229–238.

32. Howard G, Wagenknecht LE, Burke GL, et al. Cigarette smoking and progression of atherosclerosis: the Atherosclerosis Risk in Communities (ARIC) study. *JAMA.* 1998;279:119–124.

33. Blackburn H, Luepker R. Heart disease. In: Last JM, Wallace RB, eds. *Maxcy-Rosenau-Last Textbook of Public Health and Preventive Medicine.* 13th ed. Norwalk, Conn: Appleton & Lange; 1992:827–847.

34. American Heart Association. *Heart and Stroke Facts.* Dallas, Tex: National Center; 1996. AHA publication 55-0523.

35. Sempos C, Fulwood R, Haines C, et al. The prevalence of high blood cholesterol levels among adults in the United States. *JAMA.* 1989;262:45–52.

36. US Dept of Health and Human Services. *Report of the Expert Panel on Population Strategies for Blood Cholesterol Reduction.* Bethesda Md: National Heart, Lung, and Blood Institute; 1990. NIH publication 90-3047.

37. US Dept of Health and Human Services. *Report of the Expert Panel on Detection, Evaluation, and Treatment of High Blood Cholesterol in Adults.* Bethesda, Md: National Heart, Lung, and Blood Institute; 1988. NIH publication 88-2925.

38. Gardner CO, Fortmann SP, Kraus RM. Association of small low density lipoprotein particles with the incidence of coronary artery disease in men and women. *JAMA*. 1996; 276:878–881.

39. Hokanson JE, Austin MA. Plasma mycycenide level is a risk factor for cardiovascular disease independent of high-density lipoprotein cholesterol level. *J Cardiovasc Risk*. 1996;3:213–219.

40. Rifkind BM. High-density lipoprotein cholesterol and coronary artery disease: survey of the evidence. *Am J Cardiol*. 1990;66:3A–6A.

41. Kris-Etherton PM, ed. *Cardiovascular Disease: Nutrition for Prevention and Treatment*. Chicago, Ill: American Dietetic Association; 1990.

42. Sharett AL, Patsch W, Sorlie PD. Associations of lipoprotein cholesterols, apolipoproteins A-I and B, and triglycerides with carotid atherosclerosis and coronary heart disease. *Atheroscler Thromb* 1994;14: 1098–1014.

43. Nygard O, Nordrehaug JE, Refsum H, et al. Plasma homocysteine levels and mortality in patients with coronary artery disease. *New Engl J Med*. 1997; 337:230–236.

44. Stampfer MJ, Malinow MR, Willett WC, et al. A prospective study of plasma homocysteine and risk of myocardial infarction in US physicians. *JAMA*. 1992; 268:877–881.

45. Nygard O, Vollset SE, Refsum H, et al. Total plasma homocysteine and cardiovascular risk profile. *JAMA*. 1995;274:1526–1533.

46. Graham IM, Daly LE, Refsum HM, et al. Plasma homocysteine as a risk factor for vascular disease. The European Concerted Action Project. *JAMA*. 1997;277:1775–1781.

47. Mudd SH, Skouby F, Levy HL, et al. The natural history of homocystinuria due to cystathione b-synthase deficiency. *Am J Hum Gen*. 1985; 37:1–31.

48. Ma J, Stampfer MJ, Hennekens CH, et al. Methylenetetrahydrofolate reductase polymorphism, plasma folate, homocysteine, and risk of myocardial infarction in US physicians. *Circulation*. 1996;94:2410–2416.

49. Selitub J, Jaaynes PF, Wilson PWF, et al. Vitamin status and intake as primary determinants of homocysteinuria in an elderly population. *JAMA*. 1993;270: 2693–2698.

50. Ward M, McNulty H, McPartlin J, et al. Plasma homocysteine, a risk factor for cardiovascular disease, is lowered by physiological doses of folic acid. *Q J Med*. 1997;90:519–524.

51. National Research Council. *Diet and Health: Implications for*

Reducing Chronic Disease Risk.
Washington, DC: National
Academy Press; 1989.

52. Centers for Disease Control and
Prevention. *National Diabetes
Fact Sheet: National Estimates
and General Information on
Diabetes in the United States.*
Atlanta, Ga; 1997.

53. Barrett-Connor E, Orchard T.
Diabetes and heart disease. In:
*Diabetes in America: Diabetes
Data Compiled 1984.* Bethesda,
Md: US Dept of Health and
Human Services;1985:XVI1–
XVI41. NIH publication 85-1468.

54. Fisher M, Eckhart C, eds. *Guide
to Clinical Preventive Services:
An Assessment of the Effectiveness of 169 Interventions. Report
of the US Preventive Services Task
Force.* Baltimore, Md: Williams &
Wilkins; 1989.

55. Foster WR, Burton BT, eds.
National Institutes of Health
consensus conference: health
implications of obesity. *Ann
Intern Med.* 1985;103:977–1077.

56. Kuczmarski RJ, Fiedal KM,
Campbell SM, et al. Increasing
prevalence of overweight among
US adults: the National Health
and Nutrition Examination
Surveys 1960–91. *JAMA.* 1994;
272:205–211.

57. Ernst ND, Obarzanak E, Clark
MB, et al. Cardiovascular risks
related to overweight. *J Am Diet
Assoc.* 1997;97:547–551.

58. US Dept of Health and Human
Services. *Healthy People 2000:
National Health Promotion and
Disease Prevention Objectives.*
Washington, DC: Public Health
Service; 1991. DHHS publication
PHS 91-50212.

59. Hubert HB, Fenleib M,
McNamara PM, et al. Obesity as
an independent risk factor for
cardiovascular disease: a 26-year
follow-up of participants in The
Framingham Heart Study.
Circulation. 1983;67:969–977.

60. Williamson DF, Pamuk E, Thun
M, et al. prospective study of
intentional weight loss and
mortality in never-smoking
overweight US white women
aged 40–64. *Am J Epidemiol.*
1995;141:1128–1141.

61. Freedman DS, Williamson DF,
Croft JB, et al. Relation of body
fat distribution to ischemic
heart disease: the National
Health and Nutrition Examination Survey I (NHANES I)
Epidemiologic Follow-up
Study. *Am J Epidemiol.* 1995;
142:53–63.

62. Prineas RJ, Folsom AR, Kaye SA.
Central adiposity and increased
risk of coronary artery mortality
in older women. *Ann Epidemiol.*
1993;3:35–41.

63. Centers for Disease Control and
Prevention. *Surgeon General's
Report on Physical Activity and
Health.* Atlanta, Ga; July 1996.

64. Blair SN, Kohl HW, Paffenbarger RS, et al. Physical fitness and all-cause mortality: a prospective study of healthy men and women. *JAMA.* 1989;262:2395–2401.

65. Hakim AA, Petrovich H, Burchfiel CM, et al. Effects of walking on mortality among nonsmoking retired men. *New Engl J Med.* 1998;338:94–99.

66. Wannamethee SG, Shaper AG. Lifelong teetotallers, ex-drinkers and drinkers: mortality and the incidence of major coronary heart disease events in middle-aged British men. *Int J Epidemiol.* 1997;26:523–531.

67. Hanna EZ, Chou SP, Grant BF. The relationship between drinking and heart disease morbidity in the United States: results from the National Health Interview Survey. *Alcohol Clin & Exp Res.* 1997;21:111–18.

68. Keil U, Chambless LE, Doring A, et al. The relation of alcohol intake to coronary heart disease and all-cause mortality in a beer-drinking population. *Epidemiology.* 1997;8:150–156.

69. Criqui, MH. Alcohol and coronary heart disease: consistent relationship and public health implications. *Clin Chim Acta.* 1996;246:51–57.

70. Williams RB Jr. Psychological factors in coronary artery disease: epidemiologic evidence. *Circulation.* 1987; 76:117–123.

71. Greenwood DC, Muir KR, Packham CJ, et al. Coronary heart disease: a review of the role of psychosocial stress and social support. *J Pub Health Med.* 1996;18:221–231.

72. McQueen DV, Siegrist J. Social factors in the etiology of chronic disease: an overview. *Soc Sci Med.* 1982;16:353–367.

73. Kawachi I, Sparrow D, Spiro A III, et al. A prospective study of anger and coronary heart disease: The Normative Aging Study. *Circulation.* 1996; 94:2090–2095.

74. US Department of Health and Human Services. *Working Group Report on Management of Patients with Hypertension and High Blood Cholesterol.* Bethesda, Md: National Institutes of Health; 1990. NIH publication 90-2361.

75. Powell KE, Blair SN. The public health burdens of sedentary living habits: theoretical but realistic estimates. *Med Sci Sports Exer.* 1994;26:851-856.

76. Abbott RD, Donohue RP, MacMahon SW, et al. Diabetes and the risk of stroke: the Honolulu Heart Program. *JAMA.* 1987;257:949–952.

77. Kovar MG, Harris MI, Hadden WC. The scope of diabetes in the United States population. *Am J Public Health.* 1987;77:1549–1550.

78. Stamler J, Wentworth D, Neaton JD. Is relationship between serum cholesterol and risk of premature death from coronary heart disease continuous and graded? *JAMA*. 1986;256:2823–2828.

79. Centers for Disease Control. Deaths from coronary heart disease—United States, 1986. *MMWR*. 1989;38:16.

80. American Diabetes Association. Screening for diabetes. *Diabetes Care*. 1990;13:7–9.

81. Bittl JA. Advances in coronary angioplasty. *New Engl J Med.*. 1996;35:1290–1302.

82. Oldridge NB, Guyatt GH, Fischer ME. Cardiac rehabilitation after myocardial infarction: combined experience of randomized clinical trials. *JAMA*. 1988;260:945–950.

83. Hjermann I, Welve Byre K, Holme I, et al. Effect of diet and smoking intervention on the incidence of coronary heart disease: report from the Oslo Study Group of a randomized trial in healthy men. *Lancet*. 1981;2:1303–1310.

84. Multiple Risk Factor Intervention Trial Research Group. Multiple risk factor intervention trial: risk factor changes and mortality results. *JAMA*. 1982;248:1465–1477.

85. Levy RI. Primary prevention of coronary heart disease by lowering lipids: results and implications. *Am Heart J*. 1985;110:1116–1122.

86. The Lipid Research Clinics Coronary Primary Prevention Trial Results. I. Reduction in incidence of coronary heart disease. *JAMA*. 1984;251:351-364.

87. Puska P, Tuomilehto J, Nissinen A, et al. The North Karelia Project: 15 years of community based prevention of coronary heart disease. *Ann Med*. 1989; 21:169–173.

88. Farquhar JW, Maccoby N, Wood PD, et al. Community education for cardiovascular health. *Lancet*. 1977;1:1192–1195.

89. Flora JA, Maibach EW, Maccoby N. The role of media across four levels of health promotion intervention. *Ann Rev Public Health*. 1989;10:181–201.

90. Farquhar JW, Fortmann SP, Flora JA, et al. Effects of community-wide education on cardiovascular disease risk factors: the Stanford five-city project. 1990; 264:359–365.

91. Mittlemark MB, Luepker RV, Jacobs DR, et al. Community-wide prevention of cardiovascular disease: education strategies of the Minnesota Health Program. *Prev Med*. 1986; 15:1–17.

92. Lasater T, Abrams S, Artz L, et al. Lay volunteer delivery of a community-based cardiovascular risk factor change program: The

Pawtucket Experiment. In: Matarazzo JD, Weiss SM, Herd JA, Miller NE, Weiss SM, eds. *Behavioral Health: A Handbook of Health Enhancement and Disease Prevention.* New York, NY: Wiley-Interscience Publications; 1984:1166–1170.

93. Lefebvre RC, Linnan L, Sundraram S, et al. Counseling strategies for blood cholesterol screening programs: recommendations for practice. *Patient Educ Counsel.* 1990;16:97–108.

94. Schooler C, Farquhar JW, Fortmann SP, et al. Synthesis of findings and issues from community prevention trials. *Ann Epidemiol.* 1997;7S:S54–S68.

95. Killoran A, Fentem P, Caspersen C. Moving on, international perspectives on promoting physical activity. London, UK: Health Education Authority; 1994.

96. Fortmann SP, Flora JA, Winkleby M, et al. Community intervention trials: reflections on the Stanford five-city project experience. *Am J Epidemiol.* 1995;142:576–586.

97. New York State Healthy Heart Program. *Eight Approaches in Community Intervention: An Interim Report.* Albany, NY: New York State Department of Health; 1992.

98. *Final Report: The South Carolina Cardiovascular Disease Prevention (CVD) Project.* Columbia, SC: Dept of Health and Environmental Control; 1991.

99. Brownson RC, Smith CA, Pratt M, Mack NE, Jackson-Thompson J, Dean CG, Dabney S, Wilkerson JC. Preventing cardiovascular disease through community-based risk reduction: the Bootheel Heart Health Project. *Am J Public Health.* 1996;86:206–213.

100. Indian Health Service. ITHP (Inter-tribal Heart Project) Manual of Operations. Bemidji, Minn: Indian Health Service; 1992.

101. *J Health Educ.* 1992;23(3). Entire issue dedicated to descriptions and accounts of PATCH program.

102. US Dept of Health and Human Services. Evaluating community efforts to prevent cardiovascular diseases. Atlanta, Ga: Centers for Disease Control and Prevention; 1995.

103. Simons-Morton DG, Simons-Morton BG, Parcel GS, Bunker JF. Influencing personal and environmental conditions for community health: a multilevel intervention model. *Family Commun Health.* 1988;11:25–35.

104. Sallis JF, Owen N. Ecological models. In: Glanz K, Lewis FM, Rimer BK, eds. *Health Behavior and Health Education: Theory, Research, and Practice.* San Francisco, CA: Josey Bass Publishers; 1997:403–424.

105. King AC, Jeffery RW, Fidinger F, Dusenbury L, Provence S, Hedlund SA, Spangler K. Environmental and policy approaches to cardiovascular disease prevention through physical activity: issues and opportunities. *Health Educ Q.* 1995;22:499–511.

106. Schmid TL, Pratt M, Howze E. Policy as intervention: environmental and policy approaches to the prevention of cardiovascular disease. *Am J Public Health.* 1995;85:1207–1211.

107. Association of State and Territorial Chronic Disease Program Directors, AST Directors of Health Promotion and Public Health Education, AST Public Health Nutrition Directors. Physical activity issue paper. 1997.

108. Avins AL, Browner, WS. Improving the prediction of coronary heart disease to aid in the management of high cholesterol levels: What a difference a decade makes. *JAMA.* 1998; 279:445-49.

109. American Heart Association. *1992 Heart and Stroke Facts.* Dallas, Tex: National Center; 1991. AHA publication 55-0386.

110. Bronner LL, Kanter DS, Manson JE. Medical progress: primary prevention of stroke. *New Engl J Med.* 1995;333:1392–1400.

111. Laio D, Myers R, Hunt S, et al. Familial history of stroke and stroke risk. The Family Heart Study. *Stroke.* 1997;28:1908–1912.

112. Kittner SJ, Stern BJ, Feeser BR, et al. Pregnancy and the risk of stroke. *New Engl J Med.* 1996; 335:768–774.

113. Gillum RF, Ingram DD. Relation between residence in the sourtheast region of the United States and stroke incidence. The NHANES I Epidemiologic Followup Study. *J Hypertension.* 1996;14(suppl):S39–S46.

114. Sudlow CL, Warlow CP. Comparable studies of the incidence of stroke and its pathological types: results from an international collaboration. *Stroke.* 1997;28: 491–499.

115. Centers for Disease Control and Prevention. Prevention of disability and associated health conditions—United States, 1991–92. *MMWR.* 1994;43:730–731, 737–739.

116. Lanska DJ, Peterson PM. Comparison of additive and multiplicative models of regional variation in the decline of stroke mortality in the United States. *Stroke.* 1996;27:1055–1059.

117. Shahar E, McGovern PG, Pankow JS, et al. Stroke rates during the 1980s. The Minnesota Stroke Survey. *Stroke.* 1997;28: 275–279.

118. Kochanek KD, Hudson BL. *Advance Report of Final Mortal-*

ity Statistics, 1992. *Monthly Vital Statistics Report,* Washington, DC: Dept of Health and Human Services, Centers for Disease Control and Prevention, Nutrional Center for Health Statistics; 1992.

119.Cowan LD, Leviton A, Nelson KB. Neurological disorders. In: Last JM, Wallace RB, eds. *Maxcy-Rosenau-Last Textbook of Public Health and Preventive Medicine.* 13th ed. Norwalk, Conn: Appleton & Lange; 1992:929–935.

120.US Dept of Health and Human Services. *The Prevention and Treatment of Complications of Diabetes Mellitus: A Guide for Primary Care Practitioners.* Atlanta, Ga: Centers for Disease Control; 1991.

121.Cutler JA, MacMahon SW, Furberg CD. Controlled clinical trials of drug treatment for hypertension. A review. *Hypertension.* 1989;13:36–44.

122.Barnett HJM, Elasziw M, and Meldrum HE. Drug therapy: Drugs and surgery in the prevention of ischemic stroke. *New Engl J Med.* 1995;332:238–248.

123.MacMahon S. Blood pressure and the prevention of stroke. *J Hypertension.* 1996;14(suppl): S39–S46.

124.US Dept of Health and Human Services. *The Health Benefits of Smoking Cessation. A Report of the Surgeon General.* Rockville, Md: Public Health Service, Office on Smoking and Health; 1990. DHHS publication PHS 90-8416.

125.Wannamethee SG, Shaper AG, Whincup PH, et al. Smoking cessation and the risk of stroke in middle-aged men. *JAMA.* 1995;274:155–160.

126.Kawachi I, Colditz GA, Stampfer MJ, et al. Smoking cessation and decreased risk of stroke in women. *JAMA.* 1993;269:232–236.

127.Lightwood JM, Glantz SA. Short-term economics and health benefits of smoking cessation: myocardial infarction and stroke. *Circulation.* 1997;96:1089–1096.

128.Prospective Studies Collaboration. Cholesterol, diastolic blood pressure, and stroke: 13,000 strokes in 450,000 people in 45 prospective cohorts. *Lancet.* 1995;346:1647–1653.

129.Marwick C. New era for acute stroke treatment. *JAMA.* 1997; 277:199–200.

130.Harmsen P, Rosengren A, Tsipogianni A, et al. Risk factors for stroke in middle-aged men in Goteborg, Sweden. *Stroke.* 1990;20:223–229.

131.Dunbabin DW, Sandercock PAG. Preventing stroke by the modification of risk factors. *Stroke.* 1990;21:IV36–IV39.

132.Centers for Disease Control. Deaths from stroke—United

States, 1986. *MMWR.* 1989;38:12.

133. Caplan LR. Diagnosis and treatment of ischemic stroke. *JAMA.* 1991;266:2413–2418.

134. Wilterdink JL, Easton JD. Prevention and treatment of stroke. *Heart Dis Stroke.* 1992;1:51–55.

135. US Dept of Health and Human Services. State stroke belt projects take aim at high mortality rates. In: *Infomemo.* Bethesda, Md: National Institutes of Health; 1992.

SUGGESTED READING

American Heart Association. *1997 Heart and Stroke Statistical Update.* Dallas, Tex: National Center; 1996. AHA publication 55-0524.

American Heart Association. *Heart and Stroke Facts.* Dallas, Tex: National Center; 1996. AHA publication 55-0523.

Bronner LL, Kanter DS, Manson JE. Medical progress: pPrimary prevention of stroke. *New Engl J Med.* 1995;333:1392–1400.

Manson JE, Ridker PM, Gaziano JM, et al., eds. *Prevention of Myocardial Infarction.* New York, NY: Oxford University Press Inc; 1996.

Marmot M, Elliott P, eds. *Coronary Heart Disease Epidemiology:* *From Aetiology to Public Health.* New York, NY: Oxford University Press Inc; 1992.

Schooler C, Farquhar JW, Fortmann SP, et al. Synthesis of findings and issues from community prevention trials. *Ann Epidemiol.* 1997;7S:S54–S68.

RESOURCES

American Heart Association
7272 Greenville Avenue
Dallas, TX 75231-4596
(214) 373-6300
www.amhrt.org

National Center for Chronic Disease Prevention and Health Promotion
Centers for Disease Control and Prevention
1600 Clifton Road, NE, MS K-45
Atlanta, GA 30333
(770) 488-5532
www.cdc.gov/nccdphp/nccdhome.htm

National Heart, Lung, and Blood Institute
Information Center
PO Box 30105
Bethesda, MD 20824-0105
(301) 951-3260
www.nih.gov/nhlbi/nhlbi.htm

CHAPTER 12

CANCER

ICD-9 140-239

Cancer is the second leading cause of death in the United States, accounting for nearly 1.4 million new cases and 560 000 deaths in 1997 (Table 12.1).[1] The lifetime probability of developing cancer is now estimated at 1 in 3. Over the past 50 years, the death rate from cancer has increased steadily; a sharp rise in lung cancer rates is the main reason for this increase (Figures 12.1a and 12.1b). However, it appears that a slight decline in cancer mortality began in 1991, due in large part to a decline in lung cancer.[3] This could portend a progressive decline in cancer mortality in the coming decade.

Rates of cancer vary by age and sex. Although cancer occurs more frequently with advancing age, it is also the leading cause of death due to disease among US children aged 1 to 14.[1] Cancer becomes 100 times more common in men and 30 times more common in women as age increases from 25 to 75 years.[4] The

Ross C. Brownson, PhD
John S. Reif, DVM, MSc
Michael C.R. Alavanja, DrPH
Dileep G. Bal, MD, MPH

overall 1994 cancer mortality rates were 160 per 100 000 in men and 111 per 100 000 in women—a difference of 44%.[5]

Racial and ethnic groups are not affected equally by cancer (Figures 12.2a and 12.2b). Black men have the highest incidence rate of cancer and non-Hispanic White men have the next highest rate (14% lower than that of Black men).[6] Cancer mortality rates were virtually identical in Blacks and Whites 35 years ago, but since 1960, cancer death rates have increased 51% in Black men and 10% in Black women, compared with increases of 17% in White men and 2% in White women. For five cancers—larynx, oral cavity, pancreas, colorectal, and leukemia—mortality rates for Whites have been decreasing, whereas rates for Blacks have been increasing.[7] Cancer death rates for people of Hispanic origin are approximately 41% lower than those of non-Hispanic populations.[6]

Excess cancer rates among Blacks are largely attributed to factors associated with socioeconomic status.[8] Higher cancer incidence and mortality rates among the socioeconomically disadvantaged are the

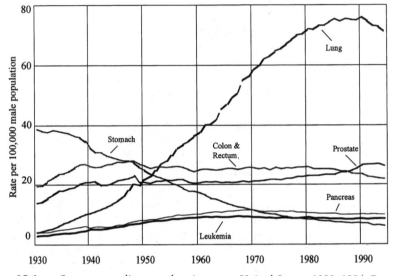

Figure 12.1.a—Cancer mortality rates by site, men, United States, 1930–1994. Rates are adjusted to the age distribution of the 1970 census population. *Sources*: National Center for Health Statistics; American Cancer Society.

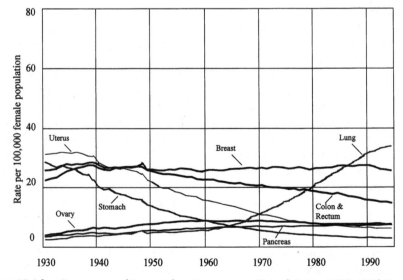

Figure 12.1.b—Cancer mortality rates by site, women, United States, 1930–1994. Rates are adjusted to the age distribution of the 1970 census population. *Sources*: National Center for Health Statistics; American Cancer Society.

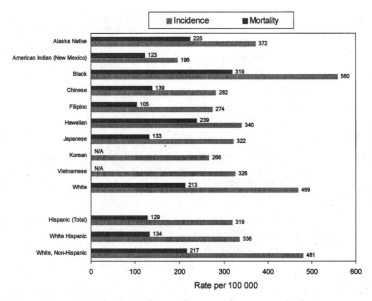

Figure 12.2.a—Cancer incidence and mortality rates by race and ethnic group, men, United States, 1988–1992. Rates are adjusted to the age distribution of the 1970 census population. *Source*: US Dept. of Health and Human Services.[6]

result of several factors. These include a higher prevalence of major cancer risk factors such as cigarette smoking, dietary factors, delays in cancer diagnosis, and lack of access to prompt and adequate treatment following diagnosis. Many of these factors are consequences of living in poverty. Twenty-eight percent of Blacks in the United States, compared with 8% of Whites, live below the poverty level.[9] Thus, being Black becomes a convenient, albeit somewhat misleading, proxy measure of confounding factors such as income, education, and social deprivation.[10]

The observed 5-year survival rate from cancer—that is, the proportion of patients alive 5 years after diagnosis—has improved over the past 50 years from 20% in the 1930s to 33% in the 1960s to 40% in the 1980s. The observed survival rate is differentiated from the usually cited relative survival rate (ie, when other causes of death are taken into account), which is currently 56% (Table 12.1).

The economic impact of cancer is enormous. The estimated direct medical costs of cancer in 1994 were more than $41.4 billion.[11] Direct costs associated with cancer increased 129% between 1985 and 1994.[11] In contrast to the huge cost of cancer treatment, the total national resources dedicated to early detection

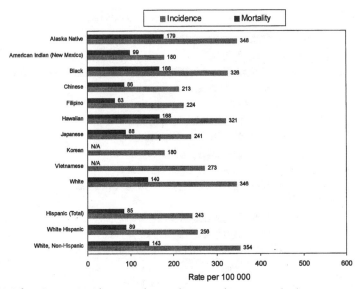

Figure 12.2.b—Cancer incidence and mortality rates by race and ethnic group, women, United States, 1988–1992. Rates are adjusted to the age distribution of the 1970 census population. *Source*: US Dept. of Health and Human Services.[6]

activities, such as screening for breast, cervical, and colorectal cancer, are estimated at only $3 to $4 billion per year.[12] The allocation of national resources to the primary prevention of cancer (eg, tobacco control, dietary intervention) is even smaller.

PATHOPHYSIOLOGY AND CANCER REGISTRATION

Cancer is a diverse group of diseases characterized by uncontrolled growth and spread of abnormal cells. Tumors, or abnormal enlargements of tissue, may be either benign or malignant. Benign tumors are generally innocuous and slow growing, whereas malignant tumors (commonly called cancers) contain abnormal genetic material and grow more rapidly. The principal danger of a cancer is its tendency to metastasize, or invade neighboring tissues or organs, and to grow in other areas of the body. If this spread remains untreated, cancer cells invade vital organs or cause dysfunction by displacing normal tissue.

Different cancer types have widely varying induction periods— that is, the time between exposure to cancer-causing agents and cancer occurrence. For example, the induction period for some types of

Table 12.1—Health Impact of Major Cancers, United States

Cancer Type (ICD-9 code)	Number of New Cases[a]	Number of Deaths[a]	Five-Year Survival[b]	Number of Hospital Days[c]
All sites (140–239)	1 382 400	560 000	56	13 225
Lung (162)	178 100	160 400	14	1 536
Colon and rectum (153, 154)	131 200	54 700	61	1 600
Breast (174)	181 600	44 190	84	525
Prostate (185)	334 500	41 800	87	585
Pancreas (157)	27 600	28 100	4	429
Non-Hodgkin's lymphoma (200, 202)	53 600	23 800	51	598
Leukemia (204–208)	28 300	21 310	42	651
Stomach (151)	22 400	14 000	21	294
Bladder (188)	54 500	11 700	81	310
Oral cavity (140–149)	30 750	8 440	53	—
Skin—melanoma (172)	40 300	7 300	87	26
Uterine corpus (182)	34 900	6 000	84	199
Uterine cervix (180)	14 500	4 800	69	94
Hodgkin's disease (201)	7 500	1 480	81	79

[a]Estimated for 1997.[1]
[b]Five-year relative survival rate for 1986–1992.[1]
[c]Hospital days in thousands, based on the 1994 National Hospital Discharge Survey.[2]

leukemia may be as short as a few years, compared with induction periods as long as 45 years for some cases of bladder cancer.

Cancers are classified according to their organ or tissue of origin (site code) and according to their histologic features (morphology code). The most widely used classification schemes are the *International Classification of Diseases, Ninth Revision, Clinical Modification* (ICD-9-CM),[13] and the *International Classification of Diseases for Oncology* (ICD-O).[14] The existence of hundreds of cancer varieties is readily apparent when 22 major sites of origin and 88 major histologic types are combined.[7]

In addition to being grouped by site and histologic features, cancers are classified according to their stage at diagnosis, or the extent to which the cancer has grown locally or invaded other tissues or organs. Cancer cells may remain at their original site (local stage), spread to an adjacent area of the body (regional stage), or spread throughout the body (distant stage).

Cancer registries collect detailed information on cancer patients through hospitals and medical clinics (also see Chapter 3). Cancer registry data have many valuable uses, such as evaluation of cancer incidence patterns, cancer risk factors, effects of prevention and early detection efforts, survival patterns, and treatment effects. In the United States, the most comprehensive cancer data are collected by the National Cancer Institute's Surveillance, Epidemiology, and End Results (SEER) Program, which was established in 1973.[7] The SEER Program collects incidence and survival information in five states and four metropolitan areas that comprise about 9.6% of the US population. The Centers for Disease Control and Prevention's recently funded National Program of Cancer Registries (Public Law 102-515) has funded 42 states and the District of Columbia to develop registries or to enhance current registries. When fully operational, this program will provide cancer incidence information on 93% of the US population.

RISK FACTORS

Several estimates of the proportion of overall cancer deaths due to various causes have been postulated.[15–19] Those of Doll and Peto,[15] Miller,[16] and the Harvard Center for Cancer Prevention[17] provide a useful benchmark on which to base preventive efforts (Table 12.2). For example, priority must be given to

eliminating tobacco use, becoming more physically active, and adopting diets that contain less fat and more fresh fruits and vegetables.

POTENTIAL FOR PREVENTION AND CONTROL

In 1985, the National Cancer Institute set a goal of reducing cancer mortality by 50% by the year 2000 through the systematic application of existing cancer control technologies.[20] Key elements in this effort include (1) reducing the prevalence of smoking; (2) reducing the percentage of total calories in the diet from fat; (3) increasing the average daily consumption of fiber; (4) increasing the percentage of women who undergo annual breast cancer screening (mammography and physical breast exam); (5) increasing the percentage of women who have annual Papanicolaou (Pap) tests; and (6) increasing adoption of state-of-the-art cancer treatments. Although this 50% goal was overly ambitious and will not be achieved, it has been extremely beneficial in focusing cancer control efforts at all levels of public health practice. In addition to these goals by the National Cancer Institute, the US Public Health Service has established a variety of objectives related to cancer prevention and control in *Healthy People 2000*.[21] These are now being revised for *Healthy People 2010*. It has been noted recently that

Table 12.2—Estimates of the Proportion of Cancer Deaths Attributed to Various Factors

Factor	Doll and Peto[15] Estimate (%)	Miller[16] Estimate (%)	Harvard[17] Estimate (%)
Tobacco	30	29	30
Diet	35	20	30
Infective processes	10	—	5[a]
Occupation	4	9	5
Family history	—	8	5
Reproductive and sexual history	7	7[b]	3
Sedentary lifestyle	—	—	5
Perinatal factors/growth[c]	—	—	5
Geophysical[d]	3	1	2
Alcohol[e]	3	6	3
Socioeconomic status	—	—	3
Pollution	2	—	2
Medication and medical procedures	1	2[f]	1
Industrial and consumer products	<1	—	
Salt/other food additives/ contaminants	—	—	1

[a]Viruses and other biologic agents.
[b]Attributed to parity (4%) and sexual activity (3%).
[c]Excess energy intake early in life and/or larger birth weight.
[d]Mainly natural background radiation and sunlight.
[e]With the exception of liver cancer, most alcohol-related cancers result from the combination of alcohol consumption and cigarette smoking.[15]
[f]Attributed to drugs (1%) and radiation (1%).
Note: Data compiled from Doll and Peto,[15] Miller,[16] and the Harvard Report on Cancer Prevention.[17]

without a stronger US commitment to cancer prevention, public health goals are unlikely to be achieved.[22]

PUBLIC HEALTH AGENCY PROGRESS IN CANCER CONTROL

As noted by Alciati and Marconi,[23] public health agencies at the federal, state, and local levels are vital entities in translating cancer control technologies into practice. The federal support for cancer control activities in state health agencies only began in 1986 when the National Cancer Institute initiated its Technical Development in Health Agencies Program. More recent cancer control demonstration projects in the public health setting include the National Cancer Institute-sponsored, American Stop Smoking Intervention Study (ASSIST), and the Centers for Disease Control and Prevention-funded, Breast and Cervical Cancer Prevention Program. Meissner et al.[24] summarized internal and external factors contributing to success in controlling cancer in the public health setting. Internal factors include (1) commitment of the organization's leadership to cancer control; (2) existence of appropriate data to monitor and evaluate programs; (3) appropriately trained staff; and (4) the ability to obtain funds for future activities. External factors include (1) successful linkages and coalitions; (2) an established cancer control plan; (3) access to outside health experts; (4) an informed state legislature; and (5) diffusion of initially successful programs to other sites.

Describing each cancer site in detail would be impractical. Therefore, we have limited this discussion to cancers that have one or more of the following characteristics: (1) they account for a major proportion of all cancer cases; (2) they can be reduced through scientifically proven prevention and control measures; or (3) they are frequently encountered in public health practice. Because of their importance, cancers of the lung, colon and rectum, breast, and cervix are discussed in detail. Shorter descriptions are provided for pros-tate cancer, lymphoma, leukemia, bladder cancer, cancer of the oral cavity, and skin melanoma.

LUNG CANCER

ICD-9 162

SIGNIFICANCE

Lung cancer is the leading cause of cancer deaths in the United States, accounting for 29% of all cancer deaths in 1997, or a total of 160 400 deaths.[1] Lung cancer is also the most common cancer worldwide.[25] This high mortality rate results from both a high incidence rate and a low survival rate: Only 14% of US lung cancer patients survive 5 years after diagnosis. We have seen little improvement in this survival rate over the past 25 years.

PATHOPHYSIOLOGY

More than 90% of lung cancers are believed to originate in the basal cells of the lung epithelium, or the lining surfaces of the lung. A series of changes, over a period of years, occurs as lung cancer develops. These involve an increase in the number of cells, structural changes in certain epithelial cells that lead to abnormal function, appearance of patient signs and symptoms, and cancer spread. The major cell types of lung cancer are squamous cell cancer (approximately 29% of cases), adenocarcinoma (approximately 25% of cases), small cell cancer (approximately 18% of cases), and large cell cancer (approximately 9% of cases).[7] Lung cancer growth rates vary based on the cell type involved. Of the major cell types, small cell cancer appears to grow and spread the most rapidly.

DESCRIPTIVE EPIDEMIOLOGY

Because lung cancer is so strongly associated with cigarette smoking, its descriptive epidemiology is largely explained by smoking patterns and trends.

High-Risk Groups

Although lung cancer mortality rates remain 2.3 times higher among men than among women, lung cancer surpassed breast cancer as the leading cause of cancer deaths in women in 1987. Mortality rates are 1.3 times higher among Blacks than among Whites. This racial difference is almost entirely the result of large differences in mortality between Black and White men.[6] Rates are nearly identical in Black and White women. Lung cancer mortality rates are approximately 50% lower among people of Hispanic origin than among non-Hispanics.[6] Lung cancer rates increase with age, with 60 years being the average age of diagnosis. Lung cancer risk is also higher for people with a family history of lung cancer and for individuals who have been previously diagnosed with a nonmalignant lung disease, such as tuberculosis or asthma.[26] People of lower socioeconomic status are at higher risk for lung cancer.

Geographic Distribution

In the United States, lung cancer rates are generally highest in the southern and lower midwestern states.[7] Kentucky has the highest lung cancer death rate, and Utah has the lowest. Worldwide, lung cancer is most common in developed countries such as the United States, Scotland, Australia, and Russia.[25] Deaths from lung cancer are relatively rare in Mexico, Central America, and South America.

Time Trends

The lung cancer mortality rate in the United States has increased dramatically over the past 50 years, from 7 per 100 000 in 1940 to 49 per 100 000 in 1989.[1, 7] The major increase in lung cancer mortality rates in men occurred from 1940 to 1979. In the 1980s, the rate of increase slowed, and now the male lung cancer mortality rate has begun to decline.[7] In contrast, a sharp increase in lung cancer mortality rates was observed among women in the 1960s, and this rapid increase continues. Female lung cancer mortality rates are not projected to decline until around the year 2010.[27]

RISK FACTORS

Magnitude of Risk Factors

The strongest risk factor for lung cancer is cigarette smoking (Table 12.3). The association between smoking and lung cancer is one of the most widely studied and clearly defined relationships in chronic disease epidemiology. The relative risk of lung cancer due to smoking is approximately 10 for men and 5 for women, although this difference has been lessening over time as women have begun smoking more cigarettes per day and have started smoking at increasingly younger ages.[28]

Certain occupational pursuits also increase lung cancer risk, although

exposures on a population basis are much lower than cigarette smoking.[19, 29] Asbestos exposure among nonsmokers accounts for a relative risk of about 5.[30] When asbestos exposure is combined with cigarette smoking, the risk increases markedly to approximately 50-fold. Occupational exposure to radon accounts for a 20-fold increase in lung cancer risk.[31] Radon also interacts with smoking to greatly increase the risk. Increases in lung cancer risk have also been documented for exposure to polycyclic hydrocarbons (eg, among gas, steel, coal, and asphalt workers) and inorganic arsenic (eg, among smelter workers and pesticide manufacturers).[19, 29, 32]

Exposure to radon gas in the home, especially in combination with cigarette smoking, may increase

Table 12.3—Modifiable Risk Factors for Lung Cancer, United States

Magnitude	Risk Factor	Best Estimate (%) of Population Attributable Risk[a] (Range)
Strong (relative risk[a] >4)	Cigarette smoking	87 (84–90)
Occupation[b]	13 (10–20)	
Moderate (relative risk 2–4)	None	—
Weak (relative risk <2)	Residential radon exposure	10 (7–25)
	Environmental tobacco smoke exposure	2 (1–6)
Possible	Diet low in b-carotene	—
	High-fat diet	—
	Urban air pollution	—

[a]Defined in Table 2.4, page 51; population attributable risk estimates do not add to 100% because they ignore the overlapping effects of some risk factors, such as cigarette smoking and occupation.
[b]Includes occupational exposures to asbestos, polycyclic hydrocarbons, arsenic, and radon gas.
Note. Data compiled from references 15, 16, 19, 25, 29, 34, 37, and 38.

the risk of lung cancer.[33] In addition, exposure to environmental tobacco smoke, or passive smoking, elevates lung cancer risk slightly in nonsmokers.[34] Numerous studies[35] have also shown that a diet low in certain fruits and vegetables (eg, those that contain b-carotene) increases lung cancer risk, although the results from a recent large clinical trial on b-carotene supplementation showed no beneficial effect on lung cancer mortality.[36]

Population-Attributable Risk

An estimated 87% of lung cancer cases are attributable to cigarette smoking (Table 12.3).[37] Occupational exposures are estimated to contribute to an additional 13% of lung cancers. Extrapolations from risks among underground miners indicate that exposure to indoor radon may account for up to 10% of lung cancer deaths,[38] although quantifying this risk factor accurately is extremely difficult. Dietary factors may account for 5% of annual lung cancer cases,[16] and exposure to environmental tobacco smoke accounts for approximately 2% of US lung cancer cases.[34]

PREVENTION AND CONTROL MEASURES

Prevention

Primary prevention through smoking reduction has tremendous potential to reduce lung cancer mortality. Smoking cessation drastically reduces the risk of lung cancer.

After 10 years of abstinence from smoking, the ex-smoker's risk of lung cancer is reduced to half that of a continuing smoker.[39] Smoking behavior is usually adopted early in life; therefore, prevention of tobacco use among youth is critical to the overall goal of reducing smoking prevalence (see Chapter 5).

Workers exposed to lung carcinogens (eg, asbestos workers, uranium miners) should also be targeted for intervention, since many of their exposures interact with smoking to increase dramatically the risk of lung cancer.[30]

Dietary changes to increase consumption of fresh fruits and vegetables may decrease lung cancer risk. These changes are consistent with dietary guidelines discussed in other sections and chapters.

Screening and Early Detection

Although the chest x-ray and examination of cells in the sputum (sputum cytology) are capable of detecting lung cancer in the early stages, the overall costs versus benefits do not currently justify recommending these tests as mass screening tools for asymptomatic individuals.[40]

Treatment, Rehabilitation, and Recovery

Lung cancer treatment is largely determined by the cell type and stage at diagnosis. Treatment options include surgery, radiation therapy, and chemotherapy. Lung cancer mortality could be reduced by an estimated 7% through early application of existing state-of-the-art treatments.[20]

EXAMPLES OF PUBLIC HEALTH INTERVENTIONS

Public health interventions that are likely to affect lung cancer rates include the National Cancer Institute's American Stop Smoking Intervention Study (ASSIST) for Cancer Prevention,[41] the Centers for Disease Control and Prevention's Initiatives to Mobilize for Prevention and Control of Tobacco Use (IM-PACT),[42] and dedicated state tobacco taxes, such as those in California and Massachusetts (see Chapter 5).[43, 44]

AREAS OF FUTURE RESEARCH AND DEMONSTRATION

First, we must determine and apply effective smoking prevention and cessation techniques that target high-risk and/or difficult-to-reach populations such as youth, minorities, the economically disadvantaged, and heavy smokers. Second, we need to further examine the roles of risk factors such as occupational exposures and residential radon exposure and their interactions with cigarette smoking. Third, we need to evaluate the possible role of dietary factors and cooking practices in the prevention of lung cancer. Finally,

we need to identify and refine efficacious methods for detecting lung cancer in its early stages.

COLORECTAL CANCER

ICD-9 153, 154

SIGNIFICANCE

Cancer of the colon and rectum, also known as colorectal cancer, is the second leading cause of cancer death in men and the third leading cause of cancer death in women.[1] It accounts for 10% of all cancer deaths in the United States. In 1997, approximately 94 100 new cases of colon cancer and 37 100 new cases of rectal cancer were diagnosed.[1] The overall 5-year survival rate for colorectal cancer is 61%, with a rate of 91% for cancers identified in the local stage.[1]

PATHOPHYSIOLOGY

The natural history of colorectal cancer is not clearly understood. Some researchers have suggested that delays in transit time for fecal material may increase contact time between carcinogens and the bowel wall, increasing the risk of colorectal cancer. These transit-time delays may be related to a diet low in fiber or to a lack of physical activity, or both. The predominant cell type seen in colorectal cancer is adenocarcinoma (over 96% of all cases).[6]

. . . .

High-Risk Groups

Colorectal cancer mortality is 44% higher for men than for women and 15% higher for Blacks than for Whites.[7] The incidence of colorectal cancer rises sharply after age 50, with two-thirds of all patients being over age 50. The mean age at diagnosis is 62 years. Several genetic and medical conditions predispose people to colorectal cancer, although these factors are relatively uncommon in the general population. A history of colorectal cancer in a first-degree relative elevates risk. A family tendency toward the development of multiple adenomatous polyps (familial polyposis) can elevate risk of colorectal cancer at a young age.[32] Recent research has also identified a specific familial gene for colorectal cancer that may result in new opportunities for early detection and treatment.[45] In addition, individuals with inflammatory bowel disease (eg, ulcerative colitis, Crohn's disease) carry an increased risk.[32] People in higher socioeconomic groups are at higher risk of colorectal cancer.

Geographic Distribution

In the United States, rates of colorectal cancer are highest in the northeastern and north central states and lowest in the western and southwestern states.[7] Worldwide, colorectal cancer rates are highest in developed countries in North America, northern and western Europe, and New Zealand.[25] Rates are extremely low in Japan, although Japanese immigrants to the United States acquire colorectal cancer rates similar to those of Americans and residents of other westernized countries.[15,25] This suggests that lifestyle risk factors are important in causing colorectal cancer.

Time Trends

From 1973 to 1990, colorectal cancer mortality rates in the United States declined by 14%.[7] This decline occurred only among Whites. Among Blacks, colorectal cancer mortality increased during the same period.

RISK FACTORS

Magnitude of Risk Factors

Few modifiable risk factors for colorectal cancer have been firmly characterized, despite many epidemiologic studies (Table 12.4). Considerable attention has focused on the relationship between diet and colorectal cancer. Although the precise dietary components and biologic mechanisms are not clearly understood, increased risk of colorectal cancer has been associated with a diet high in saturated fat (especially through meat intake).[47] In addition, an elevated risk of colorectal cancer has consistently been associated with a diet low in vegetables and low in high-fiber

Table 12.4—Modifiable Risk Factors for Colorectal Cancer, United States

Magnitude	Risk Factor	Best Estimate (%) of Population Attributable Risk[a] (Range)
Strong (relative risk[a] >4)	None	—
Moderate (relative risk 2—4)	None	—
Weak (relative risk <2)	High-fat diet	— (15–25)
	Low-vegetable diet	— (25–35)
	Physical inactivity[b]	32 (—)
Possible	Alcohol consumption	—
	Occupation[c]	—
	Aspirin use[d]	—
	Obesity	—

[a] Defined in Table 2.4, page 51.
[b] Includes occupational and recreational physical activities.
[c] Includes occupational exposures to asbestos, metal and wood dusts, and certain chemicals.
[d] Use of aspirin may decrease risk.[48]
Note: Data compiled from references 20, 25, 29, and 46.

grains.[48, 49–51] Studies of diet and colorectal cancer are confronted with many difficulties, including a high correlation between many dietary components and problems with subjects' ability to recall past dietary practices. Growing evidence suggests that a lack of either occupational or recreational physical activity increases the risk of colorectal cancer.[52]

Population-Attributable Risk

Up to half of colorectal cancer cases may be related to diet (Table 12.4).[20, 29] Within this proportion, estimates suggest that 15% to 25% of colorectal cancer may be related to fat intake and that 25% to 35% may be related to low intake of fruits and vegetables.[25] An estimated 32% of colorectal cancer may be related to physical inactivity.[46]

PREVENTION AND CONTROL MEASURES

Prevention

Although the relationship of diet to colorectal cancer is not completely understood, dietary changes have the potential to substantially reduce colorectal cancer deaths. International and migrant population data indicate that a substantial reduction in colorectal cancer incidence could be achieved in 10 years through dietary changes alone.[20] This reduction may be achieved by increasing per capita consumption of fiber from fruits and vegetables to 20 to 30 grams per day and by decreasing per capita consumption of fat to below 30% of total calories.[20] Current public health guidelines on diet, nutrition, and cancer suggest (1) eating five or more servings of fruits and vegetables each day, (2) limiting intake of high-fat foods, particularly from animal sources, (3) being physically active, and (4) limiting alcoholic beverage consumption.[53]

Multiple complementary strategies are needed to achieve diet-related cancer prevention goals. These include routine provision of nutrition education in schools as part of comprehensive school health education, improved school lunch menus, routine nutrition counseling by health professionals, and improved food labeling so that consumers can make better dietary choices.

In addition, colorectal cancer mortality may be reduced through increased physical activity in the US population (see Chapter 7).

Screening and Early Detection

The principal screening tests for early detection of colorectal cancer are the digital rectal examination, fecal occult blood testing, and sigmoidoscopy.[40] Each of these screening tests has limitations. These limitations include incomplete access to the rectal area in the digital rectal exam, the presence of false positive and false negative results in occult blood testing, and the low compliance rate and high cost associated with sigmoidoscopy.

Whether these screening tests reduce colorectal cancer mortality remains unclear,[40] although the decline in colorectal cancer death rates over time may be related to the increased use of screening tests. The American Cancer Society recommends an annual digital rectal examination for all adults beginning at age 40 and annual fecal occult blood testing beginning at age 50.[1] Sigmoidoscopy is recommended every 3 to 5 years beginning at age 50. At a physician's recommendation, people at higher risk of colorectal cancer (eg, those with familial polyposis or ulcerative colitis) may require more frequent screening, beginning at an earlier age. The US Preventive Services Task Force recommends annual fecal occult blood testing, or sigmoidoscopy, or both for all persons age 50 and older.[40]

Treatment, Rehabilitation, and Recovery

Surgery, sometimes in combination with radiation therapy, is the most effective method of treating colorectal cancer. After successful treatment, colorectal cancer patients need to be followed closely, because they are at a high risk of having recurrent or new cancers in the colon and rectum.

EXAMPLES OF PUBLIC HEALTH INTERVENTIONS

A noteworthy public health intervention to lower diet-related cancer risk is the "5 A Day—For Better Health" project from California.[54] In "5 A Day," mass media, social marketing, and a public-private sector partnership are being used to achieve the year 2000 goal of consumption of five servings of fruits and vegetables per person per day. Preliminary evaluations of this project are encouraging, and the National Cancer Institute is currently replicating this effort in other states.[55, 56]

AREAS OF FUTURE RESEARCH AND DEMONSTRATION

Additional epidemiologic and clinical research is needed to better define the risk of colorectal cancer related to specific dietary factors. Long-term prospective studies currently under way should help clarify diet-colorectal cancer associations. Further investigation is also needed to determine the efficacy of early detection measures such as fecal occult blood assays and sigmoidoscopy. In addition, the public needs consistent, scientifically based guidelines on how to change the American diet.[57]

BREAST CANCER

ICD-9 174

SIGNIFICANCE

Breast cancer is the most common cancer type among women in the United States, accounting for 180 200 new cases and 44 190 deaths in 1997.[1] Worldwide, breast cancer is the third most common cancer, after cancers of the lung and stomach. Breast cancer rarely occurs in men (1400 US cases in 1997). Approximately one of every nine women will develop breast cancer at some time during her lifetime. The overall 5-year survival rate for breast cancer is 84%, with a range of survival from 20% for distant-stage cancer to 97% for local-stage cancer.[1]

PATHOPHYSIOLOGY

The underlying biological mechanisms involved in the development of breast cancer are not clearly understood. As with other cancers, breast cancer develops through a series of stages—in situ early stages to distant-spread late stages. It is likely that hormones, either produced by the body or taken internally, play a role in breast cancer pathogenesis. For example, it is known that the presence or absence of certain receptor proteins (ie, estrogen receptor positive or negative) can influence the success of breast cancer treatment.[58] Receptor-positive women respond better to hormonal therapy and show increased survival rates. The predominant cell type of breast cancer is adenocarcinoma (approximately 95% of cases).[7]

DESCRIPTIVE EPIDEMIOLOGY

High-Risk Groups

Although the incidence of breast cancer is higher in Whites, mortality rates are 16% higher among Black women than among White women.[7] Mortality increases with age, with 54% of deaths from breast cancer occurring among women who are 65 years of age and older. An early age at menarche and late age at menopause elevate the risk of breast cancer.[59] People of higher socioeconomic status are at higher risk of developing breast cancer. The presence of a mutation in a gene (BRCA1) on chromosome 17q12-21 has been shown to greatly increase the risk of breast cancer in women. Women with germline mutations to BRCA1 are estimated to have an 80% to 90% lifetime risk of developing breast cancer.[60] The BRCA1 gene is likely to account for 5% to 7% of all breast cancers.

Geographic Distribution

Breast cancer mortality rates in the United States are generally higher in northern states and lower in southern states. Delaware has the highest, and Hawaii has the lowest breast cancer mortality rate.[7] Urban residents tend to have higher breast cancer rates. Breast cancer rates also show wide international variations, with the highest rates being in North America and western Europe.[25]

Time Trends

Mortality due to breast cancer has remained relatively stable over the past 50 years; however, between 1973 and 1990, breast cancer mortality rates increased 2% among US women overall and 21% among Black women.[7] Breast cancer incidence rates in the United States rose from 82 per 100 000 in 1973 to 109 per 100 000 in 1990.[7] This increase has occurred in both younger and older women and is related in part to the increased use of screening mammography. Larger recent increases in breast cancer incidence rather than mortality are most likely the result of diagnosis of breast cancer at progressively earlier stages and, hence, higher survival rates.

RISK FACTORS

Magnitude of Risk Factors

Through numerous epidemiologic studies, an array of modifiable breast cancer risk factors has been established (Table 12.5).[59, 61, 62] Despite the large number of risk factors, few are strongly associated with the development of breast cancer, and no single factor or combination of factors can predict the occurrence of breast cancer in any one individual.

The risk associated with reproductive variables—never having children, being of a late age at first birth, having an early menarche, having a late menopause—is related to the

Table 12.5—Modifiable Risk Factors for Breast Cancer, United States

Magnitude	Risk Factor	Best Estimate (%) of Population Attributable Risk[a] (Range)
Strong (relative risk[a] >4)	None	
Moderate (relative risk 2–4)	Large doses of chest radiation	2 (1–3)
Weak (relative risk <2)	Never being married	—
	Never having children	5 (1–9)
	First full-term pregnancy after age 30	7 (1–13)
	Oophorectomy[b]	—
	Obesity after menopause	12 (8–16)
	Alcohol consumption	—
Possible	Physical inactivity	—
	Cigarette smoking	—
	Environmental tobacco smoke exposure	—
	High caloric or high fat diet	—
	Pesticide exposure	—
	Lack of breast-feeding	—
	Use of diethylstilbestrol	—
	Long-term use of oral contraceptives or estrogen replacements	—

[a]Defined in Table 2.4, page 51.
[b]Removal of ovaries before menopause reduces risk.[59]
Note. Data compiled from references 16, 61, and 62.

hormonal environment to which the breast is exposed (during pregnancy or during a long menstrual history).[32] Moderate-to-heavy alcohol consumption is also associated with an increased risk of breast cancer.[63]

Several other breast cancer risk factors have been examined, but the results across studies are inconsistent. These include consumption of a high caloric or high-fat diet and use of exogenous hormones, notably oral contraceptives and estrogen replacements during menopause.

In spite of few well-designed studies, most that are published have shown a decreased risk of breast cancer among women who are more active.[59] There is also limited evidence of an increased breast cancer risk among women who smoke and have the genetic predisposition to be slow acetylators of aromatic amines.[64] Exposure to environmental tobacco smoke may also be a risk factor for breast cancer.[65]

Population-Attributable Risk

Several established risk factors each account for relatively small proportions of overall breast cancer incidence (Table 12.5).

PREVENTION AND CONTROL MEASURES

Prevention

None of the established risk factors for breast cancer, with the possible exception of obesity after menopause, is readily amenable to modification. Although considerable research in this area continues, opportunities for primary prevention of breast cancer are currently limited. Therefore, public health practitioners should focus their attention on secondary prevention—that is, early detection.

Screening and Early Detection

Several large studies have demonstrated that clinical breast examination by a physician or nurse and mammography screening (ie, low-dose breast x-rays) are effective methods for the early detection of breast cancer.[40] It has been suggested that failure to use mammography on a population basis may account for as much as 19% to 25% of all breast cancer deaths.[16, 20] In addition, several studies suggest that women who practice breast self-examination (BSE) may have a greater chance of detecting breast cancer in an early stage, although the effectiveness of BSE is not yet proven. Although there remains scientific controversy regarding the benefits versus the risk of screening women in their 40s, there is convincing evidence of the effectiveness of mammography for women age 50 to 69 years.[40] The decision to screen women under age 50 is commonly considered in relation to risk; for example, women with a family history of breast cancer are screened more frequently. The American Cancer Society recommends that women 20 years of age and older practice monthly breast self-examinations.[1] On the basis of data from the National Health Interview Survey,[66] the prevalence of annual mammography screening among US women age 50 and older more than doubled from 1987 (16.5%) to 1992 (35.3%). However, the prevalence of mammography screening remains lower among women with less education, living below the poverty level, or residing in rural areas.[66]

Treatment, Rehabilitation, and Recovery

Depending on the stage of cancer and the patient's medical history, breast cancer treatment may require lumpectomy (local removal of the cancer), mastectomy (surgical removal of the breast), radiation therapy, chemotherapy, or hormone therapy. Two or more treatment methods are often used in combination. Cancer support groups such as the American Cancer Society's Reach to Recovery program can provide valuable information and emotional support to breast cancer patients.

EXAMPLES OF PUBLIC HEALTH INTERVENTIONS

The Breast and Cervical Cancer Mortality Prevention Act of 1990 established the largest public health application of breast cancer control technology.[67] This initiative enables the Centers for Disease Control and Prevention to sponsor comprehensive breast cancer screening programs through state public health departments. As of 1995, all states and nine American Indian tribes had targeted mammography screening to low-income, minority, and medically underserved populations.[67] Program components include screening and follow-up, public and professional education, mammography quality assurance, and surveillance. Evaluation of this program to date has shown initial evidence of a higher percentage of early stage breast cancers among those detected in the second or later round of screening.[68]

AREAS OF FUTURE RESEARCH AND DEMONSTRATION

Several possible risk factors for breast cancer—diet, alcohol use, physical inactivity, smoking, environmental tobacco smoke exposure, and menopausal estrogen use—would be amenable to primary prevention. Therefore, future research should focus on determining their precise roles in causing breast cancer.

The drug tamoxifen has already proven effective as a therapeutic agent by preventing or delaying the recurrence of breast cancer. Currently, studies are under way (including a nationwide, multicenter trial) to determine whether tamoxifen can play a role in breast cancer prevention among healthy, asymptomatic women.

In the area of early detection, we must (1) assess the effectiveness and long-term benefits of breast self-examination; (2) determine innovative methods to encourage women to have regular mammograms; (3) apply and enforce uniform standards of mammography quality control; and (4) identify better methods to ensure initiation and completion of breast cancer treatment.

Although techniques to assess mutations in the BRCA1 gene are currently limited to a few families for research purposes, tests are likely to be available for population-based screening in the next few years. A few of the ethical considerations relevant to use of new genetic markers include the following: (1) how should information be provided to participants of a research study when there are enormous health consequences? (2) how can confidentiality be maintained? (3) would identification of a strong genetic predisposition toward a particular cancer affect an individual's ability to be employed and/or insured? and (4) how should such tests enter the clinical and public health marketplace? Consideration of a variety of ethic issues in epidemiology is provided in detail elsewhere.[69]

CERVICAL CANCER

ICD-9 180

SIGNIFICANCE

Invasive cancer of the uterine cervix, commonly known as cervical cancer, accounted for 14 500 new cases and 4800 deaths among women in the United States in 1997.[1] In situ cervical cancer—that is, detected in the earliest, premalignant stage—is much more common, accounting for about 55 000 US cases per year. Cervical cancer is the 16th most common cancer in the United States; yet, it is the second most common cancer among women worldwide.[25]

The overall 5-year survival rate for cervical cancer is 66%; however, survival approaches 100% for cervical cancers detected in situ.

Pathophysiology

It is believed that early stages of cervical cancer are characterized by dysplasia, or the presence of cells that are altered in size, shape, and organization. Preclinical, preinvasive changes in the cervix are called cervical intraepithelial neoplasia (CIN). These early cervical cancer changes can easily be detected through the Pap test. The Pap test involves collecting and analyzing a small sample of cells from the cervix. Clinical manifestations of cervical cancer may involve bleeding or other vaginal discharges. The major cell types observed for invasive cervical cancer are squamous cell cancer (approximately 76% of cases) and adenocarcinoma (approximately 13% of cases).[7]

DESCRIPTIVE EPIDEMIOLOGY

High-Risk Groups

Cervical cancer incidence increases sharply until age 45 and peaks between the ages of 45 and 55 years. The incidence of cervical cancer is twice as high among Blacks as it is among Whites, and mortality rates are approximately 2.4 times higher among Blacks. Elevated cervical cancer rates are also observed for Hispanics, American Indians, and Hawaiian natives. Women of lower socioeconomic status are at higher risk of cervical cancer. Several religious groups—Catholic nuns, Amish, Mormons, and Jews—have very low rates of cervical cancer, probably because of marital and sexual risk factors.[70]

Geographic Distribution

Cervical cancer mortality rates in the United States are generally higher in southeastern states and lower in western and midwestern states. The District of Columbia has the highest rate, and Utah has the lowest cervical cancer mortality rate.[7] Internationally, cervical cancer rates are highest in sub-Saharan Africa, Central and South America, and Southeast Asia.[25]

Time Trends

Incidence and mortality rates of invasive cervical cancer have been decreasing steadily over the past 50 years. From 1950 to 1989, cervical cancer incidence and mortality in the United States have shown a larger annual percent decrease than have any other major cancers.[7] Researchers and public health practitioners have been concerned, however, that the declines in incidence and mortality have been leveling off in recent years.[71]

RISK FACTORS

Magnitude of Risk Factors

Major risk factors for cervical cancer include socioeconomic characteristics such as low education and low income; sexual activity variables such as multiple sex partners and early age at first intercourse; and other lifestyle factors such as cigarette smoking (Table 12.6). Considerable attention has focused on the etiologic role of sexually transmitted viruses, especially the human papilloma virus (types 16 and 18). Many of these risk factors are more common among US Blacks than among Whites. These differences account for much of the large racial difference in incidence rates.[72] Researchers also have noted that a diet low in certain vitamins, such as b-carotene and vitamin C, may increase the risk of cervical cancer.[35]

Population-Attributable Risk

Estimates of attributable risk suggest the importance of multiple sex partners, cigarette smoking, early age at first intercourse, and a history of genital infection (Table 12.6). The upper range of the attributable risk estimate for genital infection may be quite large (perhaps up to 50%) due to the potential impact of human papilloma virus infection.

Table 12.6—Modifiable Risk Factors for Cervical Cancer, United States

Magnitude	Risk Factor	Best Estimate (%) of Population Attributable Risk[a] (Range)
Strong (relative risk[a] >4)	None	
Moderate (relative risk 2–4)	Multiple sex partners	38 (26-50)
	Early age at first intercourse (≤17 years)	25 (17-33)
	History of sexually transmitted diseases[b]	5 (1-50)
Weak (relative risk <2)	Cigarette smoking	32 (23-41)
	Use of barrier contraceptive[c]	—
Possible	Low dietary intake of certain vitamins[d]	—
	Use of oral contraceptives	—

[a] Defined in Table 2.4, page 51.
[b] Includes infection with human papilloma virus, types 16 and 18.
[c] Use of barrier contraceptive methods (diaphragm and condom) reduces risk.
[d] Includes vitamin A, b-carotene, and folate.
Note: Data compiled from references 29, 70, and 72.

PREVENTION AND CONTROL MEASURES

Prevention

Several behavioral changes will reduce the risk of cervical cancer. These include limiting the number of sexual partners, delaying intercourse until a later age, avoiding sexually transmitted diseases, and eliminating cigarette smoking. Use of barrier or spermicidal contraceptives may also reduce risk.

Screening and Early Detection

The principal screening test for cervical cancer is the Pap test.

Decreases in cervical cancer incidence and mortality over the past 40 years are mainly the result of early detection due to widespread use of the Pap test.[40] It is estimated that between 37% and 60% of cervical cancer deaths could be prevented by full use of the Pap test.[16] Despite the availability and frequent use of the Pap test, subgroups of high-risk women—for example, those of lower education and income—either have never been screened or are screened infrequently.[71] Pap testing is especially important in these high-risk groups and in women who no longer see a physician for obstetric needs.

A large group of health and medical organizations has adopted a consensus recommendation on Pap test guidelines.[73] The group recommended annual Pap tests for all women who are or who have been sexually active or have reached the age of 18. At the discretion of the physician, Pap testing may be conducted less frequently after three or more annual Pap tests have been normal. The US Preventive Services Task Force recommends that Pap tests should begin with the onset of sexual activity and should be repeated at least every 3 years.[40] The prevalence of Pap testing is lower among US women with less education, living below the poverty level, and residing in rural areas.[66]

Treatment, Rehabilitation, and Recovery

Depending on the stage at diagnosis, cervical cancer is usually treated by surgery or radiation or both. In situ cancers can be treated by cryotherapy (cell destruction by extreme cold), electrocoagulation (cell destruction by intense heat), or local surgery.

EXAMPLES OF PUBLIC HEALTH INTERVENTIONS

The National Cancer Institute and the Centers for Disease Control and Prevention have funded a series of cervical cancer research and application projects since 1985.[71] Most of these projects seek to increase the use of the Pap test in high-risk populations through "inreach," or increasing use in women who attend clinics, and "outreach," or offering community-wide screening programs. Unfortunately, firm evaluation data from most of these projects are not yet available.

In addition, the Centers for Disease Control and Prevention are sponsoring large-scale cervical cancer screening projects as part of the Breast and Cervical Cancer Mortality Prevention Act of 1990.[67] Early results from this program have shown higher rates of cervical intraepithelial neoplasia among younger women and invasive cervical cancer in older women.[74]

AREAS OF FUTURE RESEARCH AND DEMONSTRATION

Further research into the causes of cervical cancer will lead to increased opportunities for primary prevention. A better understanding of the interaction between multiple risk factors is also needed. Given the high rates of cervical cancer mortality among minority and economically disadvantaged women, better targeting of proven cervical cancer control technologies is clearly needed.

PROSTATE CANCER

ICD-9 185

SIGNIFICANCE

Cancer of the prostate is the most common cancer among men in the United States, accounting for 334 000 new cases in 1997.[1] Prostate cancer is the second leading cause of cancer deaths in US men, after lung cancer. Approximately 1 of every 11 men will develop prostate cancer. The incidence and age-adjusted mortality of prostatic cancer appears to be rising worldwide, but this is due at least partially to increased screening.

Descriptive Epidemiology

Black men have the highest incidence of prostate cancer in the world, with an incidence that is 19% higher than that among White men in the United States.[1, 6] The incidence of prostate cancer in Asian countries is much lower, but Asian immigrants to the United States experience rates closer to those for US men, suggesting that environmental factors, including nutrition, may play a role in etiology. The lifetime risk of prostate cancer among African-American men is now estimated at one in eight. The median age of incidence is 70 years of age, and the 5-year survival rate for prostate cancer is 76%. Latent (subclinical) prostate cancer affects an increasing

proportion of men at each decade of life.[75]

Risk Factors

The causes of prostate cancer are largely unknown. Both environmental and familial factors may contribute to increased risk. The major hypotheses that appear to play a role in prostate cancer are hormonal, family history, and nutritional. Prostate cancer is hormonally dependent, and steroid hormones such as testosterone and dihydrotestosterone are suspected to play a role in pathogenesis. Substantial epidemiologic evidence suggests that a diet high in fat, particularly animal or saturated fat, increases the risk of prostate cancer, but the mechanism for this association is unclear.[76] A family history of prostate cancer in a first-degree relative appears to double the risk,[77] suggesting that interactions between genetic factors and environmental exposures may be important in carcinogenesis in the prostate gland. In addition, suspected environmental factors include occupational exposure to cadmium and work in rubber manufacturing and farming.[29, 32]

PREVENTION AND CONTROL MEASURES

Because its causes are not clearly understood, prostate cancer is not currently amenable to primary prevention. To promote the early detection of prostate cancer, the American Cancer Society and the National Cancer Institute recommend that men undergo an annual digital rectal examination.[1] In addition, prostatic ultrasound and measurement of prostate-specific antigen in serum may be beneficial in detecting cancers that are too small to be detected by digital rectal examination. In particular, prostate specific antigen is being applied with increasing frequency in men over 50 years of age. Unfortunately, this assay is not specific for prostate cancer since concentrations increase with age and with the development of benign prostatic hypertrophy. The use of screening techniques for secondary prevention of prostate cancer remains a topic of intense investigation.[78]

LYMPHOMA

ICD-9 200-202

SIGNIFICANCE

Lymphomas are cancers that affect lymphocytes, primarily in the lymph nodes, spleen, and thymus. Lymphomas are generally classified as either Hodgkin's disease (HD) or non-Hodgkin's lymphoma (NHL). Hodgkin's disease and NHL are considered separately because they have distinct epidemiologic patterns, biological behavior, and histologic features.

DESCRIPTIVE EPIDEMIOLOGY

The US incidence rate for NHL has increased approximately 3% and the mortality rate 2% since the 1970s, making this the third most rapidly increasing cancer.[7, 79] This increase has occurred among men and women and for Blacks as well as Whites, as well as internationally.[79] In 1997, an estimated 53 600 persons were diagnosed with NHL. NHL is the sixth most common cancer in the United States, both in terms of new cases and mortality. The incidence of NHL is higher among men than among women and among Whites than Blacks. Age-specific incidence and mortality rates increase with increasing age. Although much of the increase in NHL rates is associated with AIDS-related cancers in young men, AIDS alone does not account for the overall increase in NHL.[7, 25]

In contrast, the incidence of Hodgkin's disease appears to be declining, particularly among the elderly.[80] In 1997, approximately 7500 developed Hodgkin's disease in the United States.[1] The incidence has been higher among Whites than Blacks, and among males than females. The age distribution of HD shows a bimodal distribution with two peaks; one in early adulthood, and a second after age 60.[7] The 5-

year survival rates for NHL (51%) and HD (81%) are also markedly different.

RISK FACTORS

The causes of the lymphomas are not well understood, in part because of the diversity of histologic forms of cancer in these diagnoses. Increasing evidence indicates that exposure to certain herbicides and pesticides elevates NHL risk.[81] The strongest link to date has been shown between the use of phenoxy acid-based herbicides (such as 2,4-dichloro-phenoxyacetic acid) and NHL.[82] People with immune system disorders, organ transplant patients, and persons undergoing treatment with immunosuppressive drugs are at increased risk of NHL.[834] NHL is the most common opportunistic neoplasm occurring in persons with HIV infection and acquired immuno-deficiency syndrome (AIDS); between 8% and 27% of all cases of NHL may be the result of HIV infection.[84]

An infectious origin has been suggested for Hodgkin's disease on the basis of its epidemiologic features, age at onset, and spatial clustering. The leading candidate for an infectious agent is the Epstein-Barr virus.[85] However, no causal agent has been definitely identified.

PREVENTION AND CONTROL MEASURES

Because the causes of NHL and Hodgkin's disease are not fully understood, clear prevention strategies are unavailable. Given the growing evidence of an association between pesticide use and NHL, however, prudent use of these chemicals is warranted. No screening tests are yet available for the early detection of NHL or Hodgkin's disease. Substantial progress has been shown in the treatment of Hodgkin's disease, for which 5-year survival has improved from about 40% in 1960 to the current rate of 81%.[1]

LEUKEMIA

ICD-9 204-208

SIGNIFICANCE

Leukemia comprises a variety of cancers that arise in the bone marrow. Leukemia affects both children and adults and accounts for about 33% of cancers among children (2400 new cases per year) and 2% of adult cancer cases (25 900 new cases per year).[1] There are four main types of leukemia: acute lymphocytic leukemia, acute myelocytic leukemia, chronic lymphocytic leukemia, and chronic myelocytic leukemia. In the United States, acute lymphocytic leukemia accounts for 67% of leukemia cases among children. The most common leukemia types among adults are acute myelocytic leukemia (36% of US leukemia cases) and chronic lymphocytic leukemia (29% of US leukemia cases).

From a public health standpoint, leukemia is important not only for its health impact on the population but also because of the frequency of public inquiries regarding leukemia and the emotional nature of these inquiries and the media impact.[86] These inquiries frequently concern apparent spatial clustering of childhood leukemia cases.

DESCRIPTIVE EPIDEMIOLOGY

Leukemia is 69% more common among men in the United States than among women and is slightly more common in Whites than in Blacks.[7] Among adults, leukemia mortality has declined slightly over the past 17 years.[7] In contrast, mortality among children due to acute lymphocytic leukemia has decreased dramatically since the 1960s as the result of improvements in therapy.[87]

RISK FACTORS

The major causes of leukemia are unknown; however, several risk factors have been identified, including genetic abnormalities such as Down's syndrome, exposure to ionizing radiation, and workplace exposure to benzene and other related solvents.[32] Adult T-cell leukemia is strongly associated with infection by human T-lymphotrophic virus, type I in endemic areas.[88] Increasing evidence suggests that cigarette smoking is a causative risk factor for some forms of leukemia.[89] Recent studies have suggested that residential exposure to magnetic fields among children and occupational exposure among adults may increase risk, but additional study of this association is needed.[90]

PREVENTION AND CONTROL MEASURES

Because the causes of leukemia are largely undetermined, primary prevention is difficult. Reducing occupational and environmental exposures to radiation and leukemogenic chemicals and eliminating cigarette smoking may reduce leukemia incidence. Because symptoms often appear late, diagnosing leukemia early is difficult and no routine screening test exists.

BLADDER CANCER

ICD-9 188

SIGNIFICANCE

Bladder cancer is the most common cancer of the urinary tract, accounting for 54 500 new cases in the United States in 1997.[1]

DESCRIPTIVE EPIDEMIOLOGY

Bladder cancer is more than four times more common among men than among women. Bladder cancer incidence is higher among Whites than among Blacks, particularly for males. Incidence has been increasing over the past 17 years at a rate of approximately 1% per year.[7]

RISK FACTORS

Cigarette smoking is a well-established cause of bladder cancer. Bladder cancer risk for a smoker is approximately two to three times that of a nonsmoker, and smoking is estimated to account for 48% of bladder cancers among men and 32% among women.[91] Increased risks are also associated with occupational exposures to aromatic amines and other chemicals in the textile, rubber, and leather industries. Several other occupations have been associated with an increased risk of bladder cancer, including truck drivers, painters, printers, and chemical workers.[91] Approximately 23% of bladder cancer is attributable to occupational exposures.[29] Some studies have suggested an increased risk of bladder cancer related to a history of bladder infections or to heavy consumption of coffee.[92] More recently, bladder cancer has been associated with long-term exposure to chlorine disinfection by-products

and high concentrations of arsenic in drinking water.[93]

PREVENTION AND CONTROL MEASURES

Primary prevention of bladder cancer should focus on eliminating cigarette smoking and minimizing exposure to hazardous chemicals in the workplace. Currently, no routine screening test is available for early detection of bladder cancer.

ORAL AND PHARYNGEAL CANCER
ICD-9 140-149

SIGNIFICANCE

Cancer of the oral cavity—that is, lip, salivary gland, mouth, and throat—accounted for 30 750 new cases and 8440 US deaths in 1997.[1] Although oral cancer accounts for less than 3% of cancer cases in the United States, in some parts of India, where chewing tobacco products with betal leaves, areca nut (betel), lime, and tobacco is common, it accounts for nearly half of all cancers.

DESCRIPTIVE EPIDEMIOLOGY

Oral cancer mortality rates are 2.8 times higher among men in the United States than among women and 1.8 times higher among Blacks than among Whites.[7] The overall 5-

year survival rate for oral cancer in the United States is 53%, although survival for cancer diagnosed in the local stage is 81%.[1]

RISK FACTORS

The use of tobacco in any form—cigarettes, cigars, and pipes, as well as the use of chewing tobacco and snuff—substantially elevates the risk of cancer of the tongue, mouth, and pharynx.[94] Cigarette smokers have a 3 to 13 times greater risk of oral cancer than do nonsmokers.[94] Excessive alcohol consumption is also associated with cancer of the oral cavity. Smoking and drinking are independent risk factors for oral cancer and also interact synergistically to multiply risk. For example, among heavy smokers (ie, more than 40 cigarettes per day) who consume at least 30 drinks per week, oral cancer is increased 38-fold.[95] Poor nutrition, including lack of b-carotene and vitamin C, have also been shown to increase oral cancer risk.[94] Together, smoking and alcohol account for approximately 75% of all oral cancer in the United States.[94]

PREVENTION AND CONTROL MEASURES

Oral and pharyngeal cancers are largely preventable. Oral cancer death rates could be reduced significantly through primary prevention and early detection. Eliminating-smoking and smokeless tobacco use and reducing heavy alcohol consumption would substantially reduce oral cancer incidence. In addition, measures to reduce sun exposure (see section on skin melanoma) should be taken to reduce the risk of lip cancer. For early detection, dentists, primary care physicians, and nurses should routinely examine the oral cavity for abnormal lesions as part of periodic health examinations.

MELANOMA OF THE SKIN

ICD-9 172

SIGNIFICANCE

An estimated 90 0000 cases of skin cancer occur each year; most are highly curable basal or squamous cell cancers.[1] A small fraction of the total cases, but the vast majority of deaths, is due to malignant melanoma of the skin. Melanoma accounted for 40 300 new cases and 7300 deaths in the United States in 1997.[1]

DESCRIPTIVE EPIDEMIOLOGY

Melanoma mortality increases with age, and men have a higher risk than women. Melanoma is 15 times more common among Whites than among Blacks. From 1973 to 1989, melanoma among Whites increased faster than any other major cancer type.[7]

The 5-year survival for melanoma is 87%. Melanoma incidence rates vary inversely with latitude, although the pattern is not entirely consistent due to the lack of a perfect correlation between latitude and exposure to ultraviolet B sunlight.[96]

RISK FACTORS

A contributing factor to the rapid rise in incidence is thought to be increasing voluntary sun exposure, especially intense, repeated, blistering overdoses during childhood. Depletion of the ozone layer in the earth's upper atmosphere may also be a contributor to increasing melanoma rates.[19] Risk is highest among fair-skinned people who sunburn easily. A family history of melanoma increases the risk by two to eight times. The presence of moles with irregular pigmentation and borders (ie, dysplastic nevi) also increases melanoma risk.

PREVENTION AND CONTROL MEASURES

Prevention of melanoma should include avoiding the sun's ultraviolet rays during peak exposure periods (10 AM to 3 PM), wearing protective clothing, and wearing sunscreen preparations with a sun-protective factor of 15 or greater.[97]

To detect melanoma early and increase survival, adults should perform monthly skin self-examina-

tions.[1] This is particularly important for people with heavy occupational or recreational sun exposure or with other significant risk factors. People at high risk also should undergo routine screening by a physician, nurse, or allied health professional at an interval determined by the clinician. They should evaluate suspicious skin lesions by following the "ABCD" criteria: Asymmetry, Border irregularity, Color variability, and Diameter greater than 6 mm.[40, 97]

REFERENCES

1. American Cancer Society. Cancer Facts and Figures—1997. Atlanta, Ga: American Cancer Society; 1997.
2. National Center for Health Statistics. Vital and Health Statistics. Detailed Diagnoses and Procedures, National Hospital Discharge Survey, 1994. Hyattsville, Md: US Dept. of Health and Human Services; March 1997. DHHS publication 97-1788.
3. Cole P, Rodu B. Declining cancer mortality in the United States. *Cancer.* 1996;78:2045–2048.
4. Doll R. Progress against cancer: an epidemiologic assessment. The 1991 John C. Cassel Memorial Lecture. *Am J Epidemiol.* 1991;134:675–688.
5. National Center for Health Statistics. Advance report of final

mortality statistics, 1994. *Month Vital Stat Rep.* 1996;45(3 suppl), September 30, 1996. DHHS publication 96-1120.

6. US Dept of Health and Human Services. *Racial/Ethnic Patterns of Cancer in the United States 1988–1992.* Bethesda, Md: National Cancer Institute; 1996. NIH publication 96-4104.

7. US Dept of Health and Human Services. *Cancer Statistics Review 1973–1992.* Bethesda, Md: National Cancer Institute; 1995. NIH publication 96-2789.

8. Baquet CR, Horm JW, Gibbs T, Greenwald P. Socioeconomic factors and cancer incidence among Blacks and Whites. *J Natl Cancer Inst.* 1991;83:551–557.

9. US Bureau of Census. *Current Population Reports, P-20-448, The Black Population in the United States: March 1990 and 1989.* Washington, DC: US Govt Printing Office; 1991.

10. Bal DG. Cancer in African Americans. *CA Cancer J Clin.* 1992;42:5–6.

11. Brown ML, Hodgson TA, Rice DP. Economic impact of cancer in the United States. In: Schottenfeld D, Fraumeni JF Jr, eds. *Cancer Epidemiology and Prevention.* 2nd ed. New York, NY: Oxford University Press Inc; 1996:255–266.

12. Brown ML. The national economic burden of cancer: an update. *J Natl Cancer Inst.* 1990;82:1811–1814.

13. *International Classification of Diseases, 9th Revision, Clinical Modification.* 2nd ed. Washington, DC: US Dept of Health and Human Services; 1980. DHHS publication PHS 80-1260.

14. World Health Organization. *International Classification of Diseases for Oncology.* 2nd ed. Geneva, Switzerland: World Health Organization; 1990.

15. Doll R, Peto R. *The Causes of Cancer. Quantitative Estimates of Avoidable Risks of Cancer in the United States Today.* New York, NY: Oxford University Press Inc; 1981.

16. Miller AB. Planning cancer control strategies. In: *Chronic Diseases in Canada.* Vol. 13, No. 1. Toronto, Ontario: Health and Welfare; 1992.

17. Harvard Center for Cancer Prevention. Harvard Report on Cancer Prevention. *Cancer Causes Control.* 1996;7:S55–S58.

18. Weisburger JH, Williams GM. Causes of cancer. In: Murphy GP, Lawrence W Jr, Lenhard RE Jr, eds. *American Cancer Society Textbook of Clinical Oncology.* 2nd ed. Atlanta, Ga: American Cancer Society; 1995:10–39.

19. Thomas DB. Cancer. In: Last JM, Wallace RB, eds. *Maxcy-Rosenau-Last Textbook of Public Health and Preventive Medicine.*

Norwalk, Conn: Appleton & Lange; 1992:811–826.

20. Greenwald P, Sondik EJ, eds. *Cancer Control Objectives for the Nation: 1985–2000.* National Cancer Institute Monographs, No. 2. Washington, DC: US Govt Printing Office; 1986. DHHS publication 86-2880.

21. *Healthy People 2000: National Health Promotion and Disease Prevention Objectives.* Washington, DC: US Dept of Health and Human Services; 1991. DHHS publication PHS 91-50212.

22. Bailar JC, Gornik HL. Cancer undefeated. *N Engl J Med.* 1997;336:1569–1574.

23. Alciati MH, Marconi KM. The public health potential for cancer prevention and control. In: Greenwald P, Kramer BS, Weed DL, eds. *Cancer Prevention and Control.* New York: Marcel Dekker, Inc, 1995:435–449.

24. Meissner H, Bergner L, Marconi K. Developing cancer control capacity in state and local public health agencies. *Public Health Rep.* 1992;107:15–23.

25. Tomatis L, ed. *Cancer: Causes, Occurrence and Control.* Lyon, France: International Agency for Research on Cancer; 1990.

26. Alavanja MCR, Brownson RC, Boice JD Jr, Hoch E. Preexisting lung disease and lung cancer among non-smoking women. *Am J Epidemiol.* 1992;136:623–632.

27. Brown CC, Kessler LG. Projections of lung cancer mortality in the United States: 1985–2025. *J Natl Cancer Inst.* 1988;80:43–51.

28. Garfinkel L, Silverberg E. Lung cancer and smoking trends in the United States over the past 25 years. *CA Cancer J Clin.* 1991;41:137–145.

29. Rothenberg R, Nasca P, Mikl J, Burnett W, Reynolds B. Cancer. In: Amler RW, Dull HB, eds. *Closing the Gap: The Burden of Unnecessary Illness.* New York, NY: Oxford University Press Inc; 1987:30–42.

30. Saracci R. The interactions of tobacco smoking and other agents in cancer etiology. *Epidemiol Rev.* 1987;9:175–193.

31. Lubin JH, Boice JD Jr, Edling C, et al. *Radon and Lung Cancer Risk: A Joint Analysis of 11 Underground Miners Studies.* Rockville, MD: National Institutes of Health; 1994. NIH publication 94-3644.

32. US Dept. of Health and Human Services. *Cancer Rates and Risks.* 4th ed. Bethesda, Md: National Cancer Institute; May 1996. DHHS publication 96-691.

33. Brownson RC, Alavanja MCR. Radon. In: Steenland K, Savitz DA, eds. *Topics in Environmental Epidemiology.* Oxford, UK: Oxford University Press; 1997:269–294.

34. US Environmental Protection Agency. *Respiratory Health*

Effects of Passive Smoking: Lung Cancer and Other Disorders. Washington, DC: US Environmental Protection Agency; 1992. EPA/600/6-90/006F.

35. Steinmetz KA, Potter JD. Vegetables, fruit, and cancer. I. Epidemiology. *Cancer Causes Control.* 1991;2:325–357.

36. Omenn GS, Goodman GE, Thronquist MD, et al. Effects of a combination of beta carotene and vitamin A on lung cancer and cardiovascular disease. *N Engl J Med* 1996;334:1150–1155.

37. US Dept of Health and Human Services. *Reducing the Health Consequences of Smoking—25 Years of Progress: A Report of the Surgeon General.* Rockville, Md: Office on Smoking and Health; 1989.

38. Lubin JH, Boice JD Jr. Estimating Rn-induced lung cancer in the United States. *Health Phys.* 1989;57:417–427.

39. US Dept of Health and Human Services. *The Health Benefits of Smoking Cessation.* Rockville, Md: Centers for Disease Control, Office on Smoking and Health; 1990. DHHS publication CDC 90-8416.

40. US Preventive Services Task Force. *Guide to Clinical Preventive Services.* 2nd ed. Baltimore, Md: Williams & Wilkins; 1996.

41. Manley MW, Pierce JP, Gilpin EA, et al. The impact of the American Stop Smoking Intervention Study (ASSIST) on cigarette consumption. *Tobacco Control.* In press.

42. Centers for Disease Control and Prevention. *CDC's Tobacco Use Prevention Program: Working Toward a Healthier Future. At-A-Glance 1996.* Atlanta, GA: Dept of Health and Human Services; 1996.

43. Bal DG, Kizer KW, Felten PG, Mozar HN, Niemeyer D. Reducing tobacco consumption in California: development of a statewide anti-tobacco use campaign. *JAMA.* 1990;264:1570–1574.

44. Koh HW. An analysis of the successful 1992 Massachusetts tobacco tax initiative. *Tobacco Control.* 1996;5:220–225.

45. Peltomäki P, Aaltonen LA, Sistonen P, et al. Genetic mapping of a locos predisposing to human colorectal cancer. *Science.* 1993;260:810–812.

46. Powell KE, Blair SN. The public health burdens of sedentary living habits: theoretical but realistic estimates. *Med Sci Sports Exer.* 1994;26:851–856.

47. Willett WC, Stampfer MJ, Colditz GA, et al. Relation of meat, fat and fiber intake to the risk of colon cancer in a prospective study among women. *N Engl J Med.* 1990;323:1664–1672.

48. Thun MJ, Calle EE, Namboodiri MM, et al. Risk factors for fatal

colon cancer in a large prospective study. *J Natl Cancer Inst.* 1992;84:1491–1500.

49. Trock B, Lanza E, Greenwald P. Dietary fiber, vegetables, and colon cancer: critical review and meta-analyses of the epidemiologic evidence. *J Natl Cancer Inst.* 1990;82:650–661.

50. Potter JD. Reconciling the epidemiology, physiology, and molecular biology of colon cancer. *JAMA.* 1992;268:1573–1577.

51. Howe GR, Benito E, Castelleto R, et al. Dietary intake of fiber and decreased risk of cancers of the colon and rectum: evidence from combined analysis of 13 case-control studies. *J Natl Cancer Inst.* 1992;84:1887–1896.

52. Sternfeld B. Cancer and the protective effect of physical activity: the epidemiological evidence. *Med Sci Sport Exerc.* 1992;24:1195–1209.

53. The American Cancer Society 1996 Advisory Committee on Diet, Nutrition, and Cancer Prevention. Guidelines on Diet, Nutrition, and Cancer Prevention: Reducing the Risk of Cancer with Healthy Food Choices and Physical Activity. *CA Cancer J Clin.* 1996;46:325–341.

54. Foerster SB, Bal DG. California's "5 A Day—For Better Health" campaign. *Chronic Dis Notes Rep.* 1990;3:7–9.

55. Reynolds T. "5-A-Day For Better Health" program is launched in Boston. *J Natl Cancer Inst.* 1991;83:1538–1539.

56. Foerster SB, Kizer KW, DiSogra LK, Bal DG, Krieg BK, Bunch KL. California's 5 a Day – for Better Health! Campaign: An innovative population-based effort to effect large-scale dietary change. *Am J Prev Med.* 1995;11:124–131.

57. Bal DG, Foerster SB. Changing the American diet. Impact on cancer prevention policy recommendations and program implications for the American Cancer Society. *Cancer.* 1991;67:2671–2680.

58. Stanford JL, Szklo M, Brinton LA. Estrogen receptors and breast cancer. *Epidemiol Rev.* 1986;8:42–59.

59. Kelsey JL, Bernstein L. Epidemiology and prevention of breast cancer. *Annu Rev Public Health.* 1996;17:47–67.

60. Easton DF, Bishop DT, Ford D, et al. Genetic linkage analysis in familial breast and ovarian cancer: results from 214 families. *Am J Hum Genet.* 1993;52:678-701.

61. Brinton LA, Williams RR, Hoover RN, et al. Breast cancer risk factors among screening program participants. *J Natl Cancer Inst.* 1979;62:37–43.

62. Carter CL, Jones DY, Schatzkin A, Brinton LA. A prospective

study of reproductive, familial, and socioeconomic risk factors for breast cancer using NHANES I data. *Public Health Rep.* 1989;104:45–50.

63. Longnecker MP. Alcoholic beverage consumption in relation to risk of breast cancer: meta-analysis and review. *Cancer Causes Control* 1994; 5:73–82.

64. Ambrosone CB, Freudenheim JL, Graham S, et al. Cigarette smoking, N-acetyltransferase 2 genetic polymorphisms, and breast cancer risk. *JAMA.* 1996; 276:1494–1501.

65. Morabia A, Bernstein M, Heritier S, Khatchatrian N. Relation of breast cancer with passive and active exposure to tobacco smoke. *Am J Epidemiol.* 1996; 143:918–928.

66. Anderson LM, May DS. Has the use of cervical, breast, and colorectal cancer screening increased in the United States? *Am J Public Health.* 1995;85:840–842.

67. Henson RM, Wyatt SW, Lee NC. The National Breast and Cervical Cancer Early Detection Program: A Comprehensive Public Health Response to Two Major Health Issues for Women. *J Public Health Manage Pract.* 1996;2:36–47.

68. May DS, Lee NC, Nadel MR, Henson RM, Miller DS. The National Breast and Cervical Cancer Early Detection Program: report on the first four years of mammography provided to medically underserved women. *Am J Roentgenol.* 1998;170:97–104.

69. Coughlin SS, Beauchamp TL, eds. *Ethics and Epidemiology.* New York: Oxford University Press Inc; 1996.

70. Brinton LA, Fraumeni JF Jr. Epidemiology of uterine cervical cancer. *J Chron Dis.* 1986;39: 1051–1065.

71. National Institutes of Health. *Cervical Cancer Control. Status and Directions.* Washington, DC: US Dept of Health and Human Services; 1991. NIH publication 91-3223.

72. Schairer C, Brinton LA, Devesa SS, Ziegler RG, Fraumeni JF Jr. Racial differences in the risk of invasive squamous-cell cervical cancer. *Cancer Causes Control.* 1991;2:283–289.

73. American Cancer Society. *Guidelines for the Cancer-related Checkup: An Update.* Atlanta, Ga: American Cancer Society; 1993.

74. Lawson HW, Lee NC, Thames SF, Henson R, Miller DS. Cervical cancer screening among low-income women: results from a national screening program, 1991–1995. *J Obstet Gynecol.* In press.

75. Whittemore AS, Keller JB, Betensky R. Low-grade, latent

prostate cancer volume: predictor of clinical cancer incidence. *J Natl Cancer Inst.* 1991;83:1231–1235.

76. LeMarchand L, Kolonel LN, Wilkens LR et al. Animal fat consumption and prostate cancer: a prospective study in Hawaii. *Epidemiology.* 1994;5:276–282.

77. Steinberg GD, Carter BS, Beaty TH, et al. Family history and the risk of prostate cancer. *Prostate.* 1990;17:337–347.

78. Kramer BS, Brown ML, Prorok PC et al. Prostate cancer screening: what we know and what we need to know. *Ann Int Med.* 1993;119:914–923.

79. DeVesa SS, Fears T. Non-Hodgkin's lymphoma time trends: United States and international data. *Cancer Res.* 1992; 52(suppl):5432s–5440s.

80. Glaser SL, Swartz WG. Time trends in Hodgkin's Disease incidence: The role of diagnostic accuracy. *Cancer* 1990;66:2196-2204.

81. Zahm SH, Blair A. Pesticides and non-Hodgkin's lymphoma. *Cancer Res.* 1992;52 (suppl) 5484s–5488s.

82. Hoar SK, Blair A, Holmes FF, et al. Agricultural herbicide use and risk of lymphoma and soft-tissue sarcoma. *JAMA.* 1986;256:1141–1147.

83. Scherr PA, Mueller NE. Non-Hodgkin's lymphomas. In: Schottenfeld D, Fraumeni JF Jr, eds. *Cancer Epidemiology and Prevention.* 2nd ed. New York, NY: Oxford University Press Inc; 1996:920–945.

84. Gail MH, Pluda JM, Rabkin CS et al. Projections of the incidence of non-Hodgkin's lymphoma related to acquired immunodeficiency syndrome. *J Natl Cancer Inst.* 1991;83:965–701.

85. Mueller N, Mohar A, Evans A et al. Epstein-Barr virus antibody patterns preceding diagnosis of non-Hodgkin's lymphoma. *Int J Cancer.* 1991;49:387–393.

86. Devier JR, Brownson RC, Bagby JR Jr, Carlson GM, Crellin JM. A public health response to cancer clusters in Missouri. *Am J Epidemiol.* 1990;132:S23–S31.

87. Linet MS, Devesa SS. Descriptive epidemiology of childhood leukemia. *Br J Cancer* 1991; 63:424–429.

88. Blattner WA. Human T-cell lymphotrophic viruses and cancer causation. In: deVita VT, Hellman S, Rosenberg SA, eds. *Cancer. Principles and Practice of Oncology.* Philadelphia, Pa: Lippincott; 1993.

89. Brownson RC, Novotny TE, Perry MC. Cigarette smoking and adult leukemia: a meta-analysis. *Arch Intern Med.* 1993;153:469–475.

90. Savitz DA. Overview of epidemiologic research on electric and

magnetic fields and cancer. *Am Ind Hyg Assoc J.* 1993;54:197–204.

91. Silverman DT, Morrison AS, Devesa SS. Bladder cancer. In: Schottenfeld D, Fraumeni JF Jr, eds. *Cancer Epidemiology and Prevention.* 2nd ed. New York, NY: Oxford University Press Inc; 1996:1156–1179.

92. Matanoski GM, Elliott EA. Bladder cancer epidemiology. *Epidemiol Rev.* 1981;3:202–229.

93. Morris RD, Audet AM, Angelillo IF, Chalmers TC, Mosteller F. Chlorination, chlorination by-products, and cancer: a meta-analysis. *Am J Public Health.* 1992;82:955–963.

94. Blot WJ, McLaughlin JK, Devesa SS, Fraumeni JF Jr. Cancers of the oral cavity and pharynx. In: Schottenfeld D, Fraumeni JF Jr, eds. *Cancer Epidemiology and Prevention.* 2nd ed. New York, NY: Oxford University Press Inc; 1996;666–680.

95. Blot WJ, McLAughlin JK, Winn DM et al. Smoking and drinking in relation to oral and pharyngeal cancer. *Cancer Res.* 1988; 48:3282–3847.

96. Armstrong BK, English DR. Cutaneous malignant melanoma. In: Schottenfeld D, Fraumeni JF Jr, eds. *Cancer Epidemiology and Prevention.* 2nd ed. New York, NY: Oxford University Press Inc; 1996:1282–1312.

97. US Dept of Health and Human Services. Diagnosis and treatment of early melanoma. *Consens Dev Conf Consens Statement.* 1992 Jan 27–29; 10(1).

SUGGESTED READING

American Cancer Society. Cancer Facts and Figures—1997. Atlanta, Ga: American Cancer Society; 1997.

Greenwald P, Kramer BS, Weed DL, eds. *Cancer Prevention and Control.* New York, NY: Marcel Dekker Inc.; 1995.

Schottenfeld D, Fraumeni JF Jr, eds. *Cancer Epidemiology and Prevention.* 2nd ed. New York, NY: Oxford University Press Inc; 1996.

Tomatis L, ed. *Cancer: Causes, Occurrence and Control.* Lyon, France: International Agency for Research on Cancer; 1990.

US Dept of Health and Human Services. *Cancer Statistics Review. 1973–1989.* Bethesda, Md: National Cancer Institute; 1992. NIH publication 92-2789.

US Preventive Services Task Force. *Guide to Clinical Preventive Services.* 2nd ed. Baltimore, Md: Williams & Wilkins; 1996.

RESOURCES

American Cancer Society, Inc.
1599 Clifton Road, NE
Atlanta, GA 30329-4251
(800) ACS-2345
http://www.cancer.org

Division of Cancer Prevention and
    Control
Centers for Disease Control and
    Prevention
4770 Buford Highway, MS K-52
Atlanta, GA 30341-3724
(770) 488-5496
http://www.cdc.gov

National Cancer Institute
Cancer Information Service
Building 31, Room 10A-18
9000 Rockville Pike
Bethesda, MD 20892
(800) 4-CANCER
http://www.nci.nih.gov

CHRONIC LUNG DISEASES

ICD-9 277.00, 277.01, 490-496, 500-504, 506, 507.8, 515-517, 780.51, 780.53, 780.57

The chronic lung diseases are a diverse group of disorders with varying symptoms, diagnostic criteria, and causative factors. Most of the disorders are accompanied by impairment in lung function (Table 13.1).

Chronic lung diseases were the fourth leading cause of death in 1995, responsible for approximately 4% of all deaths in the United States.[2] These diseases also require lengthy hospitalizations, ranging from an average of 4.3 days for asthma to 7.4 days for chronic bronchitis (Table 13.2). Population-based studies in the United States have demonstrated an impairment of lung function, measured with standard techniques, in approximately 4% to 6% of White men and 1% to 3% of White women. In the National Health and Nutrition Examination Survey, 4% of men and 5% of women report physician-diagnosed chronic obstructive pulmonary disease. Rates as high as 9% to 13% have been estimated in some populations.[3]

Jay M. Goldring, PhD
David S. James, MD
Henry A. Anderson, MD

The primary consequence of chronic lung diseases that contributes to morbidity is dyspnea, or pathologic breathlessness.[4] Depending on the severity, dyspnea may result in restrictions ranging from inability to climb stairs to constant breathlessness and difficulty in sleeping.[6] Impaired respiratory tract clearance mechanisms, excessive mucus production, and reduced lung capacity probably contribute to more frequent, severe, and prolonged acute viral and bacterial respiratory infections.[4] Dyspnea also occurs in other chronic nonpulmonary conditions such as heart disease, obesity, and muscle diseases. Other symptoms of lung disease include cough, excessive phlegm or sputum production, wheezing, and hemoptysis or coughing of blood. All of these symptoms, like dyspnea, can occur in different respiratory and nonrespiratory disorders.

Among clinicians, terms used to describe specific combinations of symptoms are highly variable. The disorders of chronic bronchitis, emphysema, and asthma may overlap, and it has been difficult to give each one an adequate definition

Table 13.1—Definitions of Specific Chronic Lung Diseases[a]

Disease	ICD-9 Code	Definition
Cystic fibrosis	277.00, 277.01	Genetic disease with exocrine gland dysfunction resulting in pancreatic insufficiency, chronic progressive lung disease, and elevated sweat chloride concentration
Chronic bronchitis	490-491	Excessive tracheobronchial mucus production associated with narrowing of the bronchial airways and cough
Chronic obstructive bronchitis	491.2	Same as chronic bronchitis with involvement of smaller airways; associated with airflow abnormalities
Emphysema	492	Alveolar destruction and associated airspace enlargement
Asthma	493	Reversible airway obstruction with airway inflammation and increased airways responsiveness to a variety of stimuli
Bronchiectasis	494	Destruction of bronchial wall
Allergic alveolitis	495	Immunologically induced inflammation of the lung parenchyma
Chronic airway obstruction	496	Generalized airway obstruction not classifiable as chronic bronchitis or chronic obstructive bronchitis
Other externally induced pneumoconioses	500-504, 506.4, 507.1, 507.8, 515, 516.3	Dust-, fume- or mist-induced pneumoconioses or lung injury, nonimmunologically mediated
Sleep apnea	780.51, 780.53, 780.57	Repetitive cessation of breathing during sleep

[a]Adapted from Samet.[1]

based on clinical, physiologic, or pathologic criteria (Figure 13.1). The term *chronic obstructive pulmonary disease* (COPD) has been used generically to describe a subset of these three conditions in order to overcome some of the imprecision in clinical diagnoses. However, diagnostic specificity is further confused by the term COPD, which is sometimes used by clinicians as a nonspecific catch-all term to describe chronic respiratory symptoms with or without airflow impairment. The ICD-9 codes and the definitions used in this chapter are presented in Table 13.1.

Cystic fibrosis is an example of a multisystem disorder in which the

Table 13.2—Chronic Lung Disease Morbidity and Mortality, United States, 1994, 1995

Disease	Estimated Prevalence (in thousands)[a]	Number of Deaths[b]	Death Rate[b]	Average Length of Hospital Stay (days)[c]
Chronic bronchitis	—	6 045	1.3	7.4
Emphysema	2 028	16 927	6.4	7.1
Asthma	14 562	11 274	2.1	4.3
Other COPD	14 021	77 025	29.3	6.7
Total	30 611	111 271	39.2	—

[a]Estimates from the 1994 National Health Interview Survey; chronic bronchitis was not distinguished from other forms of chronic obstructive pulmonary disease in this survey.
[b]1995 deaths and age-adjusted death rates per 100 00 population.[2]
[c]First-listed diagnosis from the 1992 National Hospital Discharge Survey.
[d]COPD indicates chronic obstructive pulmonary disease.

respiratory system is often affected disproportionately compared to other involved organs. Until recently only a disorder of childhood, approximately one-third of individuals currently affected with cystic fibrosis are adults.[7] This dramatic improvement has been attributed to improved nutritional support, greater attention to methods of increasing phlegm clearance, and vigorous treatment of lower respiratory tract infections. Obstructive sleep apnea is an additional multisystem disorder characterized by intermittent upper respiratory tract obstruction during sleep that can result in excessive daytime sleepiness. With an estimated prevalence of 2 to 4%,[7] sleep apnea is a significant public health problem.

The diagnostic tests and associated criteria for definition differ among various chronic lung diseases. Chronic bronchitis is diagnosed by clinical signs and reported symptom history. Asthma and COPD are diagnosed by clinical evaluation and spirometric tests of lung function.[3,9] Emphysema is defined in histopathologic terms (ie, study of lung tissue) and is diagnosed with certainty only with lung biopsy or autopsy, although computerized axial-tomography (CT) scanning of the chest can be informative. A further complication is that the symptoms of gastroesophageal reflux, a digestive condition, can occasionally be similar to those of various airways diseases, and the two conditions are often confused.[9] One manifestation of the occupation-related pneumoco-

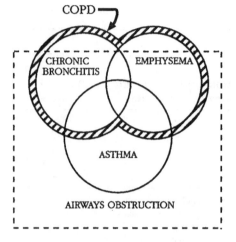

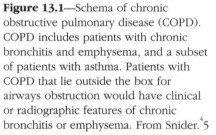

Figure 13.1—Schema of chronic obstructive pulmonary disease (COPD). COPD includes patients with chronic bronchitis and emphysema, and a subset of patients with asthma. Patients with COPD that lie outside the box for airways obstruction would have clinical or radiographic features of chronic bronchitis or emphysema. From Snider.[4,5]

nioses, or dust-induced lung conditions, is a fibrotic response to deposition of inorganic material. Diagnosis requires an exposure history and x-ray assessment.[3] In a heterogeneous group of lung disorders, interstitial lung diseases, the chest x-ray, and occasionally CT of the chest can assist in evaluation and monitoring disease status and are used in conjunction with other methods of assessing respiratory function, such as spirometry.

Spirometric testing is simple and inexpensive and is a sensitive and noninvasive method to assess obstructive lung diseases as well as different fibrotic or restrictive lung diseases. Spirometry measures the expired volume as a function of time. Forced vital capacity (FVC) and forced expiratory volume in the first 1 second (FEV1) are less variable than many other tests of lung function.[2] Using the FVC or FEV1, or the ratio of FEV1 to FVC (FEV1/FVC), lung disorders can be categorized into those with airflow obstruction (FEV1/FVC < 0.75) or restriction (FVC < 80% of predicted) or into mixed disorders (decreases in both FEV1/FVC and FVC).

In addition to spirometry, other lung function tests can include measurement of total lung capacity (TLC), functional residual capacity (FRC), carbon monoxide diffusing capacity (DLCO), and cardiopulmonary exercise testing. Assessment of lung function following broncho-provocation with methacholine or histamine may indicate airway hyperreactivity and is sometimes performed if asthma is suspected but spirometry is inconclusive.

The chest radiograph is of most help in the clinical evaluation of chronic lung diseases. However, its role in the screening or epidemiologic study of lung diseases is limited by expense, feasibility, and technical considerations. A uniform method of chest radiograph interpretation has been developed by the International

Labor Organization (ILO)[11] for use in selected clinical settings (eg, disability assessment for occupational lung disease) and for research purposes. The system categorizes opacities and pleural changes on the chest radiograph by their shape, size, location, and density.[11] Physicians who obtain additional training in ILO interpretation of the chest x-ray and pass an examination are called B-readers. Methods similar to the ILO scheme for the chest x-ray have not been developed for standardized interpretation of CT images of the chest.

This chapter not only discusses the two major chronic lung diseases, asthma and COPD, but also includes shorter descriptions of a variety of occupationally induced chronic lung diseases, including coal workers' pneumoconiosis, silicosis, asbestosis, byssinosis, and occupational asthma; lung diseases associated with exposure to organic dusts; and a diverse group of diseases resulting in fibrosis of the lung (ie, interstitial lung disease), cystic fibrosis, and obstructive sleep apnea.

ASTHMA

ICD-9 493

SIGNIFICANCE

According to results of the 1994 National Health Interview Survey (NHIS), asthma affects approximately 5.6% of the general population.[12] Because diagnostic criteria for asthma are not standardized, estimates of asthma prevalence vary with different data sources, which include both self-reports and physician reports.[9] International asthma prevalence estimates vary widely and range from 12% in New Zealand to less than 2% in Finland.[9] Estimates for the prevalence of asthma will also vary if they include individuals with a prior history of asthma as well as individuals with active asthma. In 1992, 4964 people in the United States died from asthma.[13]

Asthma was responsible for an estimated 13.7 million visits to physicians in 1993 through 1994.[14] With close medical management, asthma may not be associated with a loss of productivity; however, when the condition is severe, lost work or school days may result. In 1990, asthma was responsible for an estimated $726.1 million worth of lost work days.[15]

PATHOPHYSIOLOGY

Historically, asthma has been classified into two categories: allergic or atopic (extrinsic) and nonallergic or nonatopic (intrinsic) asthma. Atopy is defined as the propensity to produce abnormal amounts of IgE in response to environmental allergen exposure. Asthma was classified as allergic in approximately 90% of asthmatic children under 12 years of age, 70% of asthmatic adults under 30 years of age, and 50% of asthmatic adults over 30 years of age.[16] However, many individuals have asthmatic responses that are characteristic of both categories and the basis for this classification has recently been questioned. Evidence from a number of genetic and molecular biology studies, including the discovery of higher serum immunoglobulin E levels among asthmatics of all age groups,[17] has led to the proposal of a unifying hypothesis for both types of asthma involving immunoglobulin E hyperresponsiveness.[18]

The airways of patients with asthma show evidence of mucosal edema, epithelial disruption, infiltration with inflammatory cells, and an occasional airway filled with mucus.[8] An inflammatory response in the airways of patients with asthma is probably important in the development of the changes responsible for airway obstruction and hyperresponsiveness. In allergic asthma, immunoglobulin E-antigen complexes bind to the membranes of various connective tissue cells, causing the release of signaling chemical agents responsible for an asthmatic response. People classified as intrinsic asthmatics frequently respond positively to a battery of skin tests for common allergens, while those classified as extrinsic asthmatics do not.

Symptoms of asthma, such as intermittent wheezing or shortness of breath triggered by specific environmental exposures or exercise, frequently appear in children before the age of 5. Approximately one fourth of individuals with childhood asthma become totally symptom-free as adults, and one-fourth report only occasional wheezing as adults. Unfortunately, one-fourth of childhood asthma cases persist with the same degree of severity into adulthood. An additional one-fourth become symptom-free through adolescence but have recurring symptoms after age 21.[19]

DESCRIPTIVE EPIDEMIOLOGY

High-Risk Groups

Prevalence rates of asthma are consistently higher for Blacks than for Whites by approximately 50%.[20] The degree to which the racial difference in asthma prevalence can be explained by socioeconomic differences is controversial. In the United States, ecologic studies of national databases indicate that controlling for family income can diminish or decrease the racial difference in asthma prevalence,[21] and data from the National Health Interview Survey suggest a weak inverse correlation between family income and asthma prevalence. However, such a relationship is not evident when racial or ethnic groups are analyzed independently. In addition, this relationship has not been found in a number of other studies.[22] Asthma prevalence rates are higher among children under 18 years of age (6.9% of the population) than among the remainder of the population (5.1% in age groups 18-44, 45-64 and over 65).[11] Although childhood asthma appears to be slightly more prevalent among boys, asthma prevalence among females is greater among older age groups.[12]

Approximately 30% to 50% of the general population can be classified as atopic and most asthmatics fall into this category.[9] The development of atopy has a strong genetic compo-nent and associated genes are beginning to be identified.[23] Rat models with differing characteristics of airway responsiveness have been developed.[24] These lines of reasoning indicate that some aspects of asthma development may be under genetic control. Indeed, those with a family history of asthma have long been known to be at increased risk for developing the disease.[25]

Mortality rates of asthma show a substantially different pattern than prevalence rates. The 1995 death rate for females (2.6 per 100 000) was slightly higher than that for males (1.6 per 100 000).[13] The death rate for Blacks (3.8 per 100 000) was nearly twice the rate for Whites (1.9 per 100 000). Among Hispanics, death rates due to asthma are approximately 50% higher than among non-Hispanics.[26] Asthma-related death rates rise sharply after age 40. In addition to race, other risk factors for increased asthma mortality include previous life-threatening asthma exacerbations, hospital admission for asthma in the past year, inadequate general medical management, lack of access to medical care, and psychosocial problems including alcohol abuse and depression.[9] Increased use of b_2-agonist bronchodilator medication has also been associated with increased mortality from asthma, but the actual role of b_2-agonists has not been clarified.[27]

Geographic Distribution

Responses in the 1994 National Health Interview Survey suggest that asthma prevalence is highest in the West and Northeast (5.9%) followed by the South (5.5%) and Midwest (5.2%). Prevalence in the central city (6.3%) is higher than in suburban areas (5.3%) and rural areas (5.5%).

Time Trends

The prevalence of asthma in-creased approximately 38% between 1980 and 1990. This increase oc-curred among all age, sex, and race subgroups. Death rates increased by 46% over that time from 1.3/100 000 population to 1.9/100 000 population (Figure 13.2). The significant increase in prevalence may be related in part

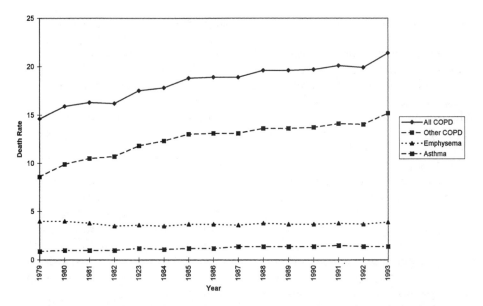

Figure 13.2—Age-adjusted chronic obstructive pulmonary disease (COPD) death rates, United States, 1979–1993

to increased awareness and more accurate diagnosis of asthma as well as to rising incidence.[28]

Seasonal trends are evident in asthma morbidity and mortality. Asthma death rates for men and women over 45 years of age are highest in February and March and lowest in July and August. Asthma hospitalization rates reflect a similar seasonal variation, with the highest rates in September through November and the lowest in June and July. These seasonal trends have not been explained fully, but researchers hypothesize that plant allergens, acute respiratory infections, cold weather, and air pollution may be contributing factors.

RISK FACTORS

Magnitude of Risk Factors

Risk factors for childhood asthma and adult-onset asthma differ. Chronic exposure to specific indoor and outdoor allergens in childhood appears to be consistently associated with development of childhood asthma (Table 13.3).[9] The most potent indoor sensitizing agents are dust mites, animal allergens, cockroach antigens, and fungi.[29] Investigators in one study found that the

Table 13.3—Modifiable Risk Factors for Developing Childhood Asthma, United States

Magnitude	Risk Factor
Strong (relative risk[a] >4)	House dust mites and cat dander
Moderate (relative risk 2–4)	None
Weak (relative risk <2)	Ambient air pollution
	Environmental tobacco smoke
Possible	Diet[b]
	Lower respiratory tract infections

[a]Relative risk is defined in Table 2.4, page 51.
[b]Consumption of "allergenic" foods (eg, milk, eggs, nuts, wheat, soya) by infants or lactating mothers.[29]

presence of more than 100 mites per gram of dust in a home was associated with a sevenfold increase in the risk of asthma development in children.[30] A significantly elevated proportion of children admitted to US emergency departments for asthma were allergic to cat dander.[31] Early childhood exposure to cockroach allergen[32] and fungal spores, particularly from Alternaria,[33] has also been associated with asthma development. Indoor concentrations of all of these allergens are higher in dark, humid, poorly ventilated environments.

Exposure to *environmental tobacco smoke* has been conclusively associated with exacerbations of childhood asthma.[34–36] Although the evidence does not conclusively show a causal association, environmental tobacco smoke is currently considered a risk factor for induction of asthma in previously asymptomatic children.[37]

Bronchoconstriction is precipitated by exposure to specific pollens in asthmatic subjects.[38] Urban exposure to particulates, sulfur dioxide, ozone, nitrogen oxides, and acidic aerosols also may be responsible for asthma exacerbation,[39] although the role of these factors in asthma development has not been established.[40]

Other suggested risk factors for childhood asthma development include respiratory tract infections in infancy[41] and low birth weight.[42]

Occupational exposure to particulate *organic dusts* and some *chemical vapors* has been associated with development of asthma in adults (discussed later under Occupational Asthma). Nonoccupational risk factors for developing adult-onset asthma have not yet been identified. Some investigators have disputed the occurrence of true "adult-onset" asthma, suggesting that the condition actually develops during childhood but is not identified at that time or is misdiagnosed.[19] There is no conclusive evidence that active smoking in adults results in a higher risk of developing asthma.[43]

Population-Attributable Risk

The relative role of genetic and environmental risk factors for asthma development cannot be quantified. Among genetic factors, progress toward identifying the specific gene or genes responsible for specific atopies is likely in the next decade. The major environmental factor responsible for asthma development appears to be exposure to indoor allergens.[9] The risk for developing asthma attributable to environmental tobacco smoke is uncertain.

PREVENTION AND CONTROL MEASURES

Prevention

Modifiable risk factors for developing childhood asthma include exposure to animal allergens and household dust. The risk of a child developing asthma may be reduced if parents minimize the presence of these allergens. Any warm-blooded pet can cause an allergic reaction; when such a reaction is suspected, the animal should be removed from the house. If this is not possible, the animal should at least be kept from the child's bedroom.[9] House dust mites can be effectively controlled by encasing mattresses and pillows in airtight covers, washing bedding every week, removing carpets, and using chemical agents to kill mites. Indoor molds can be decreased with frequent cleaning and dehumidification in moist climates.

Clean indoor air legislation, which restricts cigarette smoking in public places, has been passed in many cities and states to reduce exposure to tobacco smoke in work sites, restaurants, and shopping malls.

Exposure to ambient airborne particulates and irritants may be associated with the development of asthma or may promote episodes of bronchoconstriction. Outdoor allergens and pollutants can best be avoided by remaining indoors in an air-conditioned environment on days with high pollen or pollutant concentrations. Ongoing national programs are aimed at decreasing ambient concentrations of these pollutants and also ensuring that public health alerts are issued when pollution concentrations exceed standards. The efforts of these programs have been supported by the federal Clean Air Act Amendments of 1977 and 1990, which impose restrictions on areas of the country that fail to meet National Ambient Air Quality Standards for selected pollutants.

Screening and Early Detection

The progress of asthma cannot be arrested nor can the condition be cured, but screening programs can identify individuals with asthma. When cases are identified, effective management can minimize the frequency and severity of episodes of bronchoconstriction, making the condition less likely to progress to the point at which hospitalization is necessary.

Mild to moderate cases of asthma may be difficult to diagnose, especially among young children. The symptoms often are confused with recurrent respiratory infections or bronchitis and are not recognized as a chronic condition. Home monitoring of peak expiratory flow rates or a broncho-provocation test with methacholine or histamine may be informative if the diagnosis of asthma is uncertain. Programs to improve asthma detection should include the education of health care providers, particularly school health personnel, to recognize the condition.

Treatment, Rehabilitation, and Recovery

Effective treatment for asthma usually includes identifying and eliminating specific allergens from the environment. In most cases, however, this cannot be completely accomplished. Mild bronchospasm episodes can be controlled through the use of a self-administered inhaled beta-agonist drug. Therapy for moderately severe asthma should

include an inhaled anti-inflammatory agent, such as cromolyn or a corticosteroid, and an inhaled or oral bronchodilator.[8] Corticosteroids are very effective anti-inflammatory drugs for the treatment of asthma. Inhaled corticosteroids are safe and effective medications when prescribed in the currently recommended doses. In some instances, patients may not respond to self-administered medication and will require hospitalization with intravenous administration of medication. The total cost for asthma medications in the United States was estimated at $712.7 million in 1990.[15]

Desensitization, in which patients are given regular intramuscular injections of suspected allergens, is commonly used to treat "allergic" asthma. However, the effectiveness of this treatment is controversial.

EXAMPLES OF PUBLIC HEALTH INTERVENTIONS

Few public health interventions specifically target asthma. The National Heart, Lung, and Blood Institute and World Health Organization have recently launched the Global Asthma Initiative, which includes a multifaceted approach to reducing asthma occurrence and improving asthma management skills.[12] The program outlines six components for the care of individuals with asthma: patient education, lung function assessment, avoidance of asthma triggers, individualized medication plans for long-term management, individualized plans for addressing acute exacerbations, and regular follow-up care. Studies of asthma self-management education programs have shown that programs can decrease asthma exacerbations, missed school days, emergency room visits, and hospitalizations.[44, 45]

The program also provides recommendations for public health officials interested in reducing the costs of asthma treatment in their communities. These recommendations include surveillance of asthma in the community; formation of an asthma management team composed of government officials, health care providers, health care administrators, and community groups; the establishment of guidelines for asthma prevention and management; and institution of patient and health care provider education programs. Such programs have been instituted in a number of locations.[46]

National programs to reduce tobacco use and exposure to environmental tobacco smoke (see Chapter 5) will benefit asthma control efforts.

AREAS OF FUTURE RESEARCH AND DEMONSTRATION

Risk factors for the initiation of childhood asthma have not been

fully assessed, and animal models are beginning to be developed.[24] Further research into the genetic determinants of asthma will enable identification of high-risk individuals. Much is known about risk factors for the onset of acute bronchoconstriction episodes among individuals with asthma. Research in this area should continue, with special emphasis on the role of environmental pollutants in producing an asthma attack. The ability of pharmacologic agents, particularly anti-inflammatory agents, to alter the long-term course of asthma needs further investigation. In addition, more effective methods of community organizing, asthma self-management, and family management of childhood asthma are needed.

CHRONIC OBSTRUCTIVE PULMONARY DISEASE
ICD-9 490-492, 496

SIGNIFICANCE

Chronic obstructive pulmonary disease (COPD) has been defined as a process characterized by nonspecific changes in the lung parenchyma and bronchi that may lead to emphysema and airflow obstruction.[1, 2] The airway obstruction may not always be present, or it may be partially reversible.[47] Clinically and pathologically, chronic bronchitis, emphysema, and chronic airway obstruction can be difficult to differentiate from one another, and they are frequently grouped together under the heading of COPD (Figure 13.1).

Chronic bronchitis affects approximately 5.1% and emphysema approximately 0.8% of the general population.[11] Although asthma is nearly as prevalent in the general population as COPD, more people die from COPD. Unlike asthma, the impairment in lung function resulting from COPD is largely irreversible and progressive and occurs among older individuals who often have multiple chronic diseases that contribute to the overall disability. In 1992, COPD (ie, chronic bronchitis, emphysema, and "other COPD") accounted for 66 431 deaths in the United States (Table 13.2).

The economic costs of COPD includes both the cost of care and the loss of productivity. The findings of an 8-year prospective study suggested that disability in COPD patients progresses gradually over 7.5 years after initial diagnosis.[48] After an average of 7.5 years, most COPD patients are no longer capable of productive work.

PATHOPHYSIOLOGY

COPD is thought to result from direct interaction of environmental agents, of which tobacco smoke is the most significant, with lung tissue. Chronic exposure to cigarette smoke,

for example, is known to cause an increase in mucous gland size and goblet cell number in the large airways, as well as inflammation and microscopic fibrosis in the smaller airways.[49] Similar histopathologic changes have been noted among workers exposed to organic dusts.[50] The mechanism by which cigarette smoke causes emphysema is not known. One possibility is that cigarette smoke causes an imbalance in elastase and antielastase proteins, promoting degradation of lung tissue.[51]

Emphysema is characterized by alveolar dilation and destruction.[52] This destruction causes obstruction of expiratory airflow and the sensation of labored breathing, or dyspnea. In most patients, COPD is accompanied by emphysema and inflammation as well as narrowing of the smaller airways.

Among adults, many studies indicate that the onset of COPD begins with a moderate decline in lung function capacity before age 50. This decline can be associated with dyspnea or a moderate daily cough with sputum production. Many smokers do not recognize their "morning smoker's cough" as abnormal and indicative of disease. After age 50, the decline in lung function accelerates.[53] The damage to the lung ultimately results in inadequate oxygen delivery, and, in its advanced stages, COPD is often accompanied by heart failure.

DESCRIPTIVE EPIDEMIOLOGY

High-Risk Groups

Death rates for various forms of COPD vary by age group, beginning at ages 45 through 54 years and increasing sharply with increasing age. Mortality from COPD is higher in men than women;[54] however, higher smoking rates in men and earlier ages of initiation explain much of the difference in both mortality and prevalence.

The prevalence of chronic bronchitis is 5.5% among children under 18; 4.7% among those aged 18 through 44; 6.4% among those aged 45 through 64; and 6.1% among those over 65 years of age.[11] Chronic bronchitis is reported by approximately 50% more females than males, and prevalence of the condition is approximately 50% greater in Whites than in Blacks. The prevalence of chronic bronchitis is similar across income groups. Among a sample of nonsmokers participating in the National Health and Nutrition Examination Survey, physician-diagnosed COPD was reported by 4% of men and 5% of women with higher rates in Whites and individuals of lower socioeconomic status.[55] Death rates due to COPD are approximately 50% lower in Hispanics than in non-Hispanics.[26]

A small number of patients with COPD have a deficiency of the protein alpha1-antitrypsin.[54] Levels of alpha1-antitrypsin are genetically determined, and approximately 7% of the population has genetic traits associated with a deficiency. This protein acts to inhibit the destructive capabilities of the white blood cell elastase responsible for degradation of lung tissue, and deficiencies of alpha1-antitrypsin may be associated with emphysema. Other possible risk factors for COPD are a history of respiratory tract infections as a child, airway hyperresponsiveness,[56] air pollution, and chronic exposure to dust in occupational settings (see discussion in sections on coal workers' pneumoconiosis and silicosis).

Geographic Distribution

In general, COPD mortality rates are higher than average in the western and Rocky Mountain states (excluding Utah), as well as in Kentucky, West Virginia, and Maine. Rates differ approximately threefold between states with the highest (Wyoming, 49.1 per 100 000) and lowest (Hawaii, 16.9 per 100 000) rates. In the Tucson epidemiologic study of obstructive lung disease, migration of individuals to the city could explain only part of the higher prevalence of COPD observed in Tucson compared with other regions in the United States.[57]

Time Trends

Although death rates for emphysema have declined, overall COPD rates have increased dramatically in recent years (Figure 13.2). One reason for the increase in the prevalence of COPD is the increase in the number of older people in the United States. Changes in International Classification of Diseases coding, declining death rates for other causes, and changing diagnostic practices make long-term changes difficult to interpret.

RISK FACTORS

Magnitude of Risk Factors

The strongest risk factor for COPD development is cigarette smoking. Compared with nonsmokers, current cigarette smokers show an approximate 10-fold relative risk for COPD occurrence. The relative risk is approximately equal for men and women. The occurrence of wheezing, frequent cough, and airway hyperresponsiveness in children has been strongly associated with parental smoking (twofold to fourfold relative risks).[48]

Environmental agents, including air pollutants and occupational dusts and chemicals, may contribute to COPD incidence, either independently or in an additive fashion with cigarette smoking. Several analyses from cities with high air pollution levels indicate that hospital admissions and mortality due to COPD are associated with the presence of acidic aerosols.[56] Evidence of an association between exposure to other air pollutants and long-term lung damage remains to be fully assessed. Pollutants that may exacerbate symptoms of COPD are ozone, particulates, and cigarette smoke.[58]

Population-Attributable Risk

Almost 90% of COPD is attributable to cigarette smoking.[48] Other risk factors have not been adequately quantified to calculate attributable risk estimates.

PREVENTION AND CONTROL MEASURES

Prevention

Elimination of tobacco use is the single most important preventive activity to reduce COPD occurrence. Significant reductions in COPD morbidity and mortality can be achieved through smoking reduction. Mortality in COPD is related to the decrement in the FEV1. The normal decline in FEV1 that occurs with aging in nonsmokers is accelerated in some smokers.[1] With cessation of smoking, the rate of decline in FEV1 can approach that of nonsmokers, but the FEV1 does not appear to improve to the level of lung function seen in nonsmokers.

For COPD, risks of multiple factors appear to be additive. It is, therefore, important to identify individuals with multiple risk factors, such as smoking, occupational exposures, and ambient air pollution.

Aggravation of existing conditions such as cough or dyspnea is more likely with multiple exposures.

Screening and Early Detection

The primary mode of screening for COPD is to measure airflow obstruction with spirometry or peak airflow measurement. The patient's history, physical examination, and chest x-ray are less sensitive and more expensive and are not useful as screening methods. Screening should be limited to individuals at high risk for developing COPD, primarily cigarette smokers.

Early detection of disease allows effective intervention. Although these diseases are not generally reversible, harmful exposures such as cigarette smoking can be eliminated to slow the disease process.

Treatment, Rehabilitation, and Recovery

The most effective treatment for this group of lung diseases is avoiding exposure to the causative agent—in most cases, cigarette smoke—and to other agents (eg, ambient air pollution) that can further damage compromised lungs. Once disease is present, the goals of therapy are to decrease symptoms, decrease airflow obstruction, and prevent and treat complications. Symptoms can be alleviated with inhaled bronchodilator drugs and respiratory hygiene.[59] When the

progression of disease results in decreases of blood oxygen, supplement oxygen therapy, when given continuously, has been shown to increase survival.[60] Pulmonary rehabilitation is a multidisciplinary program composed of exercise training, education, breathing retraining, and psychosocial support. Pulmonary rehabilitation does not reverse the course of the disease as measured by lung function, but programs have been shown to decrease dyspnea, increase exercise tolerance, and improve patients' quality of life.[61] Surgical removal of emphysematous lung has been shown to improve symptoms and lung function in selected individuals.[62] The patient selection criteria and long-term outcome from this technique are being examined and the role of this technique in the overall management of individuals with COPD is being debated.[62] Preventive health maintenance under a physician's supervision is important to allow early recognition and treatment of infections. Vaccination for influenza viruses and other vaccine-preventable diseases is recommended for people diagnosed with COPD.

EXAMPLES OF PUBLIC HEALTH INTERVENTIONS

Government agencies have established maximum permissible

exposure levels to many harmful occupational air pollutants to reduce harmful on-the-job exposures.[63] The regulation of ambient outdoor air pollution in the United States began in 1955 with the Air Pollution Control Act and continued with the Clean Air Act in 1963 and its amendments in 1970, 1977, and 1990. The Clean Air Act regulates the quality of outdoor air by setting standards for emissions from vehicles and stationary sources such as power plants.

Various states and municipalities have adopted emissions limits or have passed clean indoor air acts for hazardous air pollutants to regulate, for example, smoking or pesticide applications in public buildings. Many public health departments issue alerts when air pollutant levels exceed guidelines, so that individuals with COPD can avoid activities that are likely to exacerbate their condition. (Public health interventions for reduction of cigarette smoking are discussed in detail in Chapter 5.)

AREAS OF FUTURE RESEARCH AND DEMONSTRATION

Major overall risk factors for COPD are well understood. Thus, future research should help elucidate reasons for individual susceptibility to COPD development.[64] Additional studies of the cellular basis of COPD and identification of more sensitive and specific biochemical, genetic, and molecular markers of COPD[64] should lead to better methods of control. Additional epidemiologic studies are necessary to assess the interaction between cigarette smoking and putative risk factors such as air pollution and occupational chemicals. Improved methods of secondary prevention are required to identify and intervene in at risk individuals with accelerated declines in lung function. Methods of increasing the efficacy and duration of the known benefits of pulmonary rehabilitation programs are also needed.

CYSTIC FIBROSIS

ICD-9 277.00, 277.01

SIGNIFICANCE

Cystic fibrosis is a genetic disease due to abnormal mucus and altered function of the lung, pancreas, intestine, and exocrine glands.(Cystic Fibrosis Foundation National Registry, unpublished data, 1996). It results in premature death most frequently from respiratory failure due to chronic inflammation and infection. With an emphasis on treatment of the lung disease and nutritional deficiencies, there has been a dramatic improvement in survival in the past 4 decades (Figure 13.3) (Cystic Fibrosis Foundation National Registry, unpublished data,

1996). In 1990, there were approximately 30 000 individuals with cystic fibrosis in North America.[6] In 1960, the median survival for individuals with cystic fibrosis was 5 years, and in 1995, the median survival was 30 years.[65]

DESCRIPTIVE EPIDEMIOLOGY

Cystic fibrosis is the most common lethal genetic defect in individuals of Northern European descent in North American, and has been estimated to occur in approximately 1 in 3500 births in this population.[6] In the United States, cystic fibrosis occurs in approximately 1 of 14 000 Black births, 1 in

11 500 Hispanic births, 1 in 10 500 American Indian and Alaska Native births, and 1 in 25 500 Asian births.[6] Cystic fibrosis is an autosomal recessive defect and the prevalence in individuals of Northern European decent of the heterozygote form is approximately 1 in 25. Heterozygotic individuals are not affected.

The mean age at the time of diagnosis of cystic fibrosis is 3 years, with a median age of 7 months.[6] The clinical findings or reasons for diagnosis are persistent or acute respiratory symptoms, failure to thrive and malnutrition, malabsorption, meconium ileus, other intestinal obstruction, or a positive family history for cystic fibrosis.[6] The

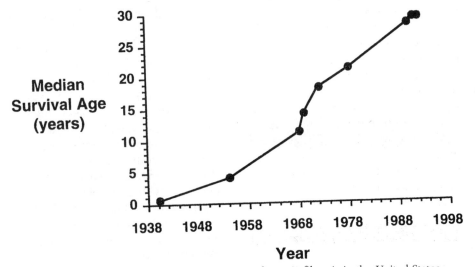

Figure 13.3—Median survival age of patients with cystic fibrosis in the United States, 1940–1994

diagnosis of cystic fibrosis occurs after 12 years in 10% of individuals.[6] The cause of death is most commonly respiratory failure.

PATHOPHYSIOLOGY

Cystic fibrosis is a manifestation of abnormal chloride movement in epithelial cells resulting in thick mucous. Over 400 genetic mutations have been identified in the cystic fibrosis gene, located on chromosome 7, that effect the function of the transmembrane conductance regulator (CFTR) protein. The most common defect, F508, accounts for about 70% of the defects in affected individuals in the United States.[6] The abnormal mucous may affect the lung, pancreas, intestines, exocrine glands, and sometimes the liver. The extent of organ involvement depends in part on the level of CFTR function in the tissues. The relationship between the pulmonary disease and CFTR is less clear and may reflect individual variations in exposure and response to respiratory irritants, compliance with therapeutic regimens aimed at improving airway clearance of excessive amounts of phlegm, and other poorly defined host factors.

RISK FACTORS

In cystic fibrosis, lung function is the strongest predictor of survival.[66]

For every 10% decrease in the percent predicted FEV1, the relative risk of death increases by 2.[67] Other factors leading to increased survival are male sex, maintenance of body weight, pancreatic sufficiency, diagnosis after the age of 2 years.[66] The worse survival for females with cystic fibrosis is related to poor weight maintenance.[66]

PREVENTION AND CONTROL MEASURES

Screening and Early Detection

In over 80% of individuals with cystic fibrosis, there is no prior family history.[68] The primary forms of screening for cystic fibrosis have been in the newborn and population-based carrier detection. The most common method used for screening is measurement of immunoreactive trypsinogen on dried blood spots.[69] Direct gene analysis has been utilized as the second test in a two-tiered screening program.[70] Older programs frequently measured albumin or protein in meconium from the newborn; however, this method was found to have a high false-positive rate.[69] With lack of studies finding significant improvement in outcome, and concerns about cost, efficacy, and potential risks from screening, it has been recommended that newborn screening should not be performed.[69] A more recent report has found improved pulmonary function in individuals detected by screening.[71] Carrier screening for cystic fibrosis of the general population has also not been recommended for many of the same reasons identified in newborn screening.[72] Screening and genetic counseling and education can be performed in family members or couples with a family history of cystic fibrosis and in women with cystic fibrosis and their spouses.[72] The majority of men with cystic fibrosis are infertile.

Prevention

The effects of cystic fibrosis on respiratory function lead to a significant amount of morbidity and is the leading cause of mortality. With the identification of the cystic fibrosis gene in 1989, there has been a tremendous growth in the understanding of the disease mechanism. Limited clinical trials have taken place examining the efficacy of gene therapy in the treatment of the lung disease.[73]

SLEEP APNEA

ICD-9 780.51, 780.53, 780.57

SIGNIFICANCE

Sleep apnea is one of several causes of excessive daytime sleepiness in adults. In the most common form of the condition, obstructive sleep apnea syndrome, the upper airway, pharynx, narrows or closes, initiating a sequence of events including a decrease in arterial oxygen saturation, arousal in sleep, and subsequent relief of the obstruction. The obstruction can occur repeatedly during sleep. The arousal frequently does not lead to complete awakening but does interfere with sleep efficiency. The excessive daytime sleepiness initially may occur with passive activities such as reading or watching television. With more severe disease, individuals may not be able to stay awake during important activities such as driving. In one study, individuals with obstructive sleep apnea were seven times more likely to have an automobile accident than individuals without the syndrome.[74] Other symptoms of sleep apnea include snoring, morning headaches, intellectual impairment, poor memory, poor judgment, or personality changes.[7]

Different definitions for obstructive sleep apnea syndrome are used. The syndrome consists of neuropsychiatric symptoms, most commonly excessive daytime somnolence, plus sleep disturbed breathing. Sleep disturbed breathing including apneas, hypopneas, and arterial oxygen desaturation is determined by laboratory or home monitoring of sleep. Apnea is defined as a total cessation of airflow and an hyponea occurs when there is a decrease in airflow at the nose and mouth.[7] The number of apneas and hypopneas considered abnormal depends on the population being tested and indications for testing. An apnea-hypnea index, the average number of apneas and hyponeas per hour of sleep, of greater than 5 to 10 is frequently used as abnormal in population studies.

Therapy of obstructive sleep apnea includes avoidance of known or suspected risk factors, alteration in sleep habits and positions, use of devices to increase the patency of the nasal cavity or pharynx, application of continuous positive airway pressure (CPAP) via a nasal mask, and tracheostomy.

DESCRIPTIVE EPIDEMIOLOGY

The incidence of obstructive sleep apnea syndrome has not been determined. The prevalence of the syndrome in a randomly tested population of working adults between the ages of 30 and 60 years was 2% in women and 4% in men.[75] Most studies have found a prevalence less than 5%.[7] Follow-up studies in untreated individuals diagnosed with moderate to severe obstructive sleep apnea have found increased mortality.[7]

RISK FACTORS

The prevalence of obstructive sleep apnea syndrome increases with age and is higher in males, habitual snorers, and obese individuals. Alcohol and sedative use can exacerbate or induce obstructive sleep apnea syndrome.[7] Obstructive sleep apnea syndrome has been associated with motor vehicle trauma,[74] systemic hypertension, renal insufficiency, cerebral infarction, and cardiovascular disease.[7]

PREVENTION AND CONTROL MEASURES

Better characterization of the epidemiology and long-term sequel of obstructive sleep apnea syndrome are required before screening can be recommended.[76] Populations that deserve further study are long-distance truck drivers, hazardous duty personnel, and certain groups of medical patients.[76]

Occupational Lung Diseases

The most common occupational lung disease, occupational chronic bronchitis (see COPD above), is the least specific response to occupational exposures and often the first indication of work-related pulmonary pathology. Given a sufficient dose and duration of exposure, nearly all respirable agents can contribute to the development or aggravation of chronic lung diseases. It is not uncommon to have multiple occupational lung diseases present in the same work force. This is especially true for occupational bronchitis and occupational asthma.

More specific chronic occupational lung diseases are defined by the agent associated with the specific disease. Several distinct syndromes associated with exposure to dusts have been defined, particularly for occupational settings. Especially for the pneumoconioses, an important hallmark of the disease process is the recognition of a "latency" period of typically 20 years between first exposure and the appearance of clinical disease.

Occupational dusts are classified as either inorganic (eg, coal dust, silica, asbestos) or organic (eg, cotton dust, grain dust, mold spores). The respiratory conditions associated with most inorganic dusts result from the direct effect of the dust on lung tissue. From 1968 to 1992, a total of 100 890 deaths from pneumoconiosis were recorded among US residents.[77] Diseases resulting from exposure to most organic dusts are immunologically mediated. One exception to this latter classification is the condition related to cotton dust exposure; cotton dust is organic, but the condition is probably not immunologically mediated.

The US Occupational Safety and Health Administration (OSHA) has established allowable exposure limits for all the inorganic dusts associated with disease.

Cigarette smoking increases the risk of lung disease in occupationally exposed workers. In most cases, the disease risks are additive—that is, the total disease risk is the sum of the risk from cigarette smoking and the risk from the occupational exposure. An exception to this is the multiplicative risk between asbestos exposure and cigarette smoking in the occurrence of lung cancer (discussed in Chapter 2).

The following sections briefly describe some important occupation-related chronic lung diseases.

COAL WORKERS' PNEUMOCONIOSIS
ICD-9 500

SIGNIFICANCE

Coal workers' pneumoconiosis (CWP), or black lung disease, is identified by a pattern of x-ray abnormalities and an exposure history. Between 1979 and 1990, 29 344 deaths occurred with CWP noted on their death certificates but less than 2000 CWP-associated deaths per year occurred between 1990 and 1992. Since 1969, approximately $10 billion has been paid in workers' compensation for CWP benefits.[78]

DESCRIPTIVE EPIDEMIOLOGY

The prevalence of CWP increases with increasing exposure to coal dust. In studies of CWP, years of mining are often used as a surrogate for dust exposure because information on dust exposure for individual miners is rarely complete.

CWP is classified as simple CWP if rounded opacities less than 1 cm are seen on the chest radiograph (ILO opacities "p," "q," or "r").[79] It is typical for the opacities to first appear in the upper lung fields of the chest x-ray and then to progress to involve all lung fields. In the United States, coal miners surveyed between 1985 and 1988 as part of the National Study of Coal Workers' Pneumoconiosis (NSCWP), 4% developed simple CWP after 15 years of coal dust exposure, and 19% of miners developed simple CWP after 30 or more years of exposure.[78, 80] It is uncommon in simple CWP for the radiographic abnormalities to progress after the individual has left the dusty environment. Complicated CWP or progressive massive fibrosis occurs when there are opacities larger than 1 cm on the chest x-ray. In the national study of CWP, complicated CWP occurred in approximately 2.5% of coal miners. Data from the national study suggest that the incidence of both simple and complicated CWP is declining, largely because dust standards in mines are being enforced.[78]

Chronic exposure to coal dust can lead to the development of chronic obstructive lung disease, even in the absence of radiographic changes.[81]

Coal miners with chronic obstructive lung disease have increased rates of dyspnea, cough, and phlegm production. The magnitude of the deficit in lung function due to chronic coal dust exposure is between 150 and 450 mL over an average lifetime of work in a coal mine, with a smaller percentage of individuals having deficits of greater than 1 liter.[82]

RISK FACTORS

Coal workers' pneumoconiosis is caused by respirable coal mine dust, or dust generally less than 5 μm in diameter. Usually, 10 or more years of exposure to coal dust must have elapsed before CWP can be diagnosed by a chest x-ray. Coal dust also may contain other harmful mineral dusts, such as silica dust, that increase the risk of other chronic lung diseases such as silicosis. The radiographic appearance of silicosis can be indistinguishable from CWP. The risk of CWP diagnosed by x-ray increases with higher rank of coal, in part explaining the higher occurrence in miners from the eastern coal producing regions of the United States compared to western areas. Underground miners are at higher risk than above ground or surface miners.

Risk factors for the development of chronic obstructive lung disease in coal miners are the duration and extent of dust exposure, prior dust exposure, and the presence of other risk factors for obstructive lung disease, especially cigarette smoking. The average lifetime coal dust exposure among coal miners with symptoms of chronic lung disease was found to result in a loss in lung function equivalent to that associated with smoking 20 cigarettes per day over a lifetime.[83] Coal miners working in jobs with higher silica exposure, such as surface coal mine drillers, are at higher risk for the development of chronic obstructive lung disease.

PREVENTION AND CONTROL MEASURES

Coal workers' pneumoconiosis can best be prevented by reducing coal dust exposure in the workplace, educating workers about disease risk and safe work practices and, when excessive exposure circumstances are unavoidable, providing respiratory protection. Medical monitoring of coal miners is required, and periodic chest radiographs are intended to identify individuals who have CWP in its preliminary phases, thus enabling them to avoid further exposure and possibly preventing the disease's progression to more advanced stages. The use of the ILO Pneumoconiosis grading system is critically important to allow quantification of changes over time.

The Federal Coal Mine Health and Safety Act passed in 1969 and its amendments sets limits on the amount of respirable coal dust levels in the United States. For coal dust with less than 5% silica, the standard is 2 mg/m^3. Although there is evidence that the current dust standards decrease the occurrence of CWP (Figure 13.4), the National Institute for Occupational Safety and Health has recommended that the respiratory dust standard be decreased to 1 mg/m^3 due to concerns that the current standard does not protect against other lung conditions.[84]

SILICOSIS

ICD-9 502

SIGNIFICANCE

Chronic inhalation of respirable particles of crystalline silica may result in silicosis. Like CWP, silicosis is characterized by a predominance of small, rounded x-ray abnormalities in the upper lung fields indicative of fibrosis. Also like CWP, silicosis can be divided into simple silicosis and complicated silicosis, or progressive massive fibrosis, based on the size of the opacities on the chest x-ray. In its initial phases, the disease is not associated with declines in lung function, although cough and phlegm production are common. Chronic exposure to silica dust can result in chronic obstructive lung

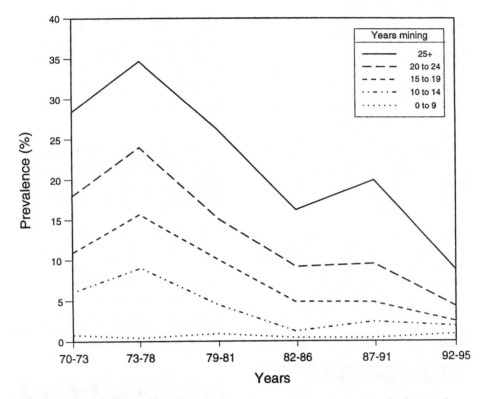

Figure 13.4—Prevalence of coal workers' pneumoconiosis, category 1 or higher, in the Coal Workers' x-ray Surveillance Program from 1970–1995, by tenure in coal mining

disease, even without x-ray changes.[85] The disease may slowly progress over 20 to 40 years to the point of respiratory failure. Individuals with silicosis are at increased risk of developing tuberculosis.[86] Silica is now categorized as a probable human carcinogen by the International Agency for Cancer Research (IARC).[87, 88] Although deaths attributed to silicosis have decreased from more than 1000 per year prior to 1971 to less than 300 in 1992,[77] an estimated 2000 cases of silicosis are diagnosed each year in the United States.[80]

DESCRIPTIVE EPIDEMIOLOGY

The prevalence of silicosis in the United States is unknown. There are no registries for the disease, and few states have surveillance requirements. By extrapolating prevalence data from a surveillance study in New Jersey to the United States, researchers have estimated that 1500 cases occur annually.[86] The US Department of Labor estimated in 1980 that 59 000 of the workers who were then exposed to silica would eventually develop silicosis.[58]

Silicosis is most prevalent among workers involved in the dry drilling or grinding of rock with a high silica content, which generates respirable particles. Silicosis is nine times more common in men than in women. The most common industrial environments where silicosis occurs among men are mines, foundries, quarries, and silica flour mills.[58] Among women, silicosis occurs most commonly in the ceramics industry.

RISK FACTORS

Silicosis is caused by chronic inhalation of crystalline silica, which is present in quartz. A more toxic form of silica may be produced when quartz is heated.[79] People such as foundry workers who are in occupations that involve both heating and grinding quartz may be at greater risk of silicosis.

PREVENTION AND CONTROL MEASURES

The most effective method for preventing silicosis is primary prevention—eliminating exposure to respirable silica. A secondary line of defense is worker education and training, use of protective equipment and enforcement of existing work site standards. Silica concentrations in the work environment should not exceed the permissible exposure limit established by the US Occupational Safety and Health Administration. As with screening for conditions associated with other inorganic dusts, x-ray screening may identify individuals who have minimal disease, enabling these people to avoid additional exposure and possibly preventing progression to more advanced phases.

ASBESTOSIS

ICD-9 501

SIGNIFICANCE

An estimated 27 500 000 workers were exposed to asbestos between 1940 and 1979.[90] Asbestos was widely used as an insulating material in many public, residential, and commercial buildings. The risk of adverse health effects from these sources of asbestos to workers or to occupants of buildings depends on many factors, including the condition of the building, the condition of the insulating material, and the duration of exposure.

Adverse health effects from exposure to asbestos include pleural effusions, pleural thickening and calcification, pleural plaques, malignant mesothelioma, lung cancer, and asbestosis.[91] Of these, asbestosis is the most prevalent chronic lung condition. Some researchers have suggested that asbestosis exposure resulting in benign pleural disease can be associated with obstructive lung disease,[92] although the findings have been the subject of debate.[93] Approximately 10 000 asbestos-related deaths (from cancer or other diseases) occur in the United States each year.[58]

In its early stages, asbestosis is often clinically characterized by dry rales, or whistling or crackling noises, at the end of each inspiration. Often clinical signs and pulmonary function abnormalities appear before chest x-ray abnormalities become apparent. Eventually, diffuse fibrosis can result in decreased lung capacity, decreased gas exchange, and severe shortness of breath. The x-ray abnormalities evident in people with asbestosis are predominantly small, irregular opacities in the lower lung fields (ILO "s," "t," and "u"). In addition, pleural thickening or pleural plaques, often with calcification, can occur alone or in combination with asbestosis. Unlike CWP or silicosis, asbestosis deaths are continuing to increase, from 1359 deaths between 1968 and 1978 to 6856 between 1979 and 1990.[94] In 1992, asbestosis was listed as the primary cause in 1992, but this may underestimate the true prevalence of this condition.[95]

DESCRIPTIVE EPIDEMIOLOGY

In various surveys, between 6% and 40% of asbestos textile or insulation workers have detectable x-ray lung abnormalities. Results from the National Health and Nutrition Examination Survey indicate that 2.3% of US males and 0.2% of US females have pleural thickening upon chest x-ray.[96] In a study of 17 800 insulation workers in the United States, asbestosis was identified as the cause of death in 7% of the workers who died.[94] Asbestos exposure may occur in a variety of occupations, including asbestos mining, asbestos milling, cement work, railroad repair work, plumbing, pipe fitting, and maintenance work.[91] While most uses of asbestos in newly manufactured products have been eliminated, many asbestos-containing products are still present in building materials and may pose a risk to workers during maintenance, repair, renovation, and demolition. A 15-year latency period usually exists between exposure and the development of asbestosis.[90]

RISK FACTORS

Asbestosis is caused by exposure to airborne asbestos fibers. The magnitude of the risk of asbestosis depends on both the duration and the intensity of the exposure to asbestos dust. The more intense and prolonged the exposure, the greater the risk of developing the disease. Brief but very heavy exposure can also cause disease.[90]

Asbestos is unique among the pneumoconiosis causing agents. Nonoccupational exposure to family members of workers bringing dust home on their clothes and residence near manufacturing facilities utilizing asbestos have been associated with the occurrence of asbestos-associated disease.[97, 98]

PREVENTION AND CONTROL MEASURES

Asbestosis can be prevented by eliminating exposure to asbestos. Asbestos has been largely eliminated from the work environment, and its release from existing materials can be controlled. Containment of asbestos in buildings may be initially less expensive than removal; however, containment may be only a temporary solution, because ongoing maintenance and repair can result in a further release of asbestos and eventual enforced removal under US EPA regulations. Recent national legislation requires accreditation of

contractors who work with asbestos and training for asbestos abatement workers to assure safety as well as prevent "bystander" exposure.[94] Safe work practices should include identifying materials that contain asbestos; implementing rigorous operating procedures, such as wetting asbestos-containing materials; and wearing a self-contained breathing apparatus. X-ray and pulmonary function screening may also help in protecting workers. Results from these examinations can encourage the workers to avoid additional exposure, make them more aware of the need for strict work practices, and encourage them to participate in special health surveillance programs.

BYSSINOSIS

ICD-9 504

SIGNIFICANCE

Byssinosis is both an acute and chronic airways disease caused by exposure to cotton dust. The acute phase of byssinosis is sometimes called "Monday morning syndrome," in which chest tightness and/or shortness of breath occurs when workers return to cotton dust exposure following a weekend or days off. Progression of the disease is characterized by chronic cough and a decline in lung function. After more than 10 years of exposure, overall pulmonary function declines. Byssinosis is similar in pathology to chronic bronchitis. A grading system has been developed for bysinnosis.[99] In the United States, approximately 500 000 workers are potentially at risk for byssinosis,[100] although the disease is rarely fatal, claiming only 15 lives in 1992.[77]

DESCRIPTIVE EPIDEMIOLOGY

The prevalence of byssinosis is approximately 20% among workers who are exposed to cotton dust and may reach more than 80% among workers with the highest exposures.[43] In 1970, it was estimated that approximately 35 000 workers in the cotton textile mills had byssinosis.[101] Since regulation of cotton dust began in 1978, the degree of lung function impairment in cotton textile workers may have decreased.[102] There is no evidence of sex or race differences in risk of byssinosis.

RISK FACTORS

Byssinosis results from exposure to the dust of cotton, flax, or hemp. The specific causal agent of byssinosis has not been identified, but bacterial endotoxins present in dust are suspected.[80] Among cotton workers, the risk is highest among workers involved in the initial stages of processing: opening,

picking, carding, stripping, and grinding.

PREVENTION AND CONTROL MEASURES

The best way to prevent byssinosis is to avoid exposure to cotton dust. Cotton dust concentrations in the workplace must be kept below the US Occupational Safety and Health Administration's permissible exposure level. Another technique known as "cotton washing" is effective but may not be feasible on a large scale. Employers must treat the acute phase of byssinosis as a sentinel health event, using it as an opportunity to reduce exposure among other workers with early symptoms.

OCCUPATIONAL ASTHMA
ICD-9 493, 506, 507.8

SIGNIFICANCE

Occupational asthma is characterized by episodes of bronchoconstriction when an individual is exposed to agents to which he or she has been sensitized. Primary occupational asthma is distinguished from exacerbations of existing asthma by the presence of a workplace sensitizing agent and diagnosis by a specific case definition.[102] The overall prevalence of occupational asthma is unknown but is estimated to be between 2% and 15% of all adults with asthma.[103] In 1986, occupational asthma exceeded asbestosis and silicosis in the total number of accepted claims for occupational lung disease by the Workers' Compensation Board in Quebec, Canada.[104] In the United States, it was estimated that 15% of all asthma cases in the 1978 Social Security Disability Survey were occupationally related.[105] Fifty percent to 90% of individuals with occupational asthma will continue to have symptoms even after being removed from the source of the exposure.[104]

It is important in diagnosing occupational asthma to establish the presence of airflow obstruction.[106] If the preliminary spirometry is normal, a repeat test, following inhalation challenge with methacholine or histamine, may be indicated. It may be difficult to establish that asthma is caused by an occupational exposure. The fact that initial symptoms may occur only at home or after work can be misleading.[104] To document a change in airflow obstruction related to work, it may be helpful to measure the peak expiratory flow rate several times a day for 2 to 3 weeks.[107] Skin testing with the suspected compound also may be of diagnostic value in selected cases. Specific inhalation challenge with the suspected compound is not performed routinely because it is expensive, time-consuming, not

widely available, and carries the risk of a potentially serious reaction.[107]

Several chronic disorders can be confused with occupational asthma. Reactive airways dysfunction syndrome occurs hours after a single exposure to high levels of irritant gases and results in cough, wheezing, and shortness of breath.[107] Reactive airways dysfunction syndrome is not usually considered a form of occupational asthma because there is no latency period between the exposure and the development of symptoms. In occupational asthma, symptoms usually do not appear until a few weeks to as long as several years after the first exposure.[104] Byssinosis is another condition that may be confused with occupational asthma.

DESCRIPTIVE EPIDEMIOLOGY

More than 200 causative agents have been associated with occupational asthma,[108] including a variety of materials of plant and animal origin, chemicals, metals, biological enzymes, and drugs (Table 13.4). Agents are classified as high molecular weight compounds (less than 1000 daltons) or low molecular weight compounds.[107] The high molecular weight compounds are proteins, polysaccharides, and peptides, which induce an allergic response by stimulating the production of specific immunoglobulin E

Table 13.4—Occupations at Risk for Occupational Asthma and the Probable Causal Agent[a]

Occupation	Causal Agent
Animal handlers, veterinarians, laboratory workers	Urine protein, dander
Bakers, millers	Wheat, rye, buckwheat, mites, hemicellulase, glucoamylase, papin, soybean
Chemical workers	Sulfonechloramides, azo dyes, ethylenediamine, anthraquinone
Coffee or tea workers	Green coffee, tea dust
Detergent workers	Proteases (*Bacillus subtilis*, esperases)
Electronics workers	Colophony, aminoethyl ethanolamine
Farm workers	Animal antigens, vegetable dusts
Fishery and oyster workers	Crab, prawns, hoya, sea squirts
Grain handlers	Grain dust, insect debris dust
Insect handlers	Bee, moth, coacroach, cricket, locust, river fly, screw worm fly, meal worm
Hairdresser	Sodium and potassium persulfate, henna
Leather workers	Formalin, chromium salts
Lumber and woodworkers, carpentry, construction, sawmill, cabinetmaking	Wood dusts (western red cedar, redwood, iroko, oak, mahogany, Douglas fir, zebrawood)
Metal workers	Platinum salts, nickle, chromium, cobalt, vanadium, tungsten carbide
Paper product workers	Natural glues
Pharmaceutical workers	Penicillins, cephalosporins, methyl dopa, spiramycin, tetracycline, pepcin, phenylglycine acid
Plastic workers, automobile repair	Diisocyanates (TDI, MDI), trimellitic anhydride, and paintersphthalic anhydride

[a]*Note:* Adapted from Alberts.[106]

and sometimes immunoglobulin G antibodies.[107] Depending on the level of exposure, the prevalence of asthma from these compounds can be high. Asthma occurs in 3% to 30% of animal handlers;[104] 10% to 45% of workers exposed to biologic enzymes that are used, for example, in laundry detergents and other cleaning agents;[107] 20% of bakers;[104] and in 70% of flight crews dispersing sterile irradiated screw worm flies.[107]

Examples of the low molecular weight compounds are isocyanates, wood dusts, metals, and drugs.[103] An allergic response involving immunoglobulin E occurs less frequently in the development of asthma from the low molecular weight compounds than from the high molecular weight compounds. Work-related asthma occurs in 4% of workers exposed to the dust of western red cedar,[104] in 5% to 10% of workers exposed to toluene diisocyanate,[108] in 29% to 40% of workers using epoxy resins,[108] and in 70% of workers exposed to platinum salts in such processes as metallurgy and photography.[107]

RISK FACTORS

Materials that have known or suspected allergic properties account for the majority of cases of occupational asthma. Occupations with a high prevalence of these agents are listed in Table 13.4. The risk of developing occupational asthma is usually related to the magnitude of exposure for many agents including western red cedar, toluene diisocyanate, baking products, and colophony fumes from soldering.[104] Atopy, or allergy, is an important risk factor for developing asthma from the high molecular weight compounds but not for the low molecular weight compounds.[104]

The risk for persistent symptoms in workers diagnosed with occupational asthma was examined in 125 western red cedar workers.[109] All workers who remained at work continued to have symptoms. Among workers who left the work, those who were older, had a longer duration of exposure, and had a longer duration of symptoms were at higher risk for having persistent symptoms.[109] Workers who develop toluene diisocyanate-related asthma and continue to be exposed to the compound have been found to have continued deterioration in pulmonary function.[108]

PREVENTION AND CONTROL MEASURES

The only way to prevent occupational asthma is to stay away from work and work sites where exposure to certain levels of agents occurs. It may be helpful to educate workers on handling materials and avoiding spills.[108] Improved ventilation and the use of respirators can decrease exposures. When sensitization occurs, the affected worker should be transferred from the area of exposure. In cases where transfer is not possible, it is debatable whether the worker should be allowed to continue working with the suspected compound, even when protective measures are instituted.[104, 107] Deaths have been recorded when sensitized individuals have been re-exposed at the workplace.[110] Desensitization prior to exposure has not been shown to be effective.[80]

CHRONIC LUNG DISEASE ASSOCIATED WITH EXPOSURE TO ORGANIC DUST

ICD-9 495, 496

SIGNIFICANCE

A variety of chronic lung conditions can develop following short-term or long-term exposure to organic dusts or gases produced from the storage or decay of organic material. It is estimated that there are 500 000 grain elevator workers in the United States.[111] Grain dust is a mixture of different grains, bacteria and fungus, mites, inorganic material, and herbicides and pesticides.[111] Grain-handlers' disease, caused by inhaling grain dust, is characterized by a drop in lung function over a work shift and by changes that persist over a harvest season.[112] Chronic grain dust exposure can result in chronic cough, phlegm, wheezing, and dyspnea and a permanent decline in lung function.[111, 113] Pulmonary fibrosis may occur but is uncommon in workers with chronic grain dust exposure.[111]

Farmer's lung is caused by inhaling spores from moldy hay and is characterized by repeated attacks of fever, chills, malaise, coughing, and breathlessness.[112] The condition is a type of hypersensitivity pneu-monitis or extrinsic allergic alveolitis that results from inhaling many different organic dusts. Most commonly, thermophilic actinomyces of other fungi are present. Testing patient serum for specific precipitating antibodies can help identify which organisms or agents may be contributing to the disease. In a well-controlled research setting, inhalation chamber challenges have been used to identify offending agents. Such testing is not a routine practice. The chronic form occurs in fewer than 5% of patients who develop the acute form of the disease.[113] Lung function is abnormal in patients with the chronic form of the disease, with a decline in the forced vital capacity (FVC) and a diffuse fibrosis on the chest x-ray.

DESCRIPTIVE EPIDEMIOLOGY

Hypersensitivity pneumonitis is a rare disease, and little is known about the distribution of the disease outside the agricultural sector. Symptoms are often similar to asthma, COPD, and bronchitis, and initial acute attacks are often mistaken for pneumonia. No single clinical or laboratory test exists to establish the diagnosis. Chronic lung disease from inhaling of grain dust is probably more common, but relatively little is known about its epidemiologic patterns.[111]

RISK FACTORS

Those at risk for disease from inhaling organic dust and gases include farmers, grain handlers, wood workers, bird breeders, mushroom workers, and animal handlers, including workers who clean pens and handle laboratory animals. Environments where water-based machining fluids are used have also been associated with hypersensitivity pneumonitis, probably due to aerosolization of bacteria or fungi growing in the fluids.

PREVENTION AND CONTROL MEASURES

Agricultural dusts are regulated in the United States; the National Institute for Occupational Safety and Health (NIOSH) has proposed a limit on grain dust of 4 mg/m³.[113] The concern over dust levels in grain handling facilities has, in part, been due to the risk of explosions.[111]

Improved design of grain elevators and livestock confinement spaces, proper ventilation, and education of farm workers and rescue services can reduce the risk from dust and toxic gases.[113] Self-contained breathing devices should be worn by workers entering closed or poorly ventilated spaces or tanks containing liquid manure.[114] Diseases caused by molds can be minimized by proper grain storage techniques. A critical factor in control of disease is worker knowledge of the circumstances where exposures are likely to occur so that preventive precautions can be taken.

INTERSTITIAL LUNG DISEASE
ICD-9 515-517

SIGNIFICANCE

Interstitial lung disease is associated with a variety of different agents and disorders (Table 13.5). Some are

Table 13.5—Causes of Interstitial Lung Diseases[a]

Known Causes	Unknown causes
Inorganic dusts	Idiopathic pulmonary fibrosis
Organic dusts	Collagen-vascular disease
Gases, fumes, vapors, aerosols	Sarcoidosis
Drugs	Histiocytosis X
Poisons	Goodpastures syndrome
Radiation	Wegener's granulomatosis
Infectious agents	Vasculitidies
Chronic pulmonary edema	Lymphocytic infiltrative disorders
Chronic uremia	

[a]Adapted from Crystal.[114]

discussed in other sections of this chapter on occupational lung diseases and lung diseases associated with inhaling organic dust and fumes. Some cases of acute interstitial lung disease, such as those caused by medications, infections, or toxic gas inhalation, can evolve into a chronic form of interstitial lung disease. The lung interstitium that is affected by this disease includes the spaces between the pulmonary capillary cells and the pulmonary alveoli, the connective tissue surrounding blood vessels and bronchi, and the connective tissue of the pleura. Pulmonary fibrosis, alveolitis, and pneumonitis are other general terms sometimes used to describe this class of lung diseases.

During the initial assessment of individuals with interstitial lung disease, it is important to look for connective tissue disease or malignancy and to consider medication use, symptom duration, and the history of exposure to different organic and inorganic dusts. Progressive dyspnea is the most common presenting complaint. Pulmonary function testing, although it may show abnormalities with a restrictive defect with decreased functional vital capacity (FVC), is more helpful in following the course of the disease than in the initial diagnostic evaluation. The location and type of opacities on the chest radiograph can be helpful in diagnosing intersti-

tial lung diseases.[115] A lung biopsy is sometimes required if the diagnosis remains in doubt or if the disease process is severe.

DESCRIPTIVE EPIDEMIOLOGY

There are few studies on the epidemiology of interstitial lung diseases. In a population-based registry in an urban county, the prevalence of interstitial lung disease in adults over the age of 18 years was 80.9 per 100 000 population in males and 67.2 per 100 000 population in females.[116] Occupational and environmental causes were the most frequent in males (20.8 per 100 000) with idiopathic pulmonary fibrosis the second most likely diagnosis (20.2 per 100 000). In women, pulmonary fibrosis was the most common diagnosis (14.3 per 100 000) with idiopathic pulmonary fibrosis second (13.2 per 100 000).[116] In the same study, the incidence of pulmonary fibrosis in males was 31.5 per 100 000 per year and in females it was 26.1 per 100 000 per year.[116] The most common incident diagnoses were pulmonary fibrosis and idiopathic pulmonary fibrosis, accounting for 46% of all diagnoses in men and 44% in women.[116] Sarcoidosis is a disease of unknown cause characterized by granulomas that most frequently affect the lung but can occur anywhere in the body. In the United States, the prevalence of sarcoidosis in Whites is 5 per 100 000; in Blacks, it is approximately 40 per 100 000.[117]

The age-adjusted mortality rates for pulmonary fibrosis in 1991 were 51 per 1 000 000 in males and 27 per 1 000 000 for females.[118] Mortality rates were highest in the West and Southeast regions of the United States and lowest in the Midwest and Northeast.[118]

RISK FACTORS

Risk factors for developing most of the interstitial lung diseases are poorly understood or are poorly understood. In an autopsy study on the risk factors for idiopathic pulmonary fibrosis, laundry workers, barbers, beauticians, painters, production metal workers, and production woodworkers were at greater risk for developing the disease.[119] Other studies on environmental factors and idiopathic pulmonary fibrosis have found increased odds ratios for exposure to wood dust, textile dust, metal dust and livestock.[120–122] Smoking has been found to be a risk factor for idiopathic pulmonary fibrosis in several studies.[119–121] In a case-control study, a history of having ever smoked increased the risk for idiopathic pulmonary fibrosis by 60%.[122] For the different inhaled agents that are known to cause interstitial lung disease (Table 13.5), it is not known why disease will develop in some individuals but not in others with similar exposures.

PREVENTION AND CONTROL MEASURES

For interstitial diseases that develop from inhaling organic or inorganic dusts or fumes, limiting or avoiding the exposure will minimize or prevent the disease. Many of the drug-induced and radiation-induced causes of interstitial disease are used in treating other, possibly life-threatening, diseases the patient may have and are, therefore, difficult to avoid. A trial of corticosteroids is often given in the initial management of the interstitial lung diseases of unknown etiology (Table 13.5), but the effectiveness of this treatment is not known.[122] For many of the interstitial diseases, treatment is primarily supportive, treating the complications of respiratory and right heart failure. Preventive care should include flu and pneumococcal vaccines.

REFERENCES

1. Samet JM. Definitions and methodology in COPD research. In: Hensley MJ, Saunders NA, eds. *Clinical Epidemiology of Chronic Obstructive Pulmonary Disease.* New York, NY: Marcel Dekker; 1989:1–22.

2. National Center for Health Statistics. 1995 Mortality Tables. Available at http://www.cdc.gov/nchswww/.

3. Higgins MW, Thom T. Incidence, prevalence, and mortality: intra- and intercountry differences. In: Hensley MJ, Saunders NA, eds. *Clinical Epidemiology of Chronic Obstructive Pulmonary Disease.* New York, NY: Marcel Dekker; 1989:22–42.

4. Levin L, Levin DC. Morbidity and quality of life in patients with COPD. In: Hensley MJ, Saunders NA, eds. *Clinical Epidemiology of Chronic Obstructive Pulmonary Disease.* New York, NY: Marcel Dekker; 1989:45–54.

5. Snider GL. Chronic bronchitis and emphysema. In: Murrary JF, Nadel JA, eds. *Textbook of Respiratory Medicine.* Philadelphia, Pa: WB Saunders Company; 1988:1069–1106.

6. Mahler DA, Tomlinson D, Olmstead EM, Tosteson AN, O'Connor GT. Changes in dyspnea, health status and lung function in chronic airway disease. *Am J Respir Crit Care Med.* 1995:151;61–65.

7. FitzSimmons SC. The changing epidemiology of cystic fibrosis. *J Pediatr.* 1993;122:1–9.

8. Bresnitz EA, Goldberg R, Kosinski RM. Epidemiology of obstructive sleep apnea. *Epidemiol Rev.* 1994;16:210–227.

9. Global Initiative for Asthma. *Global Strategy for Asthma Management and Prevention: NHLBI/WHO Workshop Report.* Bethesda, Md: National Institutes of Health; 1995. NIH Publication 95-3659. Available at www.ginasthma.com.

10. Guill, M. Respiratory manifestations of gastroesophageal reflux in children. *J Asthma.* 1995;32:173–179.

11. *Guidelines for the Use of ILO International Classification of Radiographs of Pneumoconiosis.* Geneva, Switzerland: International Labor Office; 1980.

12. *Vital and Health Statistics: Current Estimates from the National Health Interview Survey, 1994.* Series 10: Data from the National Health Interview Survey. Hyattsville, Md: Dept of Health and Human Services; 1995. DHHS publication PHS 96-1521.

13. Centers for Disease Control. Asthma—United States, 1980–1990. *MMWR.* 1992;41:733–735.

14. Burt CW, Knapp CE. *Ambulatory Care Visits for Asthma, 1993–1994.* Vol. 277. Advance Data from the National Center for Health Statistics, 1996; Available at www.cdc.gov/nchswww/default.htm. Accessed August 27, 1998.

15. Weiss KB, Gergen PJ, Hodgson TH. An economic evaluation of asthma in the United States. *N Engl J Med.* 1992;326:862–866.

16. White MV, Kaliner MA. Mast cells and asthma. In: Kaliner MA, Barnes PJ, Persson CGA, eds. *Asthma: Its Pathology and Treatment.* New York, NY: Marcel Dekker; 1991:409–440.

17. Bousquet J, Chanez P, Lacoste JY, et al. Eosinophilic inflammation in asthma. *N Engl J Med.* 1990; 323:1033–1039.

18. Vervloet D and Charpin D. Intrinsic asthma. In: Marsh DG, Lockhart A, Holgate ST, eds. *The Genetics of Asthma.* Oxford, England: Blackwell Scientific Publications; 1993: 93–101.

19. Sears MR. Epidemiological trends in bronchial asthma. In: Kaliner MA, Barnes PJ, Persson CGA, eds. *Asthma: Its Pathology and Treatment.* New York, NY: Marcel Dekker; 1991:1–49.

20. Centers for Disease Control. Asthma-United States, 1980–1990. *MMWR.* 1992;41:733–735.

21. Weitzman M, Gortmaker SL, Sobol A, Perrin JM. Recent trends in the prevalence and severity of childhood asthma. *JAMA.* 1992; 268:2673–2677.

22. Mielck A, Reitmeir R, Wjst M. Severity of childhood asthma by socioeconomic status. *Int J Epidemiol.* 1996;25:388–393.

23. Myers DA. Genetics of atopic allergy: family studies of total serum IgE levels. In: Marsh DG, Lockhart A, Holgate ST, eds. *The Genetics of Asthma.* Oxford, England: Blackwell Scientific Publications, 1993: 153–162.

24. Pauwels R, Joos G, Kips J. The genetic control of airway responsiveness in rats. In: Marsh DG, Lockhart A, Holgate ST, eds. *The Genetics of Asthma.* Oxford, England: Blackwell Scientific Publications; 1993: 113–120.

25. Lockhart A. What is bronchial asthma? The role of genetic and acquired factors. In: Marsh DG, Lockhart A and Holgate ST, eds. *The Genetics of Asthma.* Oxford, England: Blackwell Scientific Publications; 1993:3–13.

26. Maurer JD, Rosenberg HM, Keemer JB. Deaths of Hispanic origin, 15 reporting states, 1979-1981. *Vital Health Stat.* 1990; DHHS publication PHS 91-1855.

27. Spitzer WO, Suissa S, Ernst P, et al. The use of beta-agonists and the risk of death and near death from asthma. *N Engl J Med.* 1992;326:501–506.

28. Sears MR. Increasing asthma mortality—fact or artifact? *J Allergy Clin Immunol.* 1988; 82:957–960.

29. Arshad SH, Matthews S, Gant C, Hide DW. Effect of allergen avoidance on development of

allergic disorders in infancy. *Lancet.* 1992;339:1493–1497.

30. Korsgaard J. Mite asthma and residency: a case control study on the impact of exposure to house-dust mites in dwellings. *Am Rev Respir Dis.* 1983;128: 231–235.

31. Wood RA, Chapman MD, Adkinson NF, Eggleston PA. The effect of cat removal on allergen content in household-dust samples. *J Allergy Clin Immunol.* 1989;83:730–734.

32. Ausdenmoore RW, Lierl MB, Fischer TJ. Inhalant aerobiology and antigens, in Weiss EB, Stein M (eds.), *Bronchial Asthma. Mechanisms and Therapeutics.* 3rd ed. Boston, Mass: Little Brown & Co Inc; 1993;

33. O'Hollaren MT, Yuninger JW, Offord KP, Somers MJ, O'Connell EJ. Exposure to an aeroallergen as a possible precipitating factor in respiratory arrest in young patients with asthma. *N Engl J Med.* 1991;324:359–363.

34. Sporik R, Chapman MD, Platts-Mills TA. House-dust mite exposure as a cause of asthma. *Clin Exp Allergy.* 1992;22:897–906.

35. Evans D, Levison MJ, Feldman CH, et al. The impact of passive smoking on emergency room visits of urban children with asthma. *Am Rev Respir Dis.* 1987;135:567–572.

36. Chilmonczyk BA, Salmun LM, Megalithlin KN, Neveux LM, Palomaki GE, Knight GJ, Pulkkinen AJ, Haddow JE. Association between exposure to environmental tobacco smoke and exacerbations of asthma in children. *N Engl J Med.* 1993; 328:1665–1669.

37. Weitzman M. Maternal smoking and childhood asthma. *Pediatrics.* 1990; 85:505–511.

38. Suphioglu C, Singh MB, Taylor P, et al. Mechanism of grass-pollen-induced asthma. *Lancet.* 1992; 339:569–572.

39. Wardlaw AJ. The role of air pollution in asthma. *Clin Exp Allergy* 1993; 23:81-96.53.

40. Maynard RL. Air pollution: should we be concerned about it? [editorial]. *J R Soc Med.* 199; 386:63–64.

41. Busse WW, et al. The role of respiratory infections in asthma, in Holgate ST et al., eds. *Asthma: Psysiology, Immunopharmacology,* and Treatment. San Diego, Calif: Academic Press; 1993;345–352.

42. Schwartz J, Gold D, Dockery DW, Weiss ST, Speizer FE. Predictors of asthma and persistent wheeze in a national sample of children in the United States. Association with social class, perinatal events, and race. *Am Rev Respir Dis.* 1990;142: 555–562.

43. Bailey WC, Clark NM, Gotsch AR, Lemen RJ, O'Connor GT, Rosenstock IM. Asthma prevention. *Chest.* 1992;102:216S–231S.

44. Rachelefsky G. Review of asthma self-management programs. *J Allergy Clin Immunol.* 1987; 80:506–510.

45. Clark NM. Asthma self-management education: research and implications for clinical practice. *Chest.* 1989;95:1110–1113.

46. Centers for Disease Control. Asthma surveillance programs in public health departments—US. *MMWR.* 1996;45:37.

47. Edelman NH, Kaplan RM, Buist AS, et al. Chronic obstructive pulmonary disease. *Chest.* 1992;102:243S–256S.

48. The Health Consequences of Smoking. Chronic Obstructive Lung Disease: A Report of the Surgeon General. Washington, DC: US Dept of Health and Human Services; 1994. DHHS publication PHS 84-50205.

49. Pratt, PC, Vollmer RT, Miller JA. Epidemiology of pulmonary lesions in nontextile and cotton textile workers: a retrospective autopsy analysis. *Arch Environ Health.* 1980;35: 133–138.

50. Janoff A, Pryor WA, Bengali ZH. Effects of tobacco smoke components on cellular and biochemical processes in the lung. *Am Rev Respir Dis.* 1987; 136:1058–1064.

51. Thurlbeck WM, Wang NS. The structure of the lungs. In: Widdicombe JD, ed. *Respiratory Physiology.* London: Butterworth; 1974:1–30.

52. Burrows B. Natural history of chronic airflow obstruction. In: Hensley MJ, Saunders NA, eds. *Clin Epi Chron Obstructive Pulmonary Disease.* New York, NY: Marcel Dekker; 1989:99–107.

53. Feinleib M, Rosenberg HM, Collins JG, Delozier JE, Pokras R, Chevarley FM. Trends in COPD morbidity and mortality in the United States. *Am Rev Respir Dis.* 1989;140:S9-S18.

54. Redline S, Weiss ST. Genetic and perinatal risk factors for the development of chronic obstructive pulmonary disease. In: Hensley MJ, Saunders NA, eds. *Clin Epi Chron Obstructive Pulmonary Disease.* New York, NY: Marcel Dekker; 1989:139–168.

55. Whittemore AS , Perlin SA, DiCiccio Y. Chronic obstructive pulmonary disease in lifelong nonsmokers: results from NHANES. *Am J Public Health.* 1995;85(5);702–706.

56. Bates DV, Sizto R. Air pollution and hospital admissions in Southern Ontario: the acid summer haze effect. *Environ Res.* 1987;79:69–72.

57. Lebowitz MD, Burrows B. Tucson epidemiologic study of obstructive lung disease. II:

Effects of in-migration factors on the prevalence of obstructive lung diseases. *Am J Epidemiol.* 1975;102:153–163.

58. Bates DV, Gotsch AR, Brooks S, Landrigan PJ, Hankinson JL, Merchant JA. Prevention of occupational lung disease. *Chest.* 1992;102:257S–276S.

59. American Thoracic Society. Standards for the diagnosis and care of patients with chronic obstructive pulmonary disease. *Am. J. Respir Crit. Care Med.* 1995;152:S77–S120.

60. Nocturnal Oxygen Therapy Trial Group. Continuous or nocturnal oxygen therapy in hypoxemic chronic obstructive lung disease. *Ann. Intern Med.* 1980; 93:391–398.

61. Reis AL, Kaplan RM, Limberg TM, Prewitt LM. Effects of pulmonary rehabilitation on physiologic and psychosocial outcomes in patients with chronic obstructive pulmonary disease. *Ann Intern Med* 1995; 122:823-832.

62. American Thoracic Society. Lung volume reduction surgery. *Am J Respir Crit Care Med.* 1996;154: 1151–1152.

63. Petty TL, Weinmann GG. Building a national strategy for the prevention and management of and research in chronic obstructive pulmonary disease. *JAMA.* 1997;277:246–253.

64. Davis PB, Drumm M, Konstan MW. Cystic fibrosis. *Am J Respir Crit Care Med.* 1996;154:1229–1256.

65. Corey M, Farewell. Determinants of mortality from cystic fibrosis in Canada, 1970–1989. *Am J Epidemiol* 1996;143:1007–1017.

66. Kerem E, Reisman J, Corey M, Canny G, Levison H. Prediction of mortality in patients with cystic fibrosis. *N Engl J Med.* 1992;326:1187–1191.

67. Ryley H, Goodchild M, Dodge J. Screening for cystic fibrosis. *Br Med Bull.* 1992;48:805–822.

68. Farrell PM, Mischler EH, Group TCFNSS. Newborn screening for cystic fibrosis. *Adv Pediatr* 1992;39:35–70.

69. Ranieri E, Lewis BD, Gerace RL, et al. Neonatal screening for cystic fibrosis using immunoreactive trypsinogen and direct gene analysis: four years' experience. *BMJ* 1994;308:1469–1472.

70. Dankert-Roelse JE, Meerman GJt. Long term prognosis of patients with cystic fibrosis in relation to early detection detection by neonatal screening and treatment in a cystic fibrosis center. *Thorax.* 1995;50:712–718.

71. American Society of Human Genetics. Statement of the American Society Society of

Human Genetics on cystic fibrosis screening. *Am J Hum Genet.* 1992;51:1443–1444.

72. Rosenfeld MA, Collins FS. Gene therapy for cystic fibrosis. *Chest.* 1996;109:241–252.

73. Findley LJ, Unverzadt ME, Suratt P. Automobile accidents involving patients with obstructive sleep apnea. *Am Rev Respir Dis.* 1988;138:337–340.

74. Young T, Palta M, Dempsey J, Skatrud J, Weber S, Badr S. The occurrence of sleep-disordered breathing among middle-aged adults. *N Engl J Med.* 1993; 1993:1230–1235.

75. Baumel MJ, Maislin G, Pack AI. Population and occupational screening for obstructive sleep apnea: are we there yet? *Am J Respir Crit Care Med.* 1997;155: 9–14.

76. National Institute for Occupational Safety and Health. Work-related lung disease surveillance report 1996. Cincinnatti, Ohio: DHHS (NIOSH) Publication No. 96-134.

77. Attfield MD, Castellan RM. Epidemiological data on US coal miners' pneumoconiosis, 1960 to 1988. *Am J Public Health.* 1992;82:964–970.

78. International Labor Office: International Classification of radiographs of pneumoconiosis 1980.

79. Occupational Safety and Health Series 22, Geneva: ILO.

80. Weeks JL, Levy BS, Wagner GR, eds. *Preventing Occupational Disease and Injury.* Washington, DC: American Public Health Association; 1991.

81. Oxman AD, Muir DCF, Shannon HS, Stock SR, Hnizdo E, Lange HJ. Occupational dust exposure and chronic obstructive pulmonary disease. A systematic overview of the evidence. *Am Rev Respir Dis.* 1993;148:38–48.

82. Lewis S, Bennett J, Richards K, Britton J. A cross sectional study of the independent effect of occupation on lung function in British coal miners. *Occup Environ Med.* 1996;53:125–128.

83. Rogan JM, Atfeld MD, Jacobsen M, Rae S, Walker DD, Walker WH. Role of dust in the working environment in the development of chronic bronchitis in British coal miners. *Br J Ind Med.* 1973;30:217–226.

84. National Institute for Occupational Safety and Health. Occupational exposure to respirable coal mine dust. Cincinnati, Ohio: US Govt Printing Office; 1995:45.

85. Cowie RL, Mabena SK. Silicosis, chronic airflow limitation, chronic bronchitis in South African gold miners. *Am Rev Respir Dis.* 1991;143:80–84.

86. Snider DE. The relationship between tuberculosis and

silicosis. *Am Rev Respir Dis.* 1978;118:455–460.

87. Smith AH, Lopipero PA, Barroga VR. Meta-analysis of studies of lung cancer among silicotics. *Epidemiology.* 1995;6:17–24.

88. Goldsmith DF, Beaumont JJ, Morrin LA, Schenker MB. Respiratory cancer and other chronic disease mortality among silicotics in California. *Am J Ind Med.* 1995;28, 459-467.

89. American Thoracic Society. The diagnosis of nonmalignant diseases related to asbestos. *Am Rev Respir Dis.* 1986;134:363–368.

90. Mossman BT, Gee JB. Asbestos-related diseases. *N Engl J Med.* 1989;320:1721–1730.

91. Kilburn KH, Warshaw RH. Airways obstruction from asbestos exposure. Effects of asbestosis and smoking. *Chest.* 1994;106:1061–1070.

92. Jones RN, W. GH, Engr D, Weil H. Review of the Kilburn and Warshaw Chest article-Airways obstruction from asbestos exposure. *Chest.* 1995;107:1727–1729.

93. Selikoff IS, Hammond EC, Seidmon H. Mortality experience of insulation workers in the United States and Canada, 1943–1976. *Ann NY Acad Sci.* 1979; 330:91–116.

94. Asbestos School Hazard Abatement Reauthorization Act of 1990 Pub. L. 1990;101–637: 1893S.

95. Rogan WJ, Gladen BC, Ragan NB, Anderson HA. US prevalence of occupational pleural thickening: a look at chest x-rays from the first national health and nutrition examination survey. *Am J Epidemiol.* 1987;126:893–900.

96. Anderson HA, Daum SM, Fischbein AS, Selikoff IJ. Household contact asbestos neoplastic risk. *Ann NY Acad Sci.* 1976;l271: 311–323.

97. National Institute for Occupational Safety and Health. Report to Congress: Workers home contamination study conducted under the workers family protection act (29 USC 671a). Cincinnatti, OH: NIOSH, 1995.

98. Niven RM, Pickering CAC. Byssinosis: a review. *Thorax.* 1996; 51:632-637.

99. Bouhuys A, Schoenberg JB, Beck GJ, Schilling RS. Epidemiology of chronic lung disease in a cotton mill community. *Lung.* 1977;154:167-186.

100. Glindmeyer HW, Lefante JJ, Jones RN, Rando RJ, Kader HMA, Weill H. Exposure-related declines in the lung function of cotton textile workers. Relationship to current workplace standards. *Am Rev Respir Dis.* 1991;144:675-683.

101. Centers for Disease Control. Occupational disease surveil-

lance: occupational asthma. *MMWR.* 1990;39:119–123.

102. Chan-Yeung M, Lam S. Occupational asthma. *Am Rev Respir Dis.* 1986;133:686–703.

103. Chan-Yeung M. A clinician's approach to determine the diagnosis, prognosis, and therapy of occupational asthma. *Med Clin North Am.* 1990; 74:811–822.

104. Blanc P. Occupational asthma in a national disability survey. *Chest.* 1987;92:613-617.

105. Smith AB, Castallar RM, Lewis D, Matti T. Guidelines for the epidemiologic assessment of occupational asthma. *J Allergy Clin Immunol.* 1989;84:794–805.

106. Alberts WM, Brooks SM. Advances in occupational asthma. *Clin Chest Med.* 1992; 13:281–302.

107. Chan-Yeung M and Malo J. Table of the major inducers of occupational asthma. In: Bernstein I, Chan-Yeung M, Malo J, Bernstein D, eds. *Asthma in the Workplace,* New York, NY: Marcel Dekker, 1993.

108. Chan-Yeung M, Lam S, Koener S. Clinical features and natural history of occupational asthma due to western red cedar (Thuja plicata). *Am J Med.* 1982;72:411–415.

109. Chan-Yeung M. Occupational asthma. *Chest.* 1990;98:148S–161S.

110. Chan-Yeung M, Enarson DA, Kennedy SM. State of the art. The impact of grain dust on respiratory health. *Am Rev Respir Dis.* 1992;145:476–487.

111. James AL, Cookson WO, Buters G, et al. Symptoms and longitudinal changes in lung function in young seasonal grain handlers. *Br J Ind Med.* 1986;43: 587–591.

112. do Pico GA. Hazardous exposure and lung disease among farm workers. *Clin Chest Med.* 1992; 13:311–328.

113. Speizer FE. Epidemiology of environmentally induced chronic respiratory disease. *Chest.* 1981;80:21S–23S.

114. Crystal RG, Gadek JE, Ferrons VJ, Fulner JD, Line BR, Hunninghake GW. Interstitial lung disease: current concepts of pathogenesis, staging and therapy. *Am J Med.* 1981;70:542–568.

115. Coultas DB, Zumwalt RE, Black WC, Sobonya RE. The epidemiology of interstitial lung diseases. *Am J Respir Crit Care Med* 1994;150:967–972.

116. Thomas PD, Hunninghake GW. Current concepts of the pathogenesis of sarcoidosis. *Am Rev Respir Dis.* 1987;135:747–760.

117. Mannino DM, Etzel RA, Parrish RG. Pulmonary fibrosis deaths in the United States, 1979–1991. An analysis of multiple-cause

mortality data. *Am J Respir Crit Care Med.* 1996;153:1548–1552.

118. Iwai K, Mori T, Yamada N, Yamaguchi M, Hosoda Y. Idiopathic pulmonary fibrosis. Epidemiologic approaches to occupational exposure. *Am J Respir Crit Care Med.* 1994;150: 670–675.

119. Scott J, Johnston I, Britton J. What causes cryptogenic fibrosin alveolitis? A case-control study of environmental exposure to dust. *Br Med J.* 1990;301: 1015–1017.

120. Hubbard R, Lewis S, Richards K, Johnston I, Britton J. Occupational exposure to metal or wood dust and aetiology of cryptogenic alveolitis. *Lancet.* 1996; 347:284–289.

121. Baumgartner KB, Samet JM, Stidley CA, Colby TV, Waldron JA, Centers C. Cigarette smoking: a risk factor for idiopathic pulmonary fibrosis. *Am J Respir Crit Care Med.* 1997;155:242–248.

122. Mapel DW, Samet JM, Coultas DB. Corticosteroids and the treatment of idiopathic pulmonary fibrosis. *Chest.* 1996;110: 1058–1067.

SUGGESTED READING

Epler GR, ed. Occupational Lung Diseases. *Clinics in Chest Medicine.* Vol. 13. Philadelphia, Pa: WB Saunders Company; 1992.

Global Initiative for Asthma. *Asthma Management and Prevention.* Bethesda, Md: National Heart, Lung and Blood Institute; 1995. Available at: *www.ginasthma.com.*

Global Initiative for Asthma. *Global Strategy for Asthma Management and Prevention: NHLBI/WHO Workshop Report.* Bethesda, Md: National Institutes of Health; 1995. NIH publication 95-3659. Available on the Internet through *www.ginasthma.com.*

Hensley MJ, Saunders NA, eds. *Clinical Epidemiology of Chronic Obstructive Lung Disease. Lung Biology in Health and Disease.* Vol. 43. New York, NY: Marcel Dekker; 1989.

Kaliner MA, Barnes PJ, Persson CGA, eds. *Asthma: Its Pathology and Treatment. Lung Biology in Health and Disease.* Vol. 49. New York, NY: Marcel Dekker, 1991.

Landrigan PJ, Kazemi H, eds. The third wave of asbestos disease: exposure to asbestos in place, public health control. *Ann NY Acad Sci.* 1991;643.

National Asthma Education Program. *Guidelines for the Diagnosis and Management of Asthma.* Bethesda, Md: National Heart, Lung, and Blood Institute; 1991.

Rom W, ed. *Environmental and Occupational Medicine.* 2nd ed.

Boston, Mass: Little Brown & Co; 1992.

Weeks JL, Levy BS, Wagner GR, eds. *Preventing Occupational Disease and Injury*. Washington, DC: American Public Health Association; 1991.

RESOURCES

American Lung Association
1740 Broadway
New York, NY 10019
(212) 315-8700

National Heart, Lung, and Blood
    Institute Information Center
PO Box 30105
Bethesda, MD 20824-0105
(301) 951-3260

DIABETES

ICD-9 250

Approximately 15.7 million people in the United States have diabetes. A third of these are undiagnosed,[1] in part because symptoms develop gradually and it can take several years before severe symptoms occur. The prevalence rate for diagnosed cases of diabetes has risen steadily for decades, having increased eightfold since the mid-1930s from a rate of 0.37% in 1935 to 3.0% in 1994.[2, 3] Each year on average 727 000 new cases of diabetes are identified,[3] about 12 000 are among school-age children.[4] The incidence of diabetes among youth under 16 years old is about 17 cases per 100 000, which is more than the incidence of all childhood cancers combined.[5] The estimated prevalence of diabetes is about 170 per 100 000 school-age children or about 125 000 children under 19 years of age.[6, 7] The estimated prevalence of diagnosed diabetes in adults is 2900 to 3400 per 100 000.[3, 8] Between 1980 and 1994, the crude incidence of diagnosed

diabetes increased 48% from 2.5 to 3.7 per 1000.[3]

Diabetes has been ranked among the 10 leading causes of death in the United States since 1932,[8] and it is now the seventh leading underlying cause of death, with more than 61 000 deaths directly attributed to diabetes in 1996.[9] The age-adjusted death rate for diabetes, standardized to the 1990 census, was 29.9 per 100 000 in 1994. However, mortality statistics alone clearly understate the impact of diabetes. Approximately 400 000 deaths from all causes occurred in people with diabetes in 1993 or about 18% of all deaths in the United States to persons 25 years and older. Because people die of the complications of diabetes rather than the disease itself, diabetes is underreported as the underlying or even contributing cause of death. Diabetes is listed on the death certificates of only about half of the decedents who actually had diabetes.[10, 11] Death rates of middle-aged people with diabetes are twice that of people without diabetes.[12] For those who develop diabetes under age 30, more than 15% will die by age 40, 20 times the rate of the general population.[13] The leading causes of

Donald B. Bishop, PhD
Bruce R. Zimmerman, MD
Jon S. Roesler, MS

death for persons with diabetes are heart disease, 55%, diabetes, 13%, cancers, 13%, cerebrovascular disease, 10%, and pneumonia/influenza, 4%.[12] The risk of cardiovascular disease mortality is 2 to 4 times that of persons without diabetes.[12, 14]

Over the course of the disease, diabetes leads to a variety of disabling and life-threatening complications. Some of the major complications of diabetes include heart disease (80 000 deaths each year due to diabetes),[15] blindness (12 000 to 24 000 new cases each year due to diabetes),[16] and renal failure (12 000 new cases each year due to diabetes).[17] Diabetes can also lead to inadequate circulation and sensation in peripheral tissues, which can result in infection, injury, and amputation (67 000 lower extremity amputations each year due to diabetes).[1] Over 60% of those with diabetes have high blood pressure and 60% to 70% have mild to severe damage to the nervous system (neuropathy).[1] Largely because of these long-term complications, disability affects 20% to 50% of the diabetic population. Reported activity limitations and restricted activity days are 2 to 3 times higher than for persons without diabetes.[18] In 1990, in data from the National Health Interview Survey (NHIS) of those age 18 to 69 years with diabetes, 42% reported work limitations, with 28% being unable to work at all.[18]

The economic impact of diabetes is profound.[20–22] One study [23] from the American Diabetes Association estimated direct medical costs in 1997 at $44.1 billion and indirect costs at $54.1 billion, totaling over $98 billion. Another study [24] estimated the direct medical care costs of treating patients with diabetes for all medical conditions, whether or not related to diabetes, as $85.7 billion. This represents 12% of US health care expenditures attributable to 3% of the population with known diabetes.[22] Cost ratios comparing patients with confirmed diabetes to nondiabetic patients is estimated as follows: physician visit, 1.9, emergency care, 1.56, prescription drugs and durable medical equipment, 5.3, and annual health care expenditures, 4.3.[24]

Up to half the economic burden of diabetes is due to long-term complications,[25] especially coronary heart disease and end-stage renal disease.[26] In one managed care setting, the cost of poor glycemic control was found to increase exponentially; for every 1% rise to HbA1c beyond the 6% level, the cumulative increases in charges rose approximately 4%, 10%, 20%, and 30%.[27]

PATHOPHYSIOLOGY

Diabetes mellitus is a group of diseases in which the body is unable to sufficiently produce and/or properly use insulin, a hormone needed by muscle, fat, and the liver to utilize glucose. Insulin is normally secreted by the beta cells in the pancreas. Following secretion, insulin binds to specific areas on cell surfaces called receptors that allow glucose to enter the cells.

Diabetes is diagnosed through identification of elevated blood glucose concentrations. Elevated blood glucose can occur if either insulin secretion or insulin action is impaired. At one time, diabetes was felt to be a single disease, but it is now clear that many abnormalities can lead to elevated blood glucose concentrations. The American Diabetes Association (ADA) recommended new diagnostic and classification criteria for diabetes in July 1997[28] to update the previous recommendations of the National Diabetes Data Group from 1979.[29] The new recommendations modify the classification terminology to recognize the improved understanding of the pathogenesis of diabetes and change the fasting plasma glucose diagnostic level to make it concordant with the diagnosis by the 2-hour oral glucose tolerance test plasma glucose.

The new classification attempts to avoid the problem of classification by treatment rather than the underlying pathologic process. The previous terminology frequently led to confusion. It was often assumed that all patients treated with insulin had insulin-dependent diabetes mellitus (IDDM), which is not correct. Treatment is determined by the degree of hyperglycemia that can vary over time and is a reflection of the severity of the metabolic abnormality but not its cause. The terms type 1 and type 2 (using Arabic numerals) are retained, and the terms insulin-dependent diabetes mellitus (IDDM) and non-insulin-dependent diabetes mellitus (NIDDM) are no longer used.

Type 1 diabetes is defined as diabetes caused by beta cell destruction which will lead to absolute insulin deficiency and a need for insulin treatment over time. Type 1 diabetes has two subgroups, immune-mediated and idiopathic. Type 1, immune-mediated diabetes was formerly called IDDM or juvenile-onset diabetes. In the United States, this class represents about 5% to 10% of patients with diabetes.[1] The onset is usually in childhood or adolescence. The immune destruction of the beta cells may occur over several years; however, in young patients, the onset of hyperglycemia and symptoms is usually abrupt and the patient may quickly develop diabetic ketoacidosis and die without insulin treatment. It is now estimated that in 10% to 20% of Caucasians developing diabetes in adulthood the beta cell destruction may be immune mediated. In adults, the beta cell destruction may be much more gradual than in children, and there may not be an absolute requirement for insulin therapy for many years.[30]

Type 1, immune-mediated diabetes is considered an autoimmune disease--that is, it is an illness in which the immune system attacks the body's own tissues.[31] Over a period lasting from months to years, the immune system destroys the insulin-making beta cells.[32] Predisposition to type 1 diabetes is inherited as a multigenic trait with low penetrance.[33] Genetic markers have been identified as indicators of potential vulnerability to type 1, immune-mediated diabetes. At least one human leukocyte antigen (HLA) class II DR3 or DR4 antigen is found in 95% of type 1 patients.[32] DR1, DR16, and DR8 have also been linked to type 1 diabetes and DR15 and DR11 are felt to confer protection. Class II DQ genes are also closely linked to type 1 diabetes. [33,34] However, these HLA types are necessary but not sufficient for developing type 1 diabetes. That is, even though 50% to 60% of the nondiabetic White population has DR3 or DR4, fewer than 1% of all Whites have type 1 diabetes.[35] For people with both HLA-DR3 and HLA-DR4, the chance of developing type 1 diabetes is 1 in 40 compared with 1 in 500 for the general population.[6] For offspring of fathers with type 1 diabetes the lifelong risk of developing Type 1

diabetes is 8%; for children of mothers with type 1 diabetes the risk is 3%.[32] The concordance rates for type 1 diabetes in identical twins is no more than 35% to 50%, yet this is significantly greater than the rates observed for nonidentical (fraternal) twins.[36]

The trigger for the immune process leading to type 1 diabetes is unclear, but the process is identified by the presence of islet-cell antibodies (ICA), insulin autoantibodies. (IAAs), and autoantibodies to glutamic acid decarboxylase (GAD_{65}). Not all patients with these antibodies develop type 1 diabetes, but at least one of these antibodies is present in 85% to 90% of patients at the time of diagnosis of type 1 diabetes. Autoimmune-mediated beta cell destruction can be identified by low insulin release in response to intravenous glucose. The patient is persistently unable to produce sufficient insulin, and symptoms develop when beta cell destruction reaches a critical point. The process from onset to symptoms may take several years.

Type 1, idiopathic diabetes is a new classification and represents only a small subset of patients with beta cell destruction. As implied by the name, this disease is not well understood. These patients have episodic ketoacidosis and variable insulin deficiency and only intermittently require insulin treatment. This form of diabetes is strongly inherited, but it does not have HLA associations or evidence of autoimmunity. It is more common in patients of African and Asian background.

NIDDM has been relabeled type 2 diabetes, a term that was in common usage for this class of diabetes in any case.[28] Type 2 diabetes accounts for 90% to 95% of all diagnosed cases of diabetes.[1] A person with type 2 diabetes may have asymptomatic hyperglycemia (ie, an abnormally high concentration of glucose in the blood) for many years before the gradual onset of symptoms: excessive thirst, frequent urination, and weight loss. Often the diagnosis is made during routine health screening. Occasionally, the patient presents with symptoms of a chronic diabetic complication. Ketoacidosis develops only with severe physical stress.

The etiology and pathophysiology of type 2 diabetes is complex. In general, people with type 2 diabetes have insulin resistance, which means they cannot make efficient use of insulin in the muscle or liver, despite sufficient insulin production early in the course of the disease. Obesity and hyperinsulinemia are characteristic of this early phase and obesity accentuates the insulin resistance.[37] Over time the pancreas fails to increase insulin secretion enough to compensate adequately for the insulin resistance and hyperglycemia begins. Type 2 diabetes is a progressive disease and over time the response to treatment varies. Eventually, the relative beta cell deficiency and degree of hyperglycemia may become great enough that insulin treatment is required to control the hyperglycemia.[38]

The prevalence of type 2 diabetes increased in several population groups as they changed to an urbanized lifestyle of readily available food, decreased physical activity, and increased obesity. Increased physical activity results in increased insulin sensitivity of skeletal muscle. One hypothesis is that inherited insulin resistance in muscle has a selective advantage in hunter-gatherer societies exposed to periods of famine, because it blunts hypoglycemia during fasting and still allows energy storage in fat and liver during feeding following physical activity, such as a hunt.[39] Heredity has a strong influence on type 2 diabetes, although specific genetic markers have not been identified. It is felt there are many different causes for type 2 diabetes and that in the future identification of specific genetic defects will allow better classification. The risk of type 2 diabetes in siblings of patients with type 2 diabetes is up to six times that of siblings of age-matched nondiabetic controls. The risk of type 2 diabetes among the children of patients with type 2 diabetes is about twice that among the children of age-matched nondiabetic controls.[40] The concordance rate for type 2 diabetes in identical twins is as high as 90%.[41]

Gestational diabetes mellitus is usually a transient condition diagnosed in 2% to 5% of pregnancies.[1, 42] Although glucose tolerance typically reverts to normal after delivery, many women with gestational diabetes will develop type 2 diabetes in future years. Gestational diabetes can result in significant adverse outcomes for the fetus, although these are largely preventable through appropriate screening and intervention (see section on screening and early detection). Although there is controversy about the levels of plasma glucose to be used for the diagnosis of gestational diabetes mellitus the ADA does not recommend a change at this time.[28, 43]

The classification impaired glucose tolerance (IGT) has been retained and the classification impaired fasting glucose (IFG) added to the new recommendations. Both refer to the stage during which the fasting or post glucose challenge glucose levels are not normal but are not high enough to diagnose diabetes. Approximately 13.4 million people, 7% of the population, have IFG.[1]

A large number of other specific types of diabetes exist, accounting for 1% to 2% of all diagnosed cases of diabetes.[1] Of special note are the specific genetic defects of the beta cell formerly referred to as maturity-onset diabetes of the young (MODY) and elimination of the class malnutrition-related diabetes. Secondary diabetes occurs when other diseases, such as pancreatitis or pancreatic cancer, damage the pancreas or medications or other hormonal abnormalities impair insulin action. There is also a long list of other genetic syndromes sometimes associated with diabetes.

Individuals with diabetes are subject to a number of long-term complications including cardiovascular disease, microvascular disease, and neuropathy.[4] Cardiovascular complications include accelerated atherosclerosis resulting in stroke, heart disease, and peripheral vascular disease. Diabetic microvascular complications include disorders of the kidney and retina, leading to renal failure and blindness. Diabetic neuropathy, which occurs in 50% of cases within 25 years of diagnosis,[44] results in pain, weakness, and loss of sensation. The lack of blood supply caused by peripheral vascular disease and/or the nerve dysfunction of neuropathy may often result in skin ulcers, gangrene, and amputations.[45] Diabetic neuropathy is also associated with problems of sexual function as well as urinary and gastrointestinal abnormalities.

Appropriate therapy can usually be used to manage the acute symptoms and complications of diabetes, and recent research shows that therapy can address the long-term complications of the disease. Hyperglycemia appears to be of great importance in the genesis of these complications.[46] In the recently completed Diabetes Control and Complications Trial,[47] a multisite, multiyear study supported by the National Institutes of Health for patients with type 1, immune-mediated diabetes, intensive treatment that kept blood sugar levels close to normal resulted in an approximate 60% reduction in risk of diabetic damage to eyes, kidneys, and nerves.[48] Intensive therapy resulted in both a delay in onset and a major slowing in the progression of these complications, regardless of age, sex, or duration of diabetes. However, even with cooperative patients and specialized case teams, intensive therapy did not result in normoglycemia. A recently published small study in Japanese patients found similar results in type 2 patients treated with intensive insulin therapy compared to conventional therapy.[49]

DESCRIPTIVE EPIDEMIOLOGY

High-Risk Groups

Diabetes is not equally distributed in the population. Older Americans and minority populations suffer disproportionately high rates of diabetes.[50, 51] They also develop a disproportionate share of complications caused by diabetes. Aged persons with diabetes are substantially more likely to experience heart attack, stroke, vision problems, physical disability, incontinence, and nursing home stays than aged persons without diabetes.[52]

The older median age of people with diabetes contrasts sharply with the age composition of the general adult population in the United States. On the basis of the 1989 National Health Interview Survey, the median age of the adult population with diabetes is 63 years compared to 40 years for the total adult population. In addition, 58% of adults with diabetes are 60 years of age or older in contrast to 22% of all adults.[24] The mean age at diagnosis for type 1 diabetes is 16.2 years and for type 2 51.1 years.[25] For adults age 65 or older, 18.4% have diabetes.[1] Because of the increased prevalence of diabetes in older people the American Diabetes Association has recommended screening for diabetes every 3 years in those 45 years and older.[28]

The prevalence of type 1, immune-mediated diabetes is higher among Whites than among people of other races (relative risk [RR] = 1.4). In contrast, the prevalence of type 2 diabetes is higher among races other than White, such as Blacks (RR = 1.3), Hispanics (RR = 3.1), and American Indians (RR = 10.1).[53] The percentage of adults with diagnosed and undiagnosed diabetes by race and ethnicity is about 10.8% Blacks, 10.6% Mexican Americans, and 7.8% White.[1] For American Indians, the rates of diagnosed diabetes range from 5% to 50% in different tribes and population groups.[1, 23, 54] Prevalence data for Asian Americans and Pacific Islanders are limited.[55]

American Indian ancestry plays an important role in the incidence of type 2 diabetes. Mexican Americans, who have 20% to 40% American Indian ancestry, have lower incidence than people who are nearly 100% American Indian ancestry, such as the Pima.[56] However, Mexican Americans have a much higher incidence than most other populations.[57] Blacks are also at an increased risk for developing type 2 diabetes.[3, 58] There is also an increased incidence in Southeast Asians who have immigrated to the United States.[55]

The incidence of type 1, immune-mediated diabetes peaks during adolescence and declines markedly in older age groups.[4] There is little difference in the incidence between males and females. A seasonal pattern of the onset of type 1, immune-mediated diabetes has been observed, with consistently fewer cases during the summer months. The seasonal pattern is primarily attributed to the acute stress of childhood viral illnesses precipitating the clinical disease.[4]

The risk factors for gestational diabetes are similar to those that predict overt diabetes and include advanced maternal age, a family history of diabetes in a first-degree relative, obesity, and glucose in the urine (glycosuria).[42, 59] Outcomes from previous pregnancies believed predictive include stillbirth and birth of a baby weighing more than 9 pounds. Relative risk for gestational diabetes is higher for Hispanic (RR=2.45) and Black (RR=1.81) women compared with Whites.[60] Nearly 40% of the women who experience gestational diabetes develop diabetes within 20 years of the pregnancy.[61] Pregnancy, rather than being an independent risk factor, appears to be a provocative test for the development of future diabetes.[62, 63]

Geographic Distribution

The National Health Interview Survey (NHIS) reported higher prevalence rates for self-reported diabetes in the South and Northeast than in other regions of the United States,[64] although no distinction between types of diabetes was made. The highest proportion of those with type 2 diabetes live in the southeastern United States (39.2%), while those with type 1 diabetes are dispersed more evenly throughout the country.[24]

One of the most important observations related to type 1, immune-mediated diabetes is the marked geographic variability of the disease. Internationally, the risk of type 1 diabetes generally runs higher in cooler climates. The development worldwide of type 1 diabetes registries indicates a 50-fold variation in the annual incidence rates of type 1 diabetes, ranging from 0.7 per 100 000 in Shanghai to 35.3 per 100 000 in Finland.[7] In the United States rates vary from 3.3 per 100 000 for African Americans in San Diego to 20.6 per 100 000 for whites in Olmsted County, Minnesota. Approximately 40% of the variation in incidence rate in the United States is explained by racial composition.[19] Variation in regional incidence rates may also be explained in part by factors correlated with low mean temperature and the low number of sunshine hours in a day.[65] Studies have consistently shown incidence rates for type 1 diabetes to vary by season, peaking in late winter and early spring and decreasing in the summer.[66]

Time Trends

The United States is undergoing demographic shifts that are affecting diabetes and its treatments. The proportion of our population older than 65 years of age is steadily increasing, minority populations are growing at a faster rate than nonminorities, and the proportion of our population that is overweight continues to rise.[67] Self-reported diabetes among all groups has increased in prevalence from 0.37% in 1935 to 0.91% in 1958 to 3.07% in 1993.[2] From 1979 to 1981 through 1993, the number of people in the United States who reported having diagnosed diabetes increased by more than 23% to 7.8 million. During the same period, the adjusted annual prevalence rate increased from 24.9 to 30.7 per 1000 residents.[2]

Incidence rates for type 1 diabetes in the United States have been relatively stable in recent decades although subject to rapid fluctuations during certain years in certain parts of the country, for example, the Northeast, that are suggestive of epidemics.[68] In Europe and several other countries, type 1 incidence rates have been rising. Epidemics may account for this global increase.[7, 69]

The population burden of type 2 diabetes has increased enormously during the 20th century in groups such as the Pima Indians, as well as in other populations in the United States and around the world. In the United States between 1980 and 1994, the age-adjusted prevalence rate for diagnosed diabetes increased 33% (from 40.1 to 53.5 per 1000) among Blacks while increasing 11% (from 23.8 to 26.4 per 1000) among Whites.[3] Studies point to a relationship between type 2 diabetes and urbanization, or changes in lifestyle associated with modern societies in the United States, Canada, and western Europe. These changes, as well as demographic changes such as the aging of the population, have contributed to the modern epidemics of diabetes in genetically susceptible populations. Whites are perhaps unique in that they have been the least affected, but not unaffected, by whatever combination of factors is involved.[56]

While its unclear to what extent the increased prevalence of diabetes can be attributed to higher incidence rates or to better survival patterns, a recent retrospective population-based study, with cases from 1945 to 1989, is provocative. It found survival of those with diabetes, relative to the general population, had not improved.[70] This study also found that both the incidence rates of diabetes and the proportion of those with diabetes categorized as obese had risen markedly.

RISK FACTORS

Magnitude of Risk Factors

Type 1, Immune-mediated Diabetes. Although few, if any, modifiable risk factors for type 1 diabetes have been clearly established, changes in incidence over time, geographic patterns, twin studies, and seasonality are all strongly indicative of major environmental determinants of type 1, immune-mediated diabetes.[4, 68] Genetic susceptibility to type 1 diabetes appears necessary but not

sufficient to cause the disease.[71, 72] Nutrition and viruses may be important environmental triggers for those with genetic susceptibility. The most widely studied nutritional risk factors for type 1 diabetes are breast-feeding and exposure to cow's milk. A meta-analysis of selected studies found patients with type 1 diabetes were 43% more likely to have been breast-fed for less than 3 months and 63% more likely to have consumed cow's milk before age 3 to 4 months.[73] Viruses which have been linked, though not consistently, to development of type 1 diabetes include the Coxsackie B4 virus, human cytomegalovirus (CMV), and the virus causing measles during pregnancy.[71] About 20% of people born with congenital rubella have diabetes later in life.[75] Other possible risk factors include stress, maternal age at birth (older than 35), and birth order.

Type 2 Diabetes. Conditions associated with increased insulin resistance are significant risk factors for type 2 diabetes (Table 14.1). Chief among these are obesity and advancing age. The association between obesity and abnormal glucose tolerance is well recognized. Approximately 80% of people with type 2 diabetes are obese at the time of diagnosis.[4] Many studies have shown that the distribution of body fat, independent of obesity, is a risk factor for type 2 diabetes.[76] An increased central deposition of fat (ie, visceral as opposed to cutaneous), often measured as an increased waist-to-hip ratio, appears to predict type 2 diabetes.[77] Duration or years of obesity is also a risk factor, as is a high fat diet, even when adjusted for degree of obesity.[78] The evidence suggests that a lack of physical activity is an independent risk factor for type 2 diabetes, separate from obesity.[79–81] The prevalence of type 2 diabetes is consistently lower in populations where habitual physical activity is high.[76] Research also indicates that cigarette smoking may be an independent risk factor for type 2 diabetes.[82, 83] In a recent study of a Pima Indian population, those who were exclusively breast-fed in the first 2 months of life had significantly lower rates of type 2 diabetes than those who were exclusively bottle-fed (odds ratio, OR = 0.41).[74]

Among people with diabetes, a variety of factors, such as smoking and hypertension, interact to increase the risk of complications, including stroke and heart disease (Table 14.2).[53, 84]

Population-Attributable Risk

Orchard and colleagues[4] have suggested that 70% to 95% of type 1, immune-mediated diabetes may be attributed to environmental causes, including dietary practices and viral exposures. Between 20% and 90% of type 2 diabetes may be associated with obesity, although much of this may be attributable to abdominal adiposity.[77] In a 9-year follow-up of a national cohort of adults, the population-attributable risk for incidence of type 2 diabetes for weight increases of 5 kg or more was 27%.[85] In addition, approximately 24% of the incidence of type 2 diabetes may be attributable to a sedentary lifestyle.[80]

PREVENTION AND CONTROL MEASURES

Prevention

Several small clinical trials have explored the preventability of type 2 diabetes through dietary changes, increased physical activity, or drug treatment.[86–90] Some of these studies are promising but the conclusions are limited due to considerations of

Table 14.1—Modifiable Risk Factors for Type 2 Diabetes, United States

Magnitude	Risk Factor
Strong (relative risk[a] >4)	Obesity
Moderate (relative risk 2-4)	None
Weak (relative risk <2)	Physical inactivity
Possible	Cigarette smoking
	High fat/low fiber diet

[a]Defined in Table 2.4, page 51.

Table 14.2—Summary of Risk Factors for Complications of Diabetes

Complication	Age, years	Sex	Race	Obesity	Lack of Self-Management Skills and Access to Care	Hypertension	Cigarette Smoking	Hyper-lipidemia	Hyper-glycemia
Keto-acidosis	Maximum at <45	F > M	Other races > White	?	++	-	-	-	++
Congenital malformation	Increases with age of mother	F only	Other races > White	?	++	-	-	-	++
Stroke	Increases with age	F > M	Other races = White	++	+	++	+	+	+
Coronary heart disease	Increases with age	M > F	Other races = White	++	+	++	++	+	+
Peripheral vascular disease	Increases with age	M > F	Other races = White	++	+	+	++	+	+
Blindness	Maximum at >65	F > M	Other races > White	+	+	+	-	-	?
End-stage renal disease	Maximum at <45 (IDDM)	M > F	Other races > White	+	+	++	?	-	?
Amputation	Increases with age	M > F	Other races > White	+	+	+	++	+	+

Note. Adapted from Carter Center of Emory University.[53] ? = possible risk factor; ++ = major risk factor; + = risk factor; - = not a risk factor.

sample size, randomization, or intensity of the interventions.[91] The absence of results from large randomized trials on the primary prevention of diabetes limits our knowledge of effective methods for primary prevention. The National Institutes of Health (NIH) is sponsoring a prevention trial for type 1 diabetes that defines people at risk by immunologic markers and initiates insulin therapy before hyperglycemia hoping to attenuate the beta cell destruction.[92] There is also a second major prevention trial for type 2 diabetes, using diet and exercise or medications before hyperglycemia develops.[92] Until the results of these studies are available, health providers must rely in part on intervention trials for cardiovascular disease, which have produced substantial research on similar behavioral risk factors, such as physical inactivity and poor diet.

Two basic approaches to primary prevention can be used. First, the population approach seeks to alter or eliminate lifestyle and environmental characteristics that are known risk factors for diabetes from whole communities or populations. Strategies might include altering the food supply for whole populations and altering community attitudes and opportunities for exercise.[93] Second, the high-risk approach narrows the focus to particular individuals or groups with an especially high risk

for developing diabetes.[94, 95] A high-risk approach would target individuals with a family history of diabetes in combination with other metabolic and behavioral risk factors for the disease.

Strategies that can be used to prevent type 1 diabetes are different from those used to prevent type 2 diabetes. Possible approaches to prevention of type 1, immune-mediated diabetes include (1) identification of more specific genetic markers of susceptibility; (2) identification of specific immunologic markers; and (3) identification of specific environmental risk factors.[96] At present none of these approaches is feasible on a population basis and they have only been applied in a research setting to the limited subset of people with first degree relatives with type 1 diabetes. Until research identifies an effective therapy and a cost-effective screening method, primary prevention for type 1 diabetes will remain impractical. Several medications blocking the autoimmune process have been studied, but none has demonstrated long-term effectiveness without unacceptable side effects. Early administrating of insulin is being studied in the NIH trial based on animal studies demonstrating effectiveness and the safety of the treatment when injected in low doses or taken orally.

Type 2 diabetes is much more amenable to primary prevention because its pathogenesis has both strong genetic or familial markers and lifestyle components. There are no specific genetic markers from which to build prevention programs, but there are specific indicators that can be used to identify the most appropriate target groups for public health interventions. Individuals with one or more of the following characteristics are particularly at risk for developing type 2 diabetes: family history of type 2 diabetes, a history of gestational diabetes, age over 40 years old, history of hypertension, history of obesity, physical inactivity, and upper-body obesity.[95, 97–99] Primary prevention measures for these individuals should include recommendations for a nutritious, low-fat diet; weight maintenance and control; and regular physical activity.[94, 95, 97, 100]

Early in the course of type 2 diabetes, weight reduction may return the blood glucose concentrations to normal. Increased physical activity alone may decrease a person's risk of type 2 diabetes.[79–81, 90] In a recent review of epidemiologic evidence on modifiable risk factors, it was estimated that the risk of type 2 diabetes could be reduced 50% to 75% through reductions in obesity and 30% to 50% through increased physical activity.[101] Randomized clinical trial data are not yet available to confirm these estimates.

The population approach to preventing type 2 diabetes is most warranted in communities with large populations at high risk for type 2 diabetes, such as American Indians and Mexican Americans. When a population approach is used, the approach and methodology should be similar to that employed in community-based cardiovascular trials.[102–104]

Community-based interventions typically emphasize low-fat, high-fiber diets and cessation or prevention of cigarette smoking. Physical activity is often a lesser though still important priority in these programs. For communities at particular risk for diabetes, increasing physical activity will need to be an equal if not greater priority, given recent evidence that demonstrates the importance of exercise in preventing the occurrence of diabetes.[79–81, 90] Since diet and exercise patterns are frequently shared among families and friends, lifestyle interventions are potentially most effective when delivered in clusters of families or small communities.[91]

Screening and Early Detection

Population screening for type 1 diabetes is not recommended because of the infrequent occurrence of the disorder and the short time between the onset of hyperglycemia and the onset of symptoms in most patients.

The benefits of an early diagnosis of type 2 diabetes are not firmly established, but control of hyperglycemia early in the course of diabetes may prevent or delay chronic complications. At the present time, many people with overt type 2 diabetes have not had their diabetes diagnosed and will already have established diabetic complications at the time of diagnosis. Reducing hyperglycemia by diet, oral hypoglycemic agents, or insulin improves insulin secretion, at least in the short run. The degree of hyperglycemia is strongly associated with the prevalence of microvascular complications such as retinopathy.

Mass, unselective population screening for type 2 diabetes is not cost-effective,[105] even though the number of undiagnosed cases in the United States approaches the number of diagnosed cases. Screening should be limited to high-risk groups such as American Indians, Hispanics, Blacks, people with a strong family history of NIDDM, women with babies who weigh more than 9 pounds at birth or women with a morbid obstetric history, patients who are obese, patients with hypertension, and people with hypertriglyceridemia, or elevated triglyceride levels in the blood.[106] The sharp rise in the incidence of diabetes with increasing age has also lead the ADA to recommended screening every 3 years in all individuals 45 years and older.[27, 106] A successful screening program will include a written or oral questionnaire to identify risk factors for diabetes.[107] People with major risk factors for diabetes, or who indicate that they have one of the physical symptoms of diabetes (excessive thirst, hunger, or urination), should then be referred for appropriate medical evaluation.

For those most at risk of diabetes, the preferred diagnostic test is a fasting blood glucose test (no caloric consumption for at least 8 hours before testing). The new recommendations confirmed the use of fasting testing for diagnosis and stated there was no basis for concluding the 2-hour post glucose load test was more reliable. A fasting plasma glucose ≥ 126 mg/dL (7.0 mmol/L) confirmed on repeat testing a different day is considered diagnostic of diabetes. The previous diagnostic criterion for fasting plasma glucose was >140 mg/dL. If an oral glucose tolerance test (OGTT) is used the 2-hour glucose diagnostic level remains ≥ 200 mg/dL (11.1 mmol/L) If the individual has consumed food or caloric beverages shortly before testing, a random plasma glucose test may be administered. A random plasma glucose ≥ 200 mg/dL confirms the diagnosis in a patient with typical symptoms. A fasting plasma glucose level ≥ 110 mg/dL and ≤ 126 mg/dL indicates impaired fasting glucose and a 2-hour post glucose load plasma glucose between 140 and 200 mg/dL indicates impaired glucose tolerance.

Early diagnosis and aggressive treatment of gestational diabetes mellitus can also reduce fetal morbidity and mortality. This has led to the recommendation that pregnant women be screened for gestational diabetes between the 24th and 28th weeks of pregnancy.[108] In contrast to the previous recommendations, the new recommendations do not suggest screening in all pregnant women. Women at low risk of gestational diabetes are excluded from screening. The low risk group is women who are <25 years of age and of normal weight with no family history of diabetes and are not members of a high risk ethnic group. The new recommendations do not change the diagnostic methods. Different testing methods and diagnostic criteria are used for pregnant women than for men or nonpregnant women. First, a challenge test is administered using a 50-g oral glucose load. This test is positive if the plasma glucose is ≥140 mg/dL 1 hour later. When the challenge test is positive, a 100-g oral glucose load is administered on a subsequent day. This indicates gestational diabetes if any two glucose values equal or exceed these limits: fasting, 105 mg/dL; 1 hour, 190 mg/dL; 2 hour, 165 mg/dL; 3 hour, 145 mg/dL.[108]

Treatment, Rehabilitation, and Recovery

Diabetes is a chronic illness that requires lifelong care. Effective treatment should be provided by a health care team that includes a physician, a diabetes educator, a dietitian, and other health care professionals as indicated by specific problems. Nonetheless, the majority of all diabetes care is self-care, that is, delivered by patients themselves.[109] Professionals can provide advice and encouragement, but patients must deal with their diabetes on a daily basis. Therefore, treatment should include not only an initial evaluation, establishment of treatment goals, development of a management plan, cardiovascular risk factor reduction, and recognition of and care for complications but also patient education in self-management and ongoing support. Standards of medical care as well as patient education criteria have been published by the American Diabetes Association.[110, 111] They serve as guidelines to help health care professionals judge the adequacy of patient care. The American Diabetes Association also sponsors education and provider recognition programs.

The choice of treatment medications is guided by the treatment goals and type of diabetes. The patient with type 1 diabetes requires exogenous insulin. All other aspects of the treatment are secondary to the need for insulin and the need to facilitate the use of insulin. No exogenous insulin program is available that can maintain normal blood glucose levels over a long period, and this limitation of therapy must be recognized. Insulin programs capable of achieving treatment goals in people with type 1 diabetes usually consist of multiple daily injections or use of an infusion pump. Insulin action varies among individuals and by injection site; therefore, the effect of insulin must be judged individually by a trained clinician. The recent introduction of rapid acting LisPro insulin has provided an additional treatment option. Diet is an essential factor in avoiding hyperglycemia and hypoglycemia.[112] Nutritional and caloric intake must be synchronized with insulin action and distributed evenly throughout the day, with adjustments for varying levels of physical activity.[113] Current epidemiologic evidence shows a substantial benefit from maintaining a physically active lifestyle and should be an important goal of treatment.[114–120]

The recent introduction of several new medications in the United States has expanded the treatment options for people with type 2 diabetes.[121, 122] Often weight reduction alone will control hyperglycemia, particularly early in the course of the disease. Once dietary calories and fat are restricted,[123] other medications can often be withdrawn.[124] Sulfonylureas are a class of oral hypoglycemic agents that stimulate endogenous insulin release from the pancreas and are more convenient for the patient than insulin by injection. However, sulfonylureas are only useful for patients who are still capable of some endogenous insulin secretion, and there is a high secondary failure rate. Metformin belongs to the biguanide class of medications that increases insulin action in the liver and perhaps in the muscle. Metformin has been used in many areas of the world for over 20 years but only became available in the United States in 1995. Metformin can cause lactic acidosis in patients with impaired renal function and frequently has mild gastrointestinal side effects. Acarbose is an alpha-glucosidase inhibitor that blocks intestinal starch and sucrose digestion slowing the postprandial glucose rise. It is generally a safe medication but because of its mode of action has a high incidence of intolerance due to flatulence and diarrhea. Other medications in this class may be available soon. Troglitazone is a medication with a totally new mechanism of action. It lessens insulin resistance in the muscle. It was just released for general use in 1997. At that time, it was only indicated for use in patients also on insulin, but this restriction was removed thereafter. The long-term safety of troglitazone is not known, and recent reports suggest rare, severe liver toxicity.

Insulin injection therapy can control hyperglycemia in almost all cooperative patients with type 2 diabetes, although occasionally very high insulin doses are required. Often simple insulin programs are effective, and the incidence of hypoglycemia is low.

Diabetes treatment requires the active involvement of the patient, who must be knowledgeable about diabetes and diet. There is a body of well-conducted, positive research and descriptive literature on diabetes self-management.[125–128]

Self-monitoring of blood glucose (SMBG) levels by using meter-read strips has become an essential part of self-management. In the stable patient, monitoring can be done infrequently, serving merely as an indicator of progress or impending problems. In the unstable patient, it may be done several times a day to help the patient modify insulin doses.[129]

The data are now clear. Normalizing glycemic control in the diabetes patient will effectively reduce the long-term complications of retinopathy, nephropathy, and neuropathy. [48, 49, 123–134] Unfortunately, the data are not yet conclusive with regard to reduction of the macrovascular complications. Although strongly suggestive evidence that good

control will be effective in avoiding macrovascular complications is accumulating,[46, 135–138] conversely, data from the Diabetes PORT study would indicate that glycemic control and cardiovascular disease in persons with type 2 diabetes are unrelated.[139] A number of measures can be undertaken to reduce the incidence of diabetes complications,[140] including improving education and self-management skills for the patient; checking the patient's blood pressure at every visit (only 75% of diabetic patients with hypertension are treated for it); conducting annual eye exams to detect diabetic retinopathy; conducting foot exams; and encouraging patients to stop smoking, to exercise regularly, and to consume a healthy, low-fat diet. Reduction of the macrovascular complications will require aggressive treatment of dyslipidemia and hypertension. In a recent study, hypertension poorly controlled by treatment was strongly associated with the development of diabetic complications (odds ratio = 3.1).[141] In this same study, attributable risk related to avoidable risk factors (ie, uncontrolled hypertension, poor compliance with visit scheduling, inadequate diabetes education, no self-management of insulin treatment) was 0.39.

A paradigm shift in the health care model, from an acute to chronic disease focus, will be necessary for the early identification and treatment of diabetes to become standard care.[142] Presently, most health care for diabetes typically occurs late in the disease's progression, with the occurrence of end-stage complications (blindness, renal failure, amputation, and cardiovascular disease) being the norm. A focus on preventive care would shift resources to control of glycemia, dyslipidemia, hypertension, obesity, microalbuminuria, and smoking,[142] which analysis indicates would be cost-effective.[143, 144]

Continuing care is crucial in the management of diabetes, and treatment must be evaluated and modified as necessary. Education should be reinforced and patient motivation should be strengthened. Complications need to be identified and treated promptly. Proper care of the patient with diabetes is a major therapeutic challenge.[145]

EXAMPLES OF PUBLIC HEALTH INTERVENTIONS

The Division of Diabetes Translation (DDT) at the Centers for Disease Control and Prevention (CDC) supports a rapidly expanding national and state-based program to reduce the burden of diabetes in the United States. CDC's framework includes four major components: (1) defining the diabetes burden (public health surveillance), (2) developing state-based diabetes control programs, (3) conducting applied translational research, and (4) implementing the National Diabetes Education Program (NDEP).[146] The DDT appropriation from Congress has grown from $7 million in 1992 to $46 million for 1998. Over $20 million of this will be disseminated to state health department diabetes control programs now in all 50 states and 8 US territories.

Public health activities of the CDC in diabetes are guided by the following assumptions: diabetes prevention and control is linked closely to lifestyle related health behaviors concerning diet, weight management, physical activity, and vaccinations for influenza; federal, state, and local public health agencies to be maximally effective must work closely with partners in the communities they serve, including health care providers, persons and families with diabetes, payers and purchasers, and community organizations; the burden of diabetes is greater for some racial and ethnic groups; many people with diabetes are unaware they have the disease; much more is now known about the prevention of diabetes complications, but many with diabetes are not receiving adequate care; and the most important point of impact for reducing the diabetes burden is in reshaping the health care system to deliver high-quality care and services to those with diabetes.[146]

Defining the Diabetes Burden

Multiple data sources are used to determine the diabetes burden on the population, the most important data sources being the National Health and Nutrition Examination Survey (NHANES), the National Interview Survey (NHIS), and the Behavioral Risk Factor Surveillance System (BRFSS). CDC is funding state health departments to collect diabetes-related information as part of the BRFSS to develop a nationwide, state-based surveillance system.[147, 148]

The CDC through *Diabetes Surveillance Reports* and State Diabetes Fact Sheets distributes information on diabetes morbidity and mortality, use of health care services, cardiovascular disease, and other complications of diabetes. The fourth edition of *Diabetes Surveillance Reports* is now being published. CDC is also collaborating with three managed care organizations to develop a diabetes surveillance system that makes use of pharmacy, laboratory, outpatient, and inpatient data sets. Others are working on using Medicare claims data to develop national and state estimates of diabetes incidence and prevalence. In a project through the University of Minnesota, Medicaid data are being used to build a multistate surveillance system for diabetes. CDC is working with the National Center for Health

Statistics to include laboratory measurement of fasting insulins and c-peptides as well as exam measurement of peripheral vascular disease and peripheral neuropathy in NHANES IV.[146]

Routine ongoing surveillance is an important component in the public health approach to diabetes control. Surveillance data provide a factual basis for policy decisions. Because mortality data understate the impact of diabetes, surveillance efforts must rely on other data sets such as hospitalizations, blindness registries, and end-stage renal disease registries. In addition, state-based estimates of the economic cost of diabetes may be useful in formulating public health policy.[149]

State-based Diabetes Control Programs

Diabetes outcomes are determined by many environmental and social variables not readily influenced by direct clinical care.[150, 151] It's increasingly evident that the disease burden of diabetes can be reduced through primary, secondary, and tertiary prevention strategies.[152] In response, the CDC has redirected the state diabetes control programs (DCPs) to focus on population-based services and policies, reducing the role formerly taken by many of the state DCPs in the direct provision of personal health services.[150] The mission of the DCPs is to reduce the burden of diabetes by defining the diabetes burden, developing new approaches for reducing the burden, implementing effective programs to reduce the burden, and coordinating efforts in the broader community. A primary goal is to improve access to affordable, high-quality diabetes care and services, with high risk and disproportionately burdened populations seen as a priority.[143]

In 1994, 40 state DCPs initiated new 5-year funding cycles. Their proposed activities were reviewed and grouped into two large categories, health-system and community-based interventions.[150] For both types of interventions planned by the states, more than half involved information giving and technical assistance. One-third involved practice guidelines, policy development, diabetes legislation, or social action. About 10% involved developing networks or coalitions. For the health system interventions the target audience included primarily health care providers, facilities/agencies, insurance companies, and policy makers. The community interventions focused on community members, people with diabetes, and minority populations. One-third to one-half of the community interventions focused on ethnic or racial minorities.

In 1994, two states received expanded funding from CDC to develop comprehensive programs that could implement statewide, multilevel public health approaches to reduce the diabetes burden.[147] As the DCPs have expanded to include every state, the number of enhanced state programs now stands at seven. An ongoing evaluation CDC is conducting with the Battelle organization indicates that state DCPs are particularly successful at defining the burden of diabetes in their jurisdictions and at coordinating the activities of the larger diabetes community to maximize the reach and effectiveness of the DCPs.[142]

One of the seven enhanced states is North Carolina, which has a program known as Project DIRECT (Diabetes Intervention Reaching and Educating Communities Together). The goal of this multiyear project is to develop, implement, and evaluate strategies for reducing the burden of diabetes mellitus in communities with large Black populations. The mission is to improve the health-related quality of life of a Black community in Raleigh, North Carolina, by reducing diabetes complications through a community-based multicomponent intervention. For the Black community in Raleigh, Project DIRECT is working: (1) to improve access to care, quality of care, and self-care; (2) to improve detection of undiagnosed diabetes; and (3) to reduce risk factors in the entire Black community related to diabetes, especially physical inactivity and fat intake.

Another enhanced state DCP, Minnesota, has partnered with a large health maintenance organization (HMO) to form Project IDEAL (Improving care for Diabetes through Empowerment, Active collaboration, and Leadership).[153] The goal of this DCP/HMO partnership[154] is to improve diabetes care in managed care systems using a quality improvement process (QI). The QI process introduced into a large health plan has both a system and clinic level focus. System barriers, inefficient processes, and variation in practice are the targets for improvement activities. Committed leadership, collaborative teams within the clinic, and a focus on the needs of patients are key to maintaining a continuous cycle of improvement and innovation. Birch and Davis Associates are working with CDC to produce an innovative practices guide and tool kit based on the work of states like Minnesota, Washington and Texas to assist other state DCPs in the transition from patient-based to a clinic- and a systems-based focus.[146]

In recent years, many state DCPs have been actively involved with local chapters of the American Diabetes Association developing state legislation mandating health insurance coverage of diabetes supplies and education. Twenty-three states now have such legislation. Wisconsin was the first in 1991 with 20 states enacting new legislation in 1996 and 1997.

The National Diabetes Education Program

The National Diabetes Education Program (NDEP) is a joint initiative of NIH and CDC launched in June 1997 in response to the rising costs and prevalence of diabetes.[155] Additional partners include the American Diabetes Association, the Juvenile Diabetes Foundation International, the American Association of Diabetes Educators, and the American Dietetic Association.

The objectives of NDEP are to increase public awareness of the seriousness of diabetes and its risk factors and potential strategies for prevention of diabetes and its complications; to promote healthy behaviors (diet and exercise); to improve health care providers' understanding of the disease and its control; to promote an integrated (team) approach to care; and to promote health care policy activities that improve quality and access to diabetes care.[156] In 1998, NDEP will launch a national public awareness campaign to alert the general public, health care providers, payers and purchasers of health care, and policy makers as to the seriousness and commonness of diabetes.

Other Public Health Programs

Some excellent examples of public health prevention programs for diabetes are found outside the state public health systems. Two such programs—"Paso a Paso" in El Paso, Texas, and the Hispanic Diabetes Detection and Education Program in Toledo, Ohio—encouraged diabetes prevention in Hispanic populations. Both programs targeted high-risk populations using community-based tools and strategies such as posters, brochures, neighborhood fitness activities, nutrition clubs, and Spanish-language radio announcements.[157]

Since 1983 the Indian Health Service has supported a community-based physical activity program to prevent and control type 2 diabetes at Zuni Pueblo, New Mexico. In addition to regular fitness programs, classes are offered that target individuals with diabetes, high blood pressure, obesity, and gestational diabetes. Initial acceptance of the program was slow, but today the Zuni Wellness Center consistently reports monthly participation rates of 500 to 1000 in a community with a population of 8000.[157, 158] Those with type 2 diabetes participating in an exercise program at the 2-year follow-up had lost weight, lowered blood glucose values, and reduced their use of hypoglycemic medication in comparison to nonparticipants. In a weight loss competition,

45% of enrollees lost more than 2.3 kg. These studies demonstrate that participation in a community-based exercise program can produce significant weight loss and improved glycemic control in a high-risk population.[159]

The Kahnawake Schools Diabetes Prevention Project is a 3-year community-based, primary prevention program for type 2 diabetes in a Mohawk community near Montreal, Canada.[160] The objectives are to improve healthy eating and increase physical activity in elementary school children. With funding from NIDDK and support from the state legislature, a similar, school-based program called WOLF (Work Out, Low Fat) has been developed in Minnesota for the American Indian elementary school student population.[161, 162]

Recognizing the difficulties of addressing chronic illness in the primary care setting, Group Health Cooperative of Puget Sound, a managed care organization with 13 000 patients with diabetes, has adopted population-based management for patients with diabetes.[163] Under this model, clinical guidelines and epidemiological data and techniques are used to plan, organize, deliver, and monitor care to patients with diabetes. Current practice is reviewed, problems identified, and new intervention plans are introduced based on developed guidelines and monitored patient outcomes. Population-based care occurs both centrally and at the clinic level.

The six Diabetes Research and Training Centers (DRTC) established by the National Institutes of Health are an important element in the development and translation of new behavioral and education programs for diabetes. The Michigan DRTC, for example, has conducted several community-based projects using community advisory councils.[164, 165] The DRTCs also play an important role for the health professional by providing continuing education, seminars, and workshops in current diabetes management. The DRTCs also provide an array of tested evaluation and assessment instruments and professional expertise for development and implementation of diabetes programs.

AREAS OF FUTURE RESEARCH AND DEMONSTRATION

Since 1980 there have been a number of advances that have provided better tools for the treatment of diabetes. These include new forms of purified insulin, better ways to monitor blood glucose including self-monitoring at home, development of external and implantable insulin pumps that deliver insulin in a more natural pattern that replaces daily injections, laser treatment for diabetic eye disease, successful kidney transplants, improved management of diabetic pregnancies, new drugs to treat type 2 diabetes and better management through weight control, evidence from the DCCT that intensive management of blood glucose reduces and may prevent development of microvascular complications, and development of antihypertensive drugs to prevent or delay kidney failure.[166] Despite these advances, there are several studies[167–171, 145] to indicate that health systems often fail to meet current guidelines for diabetes care.[172] There are also positive circumstances where the average level of glycemia in patient populations has been declining due largely to increased frequency of monitoring and of insulin injections.[173]

Future research that provides a better understanding of both insulin deficiency and insulin resistance will enable the development of targeted pharmacological therapy.[191, 192] Pharmacological therapy to prevent type 2 diabetes in those at high-risk will necessitate research that identifies improved biological markers to identify susceptibility to diabetes, which could then make it possible to develop safer pharmacological agents to be used by all patients, including those likely to become pregnant. Drugs to reverse microvascular complications will be a great challenge, but, because of diabetes heterogeneity, the greatest challenge will be development of a therapy to correct the genetic abnormalities in those susceptible to diabetes.[193]

For both type 1 and 2 diabetes, further research is needed to better understand the causes of these diseases and to find ways to prevent and cure them. Transplantation of the pancreas or insulin producing islets of the pancreas presents one hope for cure for type 1 diabetes.[194] Unfortunately, such transplants are rejected by the human body without the use of expensive and powerful medications that could eventually cause serious health problems. Future investigations will attempt to develop less harmful drugs and to create artificial islet cells that secrete insulin in response to sugar levels in the blood.[166]

As the science begins to determine effective prevention strategies for diabetes, models are also being developed to examine the cost utility of primary, secondary, and tertiary prevention based on quality-adjusted life years (QALY) (see also Chapter 1).[141, 174] There are models that suggest cost-effectiveness of intensive therapy (ie, the DCCT[144]) is approximately $20 000 per QALY for type 1 diabetes and $16 000 for type 2 diabetes,[25, 174] which is within the general range of intervention considered cost-effective in economic models. There is also limited evidence suggesting the cost utility of behavioral interventions (ie, diet plus

exercise) for patients with type 2 diabetes.[175]

One of the major areas of research that has been needed is the prevention of type 2 diabetes and its complications. Recently, the National Institutes of Health initiated the Diabetes Prevention Program (DPP), a full-scale, multicenter, randomized clinical trial to evaluate the efficacy of interventions designed to delay or prevent onset of type 2 diabetes in high-risk individuals. Prior studies suggest up to 40% of people with IGT eventually progress to type 2 diabetes at a rate of 1% to 5% per year.[176]

The DPP is recruiting 3900 individuals with IGT at high risk for type 2 diabetes. Approximately half the study population will be composed of minorities and 20% will be 65 or older. To recruit the necessary 3900 individuals, between 66 000 and 186 000 people will be screened. The 3900 participants identified for the study are then randomly assigned to one of two drug arms (metformin and troglitazone), an intensive lifestyle intervention, or a control group. Begun in 1996, the recruitment period is three years. To date 56 000 individuals have been screened and 900 have been randomized into the study, with 43% being non-Caucasian.[92]

The DPP is being conducted in 25 medical centers throughout the nation, with all participants being followed for 3 to 6 years. Results will be reported in 2002. If the DPP is successful in either preventing or delaying the occurrence of type 2 diabetes and its complications, this would most likely result in a national diabetes screening program for much of the US population.

A second major study, also currently engaged in patient recruitment and sponsored by NIDDK, is the Diabetes Trial Type-1 (DPT-1). The DPT-1 aims to determine whether type 1 diabetes can be delayed or prevented by daily dose of insulin in individuals at genetic, immunologic, and metabolic risk. Over 300 clinics are participating in the study that began in 1994. Patient screening and recruitment runs through 1998. Some 15 000 nondiabetic relatives of individuals with type 1 diabetes are screened annually (60 000 overall) to detect the presence of islet cell antibodies (ICA). Those found to have ICA, depending on degree of risk, are randomized to receive insulin either parenterally or orally, or to be monitored closely but without receiving insulin. Study participants are followed for 3 to 6 years. As of November 1998, 49 000 individuals had been screened and 1600 found ICA positive. Of these, 187 have already developed diabetes and 304 were considered at high risk and are participating in the study.[92]

Another major area for research involves the importance and effect of normalizing blood glucose levels to provide protection from macrovascular complications of diabetes.[46, 135] Future research on the relationship between macrovascular disease and diabetes needs to address three questions.[177] First, does macrovascular disease begin years before the onset of "clinical diabetes," (ie, hyperglycemia) and what is the relationship between "early" macrovascular disease and the insulin resistance syndrome?[178] Second, why do women with diabetes lose their "gender protection" against macrovascular disease, even before menopause?[179] Third, what is the efficacy of risk factor reductions for diabetic macrovascular disease? The Epidemiology of Diabetes Intervention and Complications Study, a 10-year follow-up of the participants in the DCCT, is focusing on development of macrovascular and renal complications.

Low-cost, practical methods for achieving blood glucose control need to be developed and the findings from the DCCT need to be disseminated and made practical for persons with diabetes and their health care teams.[180–183] More research will soon be reported that addresses the relevance of the DCCT findings to type 2 diabetes.[184] Given the well-documented fact that health care for diabetes patients frequently falls short of what's recommended in modern practice care guidelines, longitudinal observational studies like that conducted by the Diabetes Patient Outcome Research Team (PORT)[185] are needed to assess how well prevailing treatments work in clinical practice settings. Because of the increasing emphasis on primary care within the health care system, studies are needed that examine referral patterns between primary care and the diabetes specialty team to identify the essential "break points" where and when patients should move between them.[186] Increasingly, patient management decisions in a managed care environment are likely to be dependent on a centralized information system that directs the collection of patient data relevant to diabetes care and provides a powerful tool for framing clinical decisions for appropriate diabetes care.[187, 188] The continuous quality improvement (CQI) process is a methodology which builds a continuous feedback loop into clinic settings and should be explored for its potential utility in enhancing patient referral patterns and ability to respond to and make use of a centralized communication system.[153, 189, 190]

Scientists will continue looking for those genes involved in type 1 and type 2 diabetes. Better genetic identification of high-risk asymptomatic people would make it possible to target screening and preventive strategies most effectively.[192] Investigations on the link between low birth weight and later diabetes may afford new prevention and treatment options.[196] Overcoming environmental factors, mainly the growing obesity, sedentary behavior, and changing demographics of our society, with require continued close, ongoing collaboration between the medical, academic, and public health sectors of our society within a framework of strong community partnership.

REFERENCES

1. Centers for Disease Control. *National diabetes fact sheet: National estimates and general information on diabetes in the United States.* Atlanta, Ga: US Department of Health and Human Services; 1997.

2. Kenny SJ, Aubert RE, Geiss LS. Prevalence and incidence of non-insulin-dependent diabetes. In: Harris MI, Cowie CC, Stern MP et al., eds. *Diabetes in America.* 2nd ed. National Institutes of Health, National Institute of Diabetes and Digestive and Kidney Diseases; 1995:4:47–67. NIH publication 95-1468.

3. Centers for Disease Control and Prevention. Trends in the prevalence and incidence of

self-reported diabetes mellitus—United States, 1980–1994. *MMWR.* 1997;46:1027–1028.

4. Orchard TJ, LaPorte RE, Dorman JS. Diabetes. In: Last JM, Wallace RB, eds. *Maxcy-Rosenau-Last Textbook of Public Health and Preventive Medicine.* 13th ed. Norwalk, Conn: Appelton & Lange; 1992:873–883.

5. Libman I, Singer T, LaPorte R. How many people in the U.S. have IDDM? *Diabetes Care.* 1993;16:841.

6. LaPorte RE, Tajima N, et al. Geographic differences in the risk of insulin-dependent diabetes mellitus: the importance of registries. *Diabetes Care.* 1985;8:101–107.

7. LaPorte RE, Matsushima M, Yue-Fang C. Prevalence and incidence of insulin-dependent diabetes. In: Harris MI, Cowie CC, Stern MP et al., eds. *Diabetes in America.* 2nd ed. National Institutes of Health, National Institute of Diabetes and Digestive and Kidney Diseases; 1995:3:37–46. NIH publication 95-1468.

8. Harris MI. Undiagnosed NIDDM: clinical and public health issues. *Diabetes Care.* 1993;16:642–652.

9. Centers for Disease Control. Mortality patterns—Preliminary data, United States, 1996. *MMWR.* 1997;46:941–944.

10. Brosseau JD. Occurrence of diabetes among decedents in North Dakota. *Diabetes Care.* 1987;10:542–543.

11. Andresen EM, Lee JA, Pecoraro RE, Koepsell TD, Hallstrom AP, Siscovick DS. Under reporting of diabetes on death certificates, King County, Washington. *Am J Public Health.* 1993;83:1021–1024.

12. Geiss LS, Herman WH, Smith PJ. Mortality and non-insulin-dependent diabetes. In: Harris MI, Cowie CC, Stern MP et al., eds. *Diabetes in America.* 2nd ed. National Institutes of Health, National Institute of Diabetes and Digestive and Kidney Diseases; 1995:11:233–257. NIH publication 95-1468.

13. Portuese E, Orchard T. Mortality in insulin-dependent diabetes. In: Harris MI, Cowie CC, Stern MP et al., eds. *Diabetes in America.* 2nd ed. National Institutes of Health, National Institute of Diabetes and Digestive and Kidney Diseases; 1995:10:221–232. NIH publication 95-1468.

14. Escobedo LG, Caspersen CJ. Risk factors for sudden coronary death in the United States. *Epidemiology.* 1997;8(2):175–180.

15. Herman WH, ed. *The Prevention and Treatment of Complications of Diabetes.* Atlanta, Ga:

Centers for Disease Control; 1991.

16. Will JC, Geiss LS, Wetterhall SF. Diabetic retinopathy. *N Engl J Med.* 1990;323:613. Letter.

17. Rettig RA, Levinsky NG, eds. *Kidney Failure and the Federal Government.* Washington, DC: National Academy Press; 1991.

18. Songer TJ. Disability in diabetes. In: Harris MI, Cowie CC, Stern MP et al., eds. *Diabetes in America.* 2nd ed. National Institutes of Health, National Institute of Diabetes and Digestive and Kidney Diseases; 1995:12:259–282. NIH publication 95-1468.

19. Centers for Disease Control, Division of Diabetes Translation: Disability. In: *Diabetes Surveillance, 1993.* Atlanta, Ga: November 1993.

20. Glauber H, Brown J. Impact of cardiovascular disease on the health care utilization in a defined diabetic population. *J Clin Epidemiol.* 1994;47:1133–1142.

21. Javitt JC, Aiello LP, Chiang Y, Ferris FL III, Canner JK, Greenfield S. Preventive eye care in people with diabetes is cost-saving to the federal government: Implications for health-care reform. *Diabetes Care.* 1994;17:909–917.

22. Rubin RJ, Altman WM, Mendelson DN. Health care expenditures for people with diabetes mellitus 1992. *J Clin Endocrinol Metab.* 1994;78: 809A-809F.

23. American Diabetes Association. Economic consequences of diabetes mellitus in the U.S. in 1997. *Diabetes Care.* 1993;21(2): 296–309.

24. Cowie CC, Eberhardt MS. Sociodemographic characteristics of persons with diabetes. In: Harris MI, Cowie CC, Stern MP et al., eds. *Diabetes in America.* 2nd ed. National Institutes of Health, National Institute of Diabetes and Digestive and Kidney Diseases; 1995:6:85–101. NIH publication 95-1468.

25. Herman WH, Eastman RC, Songer TJ, Dasbach EJ. The cost-effectiveness of intensive therapy for diabetes mellitus. *Endocrinol Metab Clin North Am.* 1997; 26(3):679–695.

26. Selby JV, Thomas Ray G, Zhang D, Colby CJ. Excess costs of medical care for patients with diabetes in a managed care population. *Diabetes Care.* 1997;20(9):1396–1402.

27. Gilmer TP, O'Connor PJ, Manning WG, Rush WA. The cost to health plans of poor glycemic control. *Diabetes Care* 1997; 20(12):1847–1853.

28. The Expert Committee on the Diagnosis and Classification of Diabetes Mellitus. Report of the

expert committee on the diagnosis and classification of diabetes mellitus. *Diabetes Care.* 1997;20: 1183-1197.

29. National Diabetes Data Group. Classification and diagnosis of diabetes mellitus and other categories of glucose intolerance. *Diabetes.* 1979;28:1039–1057.

30. Zimmet PZ, Tuomi T, Mackay R, Rowley MJ, Knowles W, Cohen M, Lang DA. Latent autoimmune diabetes mellitus in adults (LADA): The role of antibodies to glutamic acid decarboxylase in diagnosis and prediction of insulin dependency. *Diabet Med.* 1994;11:299–303.

31. Palmer JP, McCulloch DK. Prediction and prevention of IDDM, 1991. *Diabetes.* 1991; 40:943–947.

32. Atkinson MA, Maclaren NK. The pathogenesis of insulin dependent diabetes. *N Engl J Med.* 1994;331:1428–1436.

33. Muir A, Schatz DA, Maclaren NK. The pathogenesis, prediction, and prevention of insulin dependent diabetes mellitus. *Endocrinol Metab Clin North Am.* 1992;21:199–219.

34. Bertrams J, Baur M. Insulin-dependent diabetes mellitus. In: Albert ED, Baur MP, Mayr WR, eds. *Histocompatibility Testing 1984.* New York, NY: Springer-Verlag; 1984:348–358

35. Skyler J, Fabinovitch A. Etiology and pathogenesis of insulin dependent diabetes mellitus. *Pediatr Ann.* 1987;16:682–692.

36. Reece EA, Hagay Z, Hobbins JC. Insulin-dependent diabetes mellitus and immunogenetics: maternal and fetal considerations. *Obstet Gynecol Surv.* 1991;46:255-263.

37. Haffner SM, Stern MP, Hazuda HP, Mitchell BD, Patterson JK. Cardiovascular risk factors in confirmed prediabetic individuals: does the clock for coronary heart disease start ticking before the onset of clinical diabetes? *JAMA.* 1990;263:2893-2898.

38. Saad MF, Knowler WC, Pettitt DJ, Nelson RG, Charles MA, Bennett PH. A two-step model for development of non-insulin-dependent diabetes. *Am J Med.* 1991;90:229-235.

39. Wendorf M, Goldfine ID. Archeology of NIDDM: excavation of the "thrifty" genotype. *Diabetes.* 1991;40:161-165.

40. Kobberling J, Tillil H. Empiric risk figures for first degree relatives of non-insulin-dependent diabetics. In: Kobberling J, Tattersall R, eds. Serono Symposium no. 47, *The Genetics of Diabetes Mellitus.* New York, NY: Academic Press; 1982:201–209.

41. Barnett AH, Eff C, Leslie RDG, Pyke DA. Diabetes in identical

twins. *Diabetologia.* 1981;70: 87-93.

42. Coustan DR. Gestational diabetes. In: Harris MI, Cowie CC, Stern MP et al., eds. *Diabetes in America.* 2nd ed. National Institutes of Health, National Institute of Diabetes and Digestive and Kidney Diseases; 1995:35:703–717. NIH publication 95-1468.

43. Metzger BE, Organizing Committee: Summary and recommendations of the Third International Workshop-Conference on Gestational Diabetes Mellitus. *Diabetes.* 1991; 40:197–201.

44. Bild D, Selby JV, Sinnock P, Browner W, Braveman P, Showstack J. Lower extremity amputation in persons with diabetes: epidemiology and prevention. *Diabetes Care.* 1989;12:24–31.

45. Reiber GE, Pecoraro RE, Koepsell TD. Risk factors for amputation in patients with diabetes mellitus. *Ann Intern Med.* 1992;117:97-105.

46. Moss SE, Klein R, Klein BE, Meuer SM. The association of glycemia and cause-specific mortality in a diabetic population. *Arch Intern Med.* 1994; 154:2473–2479.

47. DCCT Research Group. The Diabetes Control and Complications Trial (DCCT): design and methodologic considerations for the feasibility phase. *Diabetes.* 1986;35:530–545.

48. DCCT Research Group. The effect of intensive treatment of diabetes on the development and progression of longterm complications in insulin-treated diabetes mellitus. *N Engl J Med.* 1993;329:977–986.

49. Ohkubo Y, Kishikama H, Araki E, Miyata T, Isami S, Motoyoshi S, Kojimi Y, Furuyoshi N, Shichiri M. Intensive insulin therapy prevents the progression of diabetic microvascular complications in Japanese patients with noninsulin dependent diabetes mellitus: a randomized prospective 6 year study. *Diabetes Res Clin Pract.* 1995;28:103–117.

50. Harris, MI. Summary. In: Harris MI, Cowie CC, Stern MP et al., eds. *Diabetes in America.* 2nd ed. National Institutes of Health, National Institute of Diabetes and Digestive and Kidney Diseases; 1995:1:1–14. NIH publication 95-1468.

51. Carter JS, Pugh JA, Monterrosa A. Non-insulin-dependent diabetes mellitus in minorities in the United States. *Ann Intern Med.* 1996;125(3):221–232.

52. Moritz DJ, Ostfeld AM, Blazer D II, Curb D, Taylor JO, Wallace RB. The health burden of diabetes for the elderly in four

communities. *Public Health Rep.* 1994;109:782-790.

53. Carter Center of Emory University. Closing the gap: the problem of diabetes mellitus in the United States. *Diabetes Care.* 1985;8:391-406.

54. Gohdes D. Diabetes in North American Indians and Alaska Natives. In: Harris MI, Cowie CC, Stern MP et al., eds. *Diabetes in America.* 2nd ed. National Institutes of Health, National Institute of Diabetes and Digestive and Kidney Diseases; 1995:34:683–702. NIH publication 95-1468.

55. Fujimoto WY. Diabetes in Asian and Pacific Island Americans. In: Harris MI, Cowie CC, Stern MP et al., eds. *Diabetes in America.* 2nd ed. National Institutes of Health, National Institute of Diabetes and Digestive and Kidney Diseases; 1995:33:661–681. NIH publication 95-1468.

56. Bennett PH, Stern MP. Patient population and genetics: role in diabetes. *Am J Med.* 1991;90:76S–79S.

57. Stern MP, Mitchell BD. Diabetes in Hispanic Americans. In: Harris MI, Cowie CC, Stern MP et al., eds. *Diabetes in America.* 2nd ed. National Institutes of Health, National Institute of Diabetes and Digestive and Kidney Diseases; 1995:32:631–660. NIH publication 95-1468.

58. Tull ES, Roseman JM. Diabetes in African Americans. In: Harris MI, Cowie CC, Stern MP et al., eds. *Diabetes in America.* 2nd ed. National Institutes of Health, National Institute of Diabetes and Digestive and Kidney Diseases; 1995:31:613–630. NIH publication 95-1468.

59. Coustan DR, Carpenter MW, O'Sullivan PS, Carr SR. Gestational diabetes: predictors of subsequent disordered glucose metabolism. *Am J Obstet Gynecol.* 1993;168:1139-1144.

60. Dooley SL, Metzenger BE, Cho NH. Gestational diabetes mellitus: Influence of race on disease prevalence and perinatal outcomes in a US population. *Diabetes Care.* 1991;40(suppl. 2):25-29.

61. O'Sullivan JB. Subsequent morbidity among GDM women. In: Sutherland HW, Stowers JM, eds. *Carbohydrate Metabolism in Pregnancy and the Newborn.* New York, NY: Churchhill Livingstone. 1984:174–180.

62. Boyko EJ, Alderman BW, Keane EM, Baron AE. Effects of childbearing on glucose tolerance and NIDDM prevalence. *Diabetes Care.* 1990;13:848–854.

63. Collins VR, Dowse GK, Zimmet PZ. Evidence against association between parity and NIDDM from five population groups. *Diabetes Care.* 1991;14:975–981.

64. Geiss LS, ed. *Diabetes Surveillance*. Atlanta, Ga: Centers for Disease Control; 1992.
65. Dahlqurst G, Mustonen L. Childhood onset diabetes—time trends and climatological factors. *Int J Epidemiol.* 1994;6:1234–1241.
66. Karvonen M, Tuomilehto J, Libman I, LaPorte R for WHO DiaMond Project Group: A review of the recent epidemiological data on incidence of type 1 (insulin-dependent) diabetes mellitus worldwide. *Diabetologia.* 1993;36:883–892.
67. Kuczmarski RJ, Flegal KM, Campell SM et al. Increasing prevalence of overweight among U.S. adults: the National Health and Nutrition Examination Surveys, 1960 to 1991. *JAMA.* 1994;272:205–211.
68. Krolewski AS, Warram JH, Rand LI, Kahn CR. Epidemiologic approach to the etiology of type I diabetes mellitus and its complications. *N Engl J Med.* 1987;317:1390–1398.
69. Diabetes Epidemiology Research International Group. Geographic patterns of childhood insulin-dependent diabetes mellitus. *Diabetes.* 1988;37:1113–1119.
70. Leibson CL, O'Brien PC, Atkinson E, Palumbo PJ, Melton LJ III. Relative contributions of incidence and survival to increasing prevalence of adult-onset diabetes mellitus: A population-based study. *Am J Epidemiol.* 1997;146(1):12–22.
71. Dorman JS, McCarthy BJ, O'Leary LA, Koehler AN. Risk factors for insulin-dependent diabetes. In: Harris MI, Cowie CC, Stern MP et al., eds. *Diabetes in America.* 2nd ed. National Institutes of Health, National Institute of Diabetes and Digestive and Kidney Diseases; 1995:8:165–177. NIH publication 95-1468.
72. Leslie DG, Elliott RB. Early environmental events as a cause of IDDM: evidence and implications. *Diabetes.* 1994;43;843–850.
73. Gerstein HC. Cow's milk exposure and Type 1 diabetes mellitus: A critical overview of the clinical literature. *Diabetes Care.* 1994;17:13–19.
74. Pettitt DJ, Bennett PH, Knowler WC, Hanson RL, Forman MR. Breastfeeding and incidence of non-insulin-dependent diabetes mellitus in Pima Indians. *Lancet* 1997;350(9072):166–168.
75. Eisenbarth GM. Type I diabetes mellitus. *N Engl J Med.* 1986;314:1360–1368.
76. Rewers M, Hamman RF. Risk factors for non-insulin-dependent diabetes. In: Harris MI, Cowie CC, Stern MP et al., eds. *Diabetes in America.* 2nd ed.

National Institutes of Health, National Institute of Diabetes and Digestive and Kidney Diseases; 1995:9:179–220. NIH publication 95-1468.

77. Kaye SA, Folsom AR, Sprafka JM, Prineas RJ, Wallace RB. Increased incidence of diabetes mellitus in relation to abdominal adiposity in older women. *J Clin Epidemiol.* 1991;44:329–334.

78. Everhart JE, Pertitt DJ, Bennett PH, Knowler WC. Duration of obesity increases the incidence of NIDDM. *Diabetes.* 1992; 41:235–240.

79. Helmrich SP, Ragland DR, Leung RW, Paffenbarger RS Jr. Physical activity and reduced occurrence of non-insulin-dependent diabetes mellitus. *N Engl J Med.* 1991;325:147–152.

80. Manson JE, Nathan DM, Krolewski AS, Stampfer MJ, Willett WC, Hennekens CH. A prospective study of exercise and incidence of diabetes among US male physicians. *JAMA.* 1991;268:63–67.

81. Manson JE, Rimm EB, Stampfer MJ, et al. Physical activity and incidence of non-insulin-dependent diabetes in women. *Lancet.* 1991;338:774–778.

82. Rimm EB, Manson JE, Stampfer MJ, et al. Cigarette smoking and the risk of diabetes in women. *Am J Public Health.* 1993;83: 211–214.

83. Rimm EB, Chan J, Stampher MJ, Colditz GA, Willett WC. Prospective study of cigarette smoking, alcohol use, and the risk of diabetes in men. *BMJ.* 1995; 310(6979):555–559.

84. Molitch ME. Diabetes mellitus: control and complications. *Postgrad Med.* 1989;85:182–194.

85. Ford ES, Williamson DF, Liu S.Weight change and diabetes incidence: findings from a national cohort of U.S. adults. *Am J Epidemiol.* 1997;14(3):214–222.

86. Keen H, Jarrett RJ, McCartney P. The 10 year follow-up of the Bedford survey (1962–1972); glusose tolerance and diabetes. *Diabetologia.* 1982;22:73–78.

87. Jarrett RJ, Keen H, Fuller JH, McCartney M. Worsening to diabetes in men with impaired glucose tolerance ("borderline diabetes"). *Diabetologia.* 1979; 16:25–30.

88. Sartor G, Schersten B, Carlstrom S, Melander A, Norden A, Persson G. Ten-year follow-up of subjects with impaired glucose tolerance: Prevention of diabetes by tolbutamide and diet regulation. *Diabetes.* 1980;29:41–44.

89. Eriksson K-F, Lindgarde F. Prevention of type 2 (non-insulin-dependent) diabetes mellitus by diet and physical exercise: the 6-year Malmo

feasibility study. *Diabetologia.* 1991;34:891–898.

90. Pan XR, Li GW, Hu YH, et al. Effects of diet and exercise in preventing NIDDM in people with impaired glucose tolerance. The Da Qing IGT and Diabetes Study. *Diabetes Care.* 1997; 20(4):537–544.

91. Knowler WC, Narayan KMV, Hanson RL, et al. Preventing non-insulin-dependent diabetes. *Diabetes.* 1995;44(5):483–488.

92. Bloomgarden ZT. American Diabetes Association Annual Meeting, 1997: obesity, diabetes prevention, and type 1 diabetes. *Diabetes Care.* 1997;20(12):1913–1917.

93. Simmons D, O'Dea K, Swinburn B, Voyle J. Community-based approaches for the primary prevention of non-insulin-dependent diabetes mellitus. *Diabet Med.* 1997;14(7):519–526.

94. Zimmet PZ. Primary prevention of diabetes mellitus. *Diabetes Care.* 1988;11:258–262.

95. Tuomilehto J, Wolf E. Primary prevention of diabetes mellitus. *Diabetes Care.* 1987;10:238–248.

96. Tuomilehto J, Wolf E. The challenge in the future: primary prevention of diabetes mellitus. In: Larkins R, Zimmet P, Chisholm D, eds. *Prevention of Diabetes and Its Complications: International Conference Proceedings.* 1988;993–999. Abstract 800.

97. Zimmet PZ. Challenges in diabetes epidemiology: from West to the rest. *Diabetes Care.* 1992;15:232–252.

98. Tuomilehto J. Strategies for the primary prevention of non-insulin-dependent diabetes mellitus. *Adv Exp Med Biol.* 1988;246:403–411.

99. Stern MP. Primary prevention of type II diabetes mellitus. *Diabetes Care.* 1991;14:399–410.

100. King H, Dowd JE. Primary prevention of Type 2 (non-insulin-dependent) diabetes mellitus. *Diabetologia.* 1990; 33:3–8.

101. Manson JE, Spelsberg A. Primary prevention of non-insulin-dependent diabetes mellitus. *Am J Prev Med.* 1994;10(3):172–184.

102. Farquhar JW, Fortmann SP, Maccoby N, et al. The Stanford Five City Project: an overview. In: Matarazzo JD, Weiss SM, Herd JA, Miller NE, eds. *Behavioral Health: A Handbook of Health Enhancement and Disease Prevention.* New York, NY: John Wiley & Sons; 1984: 1154–1165.

103. Blackburn H, Luepker RV, Kline FG, et al. The Minnesota Heart Health Program: a research and demonstration project in cardiovascular disease prevention. In: Matarazzo JD, Weiss SM, Herd JA, Miller NE, Weiss

SM, eds. *Behavioral Health: A Handbook of Health Enhancement and Disease Prevention.* New York, NY: John Wiley & Sons; 1984: 1171–1178.

104. Lasater T, et al. Lay volunteer delivery of a community-based cardiovascular risk factor change program: The Pawtucket Experiment. In: Matarazzo JD, Weiss SM, Herd JA, Miller NE, Weiss SM, eds. *Behavioral Health: A Handbook of Health Enhancement and Disease Prevention.* New York, NY: John Wiley & Sons; 1984:1166–1170.

105. Fisher M, Eckhart C, eds. Guide to Clinical Preventive Services. An Assessment of the Effectiveness of 169 Interventions. Report of the US Preventive Services Task Force. Baltimore, Md: Williams & Wilkins; 1989.

106. American Diabetes Association. Position statement: Screening for type 2 diabetes. *Diabetes Care.* 1998;21(suppl 1):S20–S22.

107. American Diabetes Association. Position statement: office guide to diagnosis and classification of diabetes mellitus and other categories of glucose intolerence. *Diabetes Care.* 1995;18(suppl 1):4.

108. American Diabetes Association. Position statement: Gestational diabetes mellitus. *Diabetes Care.* 1998;21(suppl 1):S60–S61.

109. Anderson RM. The challenge of translating scientific knowledge into improved diabetes care in the 1990s. *Diabetes Care.* 1991;14:418–421.

110. American Diabetes Association. Position statement: standards of medical care for patients with diabetes mellitus. *Diabetes Care.* 1998;21(suppl 1):S23–S31.

111. American Diabetes Association. National standards for diabetes self-management education programs and American Diabetes Association review criteria. *Diabetes Care.* 1998;21(suppl 1):S95–S98.

112. Galuk D. Diabetes mellitus types I and II. *Adv Clin Care.* 1991;March/April:5–7.

113. American Diabetes Association. Position statement: Nutritional recommendations and principles for people with diabetes mellitus. Diabetes Care. 1998; 21(suppl 1):

114. Spelsberg A, Manson JE. Physical activity in the treatment and prevention of diabetes. *Comprehensive Therapy.* 1995;21(10):559–564.

115. Barnard J, Jung T, Inkeles SB. Diet and exercise in the treatment of NIDDM: the need for early emphasis. *Diabetes Care.* 1994;17(12):1469–1472.

116. Yamanouchi K, Shinozaki T, Chikada K, et al. Daily walking combined with diet therapy is a

useful means for obese NIDDM patients not only to reduce body weight but also to improve insulin sensitivity. *Diabetes Care.* 1995;18(6):775–778.

117. American Diabetes Association. Position statement: diabetes mellitus and exercise. *Diabetes Care.* 1998;21(suppl 1):S40–S44.

118. Wallberg-Henriksson H, Ricon J, Zierath JR. Exercise in the management of non-insulin-dependent diabetes mellitus. *Sports Med.* 1998;25(1):25–35.

119. Mayer-Davis EJ, D'Agostino R Jr, Karter AJ, et al. Intensity and amount of physical activity in relation to insulin sensitivity: the Insulin Resistance Atherosclerosis Study. *JAMA.* 1998;279(9): 669–674.

120. Ivy JL. Role of exercise training in the prevention and treatment of insulin resistance and non-insulin-dependent diabetes mellitus. *Sports Med.* 1997;24(5): 321–336.

121. Zimmerman BR. Practical aspects of intensive insulin therapy. *Mayo Clin Proc.* 1986;61:806–812.

122. Hirsch IB, Forkas-Hirsch R, Skyler JS. Intensive insulin therapy for treatment of type I diabetes. *Diabetes Care.* 1990; 13:1265–1283.

123. Bantle JP. The dietary treatment of diabetes mellitus. *Med Clin North Am.* 1988;72:1285–1300.

124. Zimmerman BR, Service FJ. Management of non-insulin-dependent diabetes mellitus. *Med Clin North Am.* 1988;72: 1355–1364.

125. Haire-Joshu D, ed. *Management of Diabetes Mellitus: Perspectives of Care Across the Life Span,* 2nd ed. St. Louis, Mo: Mosby, 1996.

126. Clement S. Diabetes self-management education. *Diabetes Care.* 1995;18:1204–1214.

127. Brown SA. Studies of educational interventions and outcomes in diabetic adults: a meta-analysis revisited. *Patient Educ Counsel.* 1990;16:189–215.

128. Anderson BJ, Rubin RR. *Practical psychology for diabetes clinicians: how to deal with the key behavioral issues faced by patients and health care teams.* Alexandria, Va: American Diabetes Association; 1996.

129. Burritt MF, Hanson E, Munene N, Zimmerman BR. Portable blood glucose meters. *Postgrad Med.* 1991;89:75.

130. Reichard P, Nilsson B-Y, Rosenquist U. The effect of long-term intensified insulin treatment on the development of microvascular complications of diabetes mellitus. *N Engl J Med.* 1993;329:304–309.

131. The Diabetes Control and Complications Trial Research Group. The relationship of glycemic exposure (HbA1c) to

the risk of development and progression of retinopathy in the diabetes control and complications trial. *Diabetes*. 1995;44:968.

132. Hellman R, Regan J, Rosen H. Effect of intensive treatment of diabetes of the risk of death or renal failure in NIDDM and IDDM. *Diabetes Care*. 1997;20(3):258–264.

133. Nakagami T, Omori Y, Hori S, Kawahara R. Glycemic control and prevention of retinopathy in Japanese NIDDM patients. A 10-year follow-up study. *Diabetes Care*. 1997;20(4):621–622.

134. American Diabetes Association. Position statement: implications of the Diabetes Control and Complications Trial. *Diabetes Care*. 1998;21(suppl 1):S88–S90.

135. Klein R. Hyperglycemia and microvascular and macrovascular disease in diabetes. *Diabetes Care*. 1995;2:258.

136. Butler WJ, Ostrander LD Jr, Carman WJ, Lamphiear DE. Mortality from coronary heart disease in the Tecumseh study: long-term effect of diabetes mellitus, glucose tolerance and other risk factors. *Am J Epidemiol*. 1985;121:541–547.

137. Caixas A, Perez A, Homs R, Payes A, de Leiva A, Ordonez-Llanos J. Optimization of glycemic control by insulin therapy decreases the propor-tion of small dense LDL particles in diabetic patients. *Diabetes*. 1997;46(7):207–213.

138. Laakso M. Glycemic control and the risk for coronary heart disease in patients with non-insulin-dependent diabetes mellitus. The Finnish studies. *Ann Intern Med*. 1996;124(1 pt 2):127–130.

139. Meigs JB, Singer DE, Sullivan LM, et al. Metabolic control and prevalent cardiovascular disease in non-insulin-dependent diabetes mellitus (NIDDM): The NIDDM Patient Outcome Research Team. *Am J Med* 1997;102(1):38–47.

140. Herman WH, Teutsch SM, Geiss LS. Diabetes mellitus. In: Amler RW, ed. *Closing the Gap: The Burden of Unnecessary Illness*. New York, NY: Oxford University Press Inc; 1987:72–82.

141. Nicolucci A, Cavaliere D, Scorpiglione N, Carinci F, Capani F, Tognoni G, Benedetti MM, The SID-AMD Italian Study Group for the Implementation of the St. Vincent Declaration. A comprehensive assessment of the avoidability of long-term complications of diabetes. *Diabetes Care*. 1996;19(9):927–933.

142. Harris M, Eastman R. Early detection of undiagnosed non-insulin-dependent diabetes mellitus. *JAMA*. 1996;276:1261–1262.

143. Eastman RC, Javitt JC, Herman WH, Dasbach EJ, Harris MI. Prevention strategies for non-insulin-dependent diabetes mellitus: An economic perspective. In: LeRoith D, Taylor SI, Olefsky JM. eds. *Diabetes Mellitus: A Fundamental and Clinical Text*. Philadelphia, Pa: Lippincott-Raven Publishers; 1996:621–630.

144. The Diabetes Control and Complications Trial Research Group. Lifetime benefits and costs of intensive therapy as practiced in the Diabetes Control and Complications Trial. *JAMA*. 1996;276:1409–1415.

145. Harris MI. Medical care for patients with diabetes: epidemiologic aspects. *Ann Intern Med*. 1996;124(1 pt 2):117–122.

146. CDC. National Center for Chronic Disease Prevention and Health Promotion Division of Diabetes Translation 1997 Program Review.

147. Bell RA, Passaro K, Lengerich E, Norman M. Preventive-care knowledge and practices among persons with diabetes mellitus—North Carolina, Behavioral Risk Factor Surveillance System, 1994-1995. *MMWR*. 1997;46(43): 1023–1027.

148. Calonge N, Berman D, Dunn T, et al. Diabetes-specific preventive-care practices among adults in a managed-care population—Colorado Behavioral Risk Factor Surveillance System, 1995. *MMWR*. 46(43);1018–1023.

149. Roesler J, Bishop D, Walseth J. Economic cost of diabetes mellitus-Minnesota, 1988. *MMWR.*. 1991;40:229–231.

150. Anderson LA, Bruner LA, Satterfield D. Diabetes Control Programs: new directions. *Diabetes Educ*. 1995;21(5):432–438.

151. Glasgow RE. A practical model of diabetes management and education. *Diabetes Care*.1995; 18:117–126.

152. Vinicor F. Is diabetes a public-health disorder? *Diabetes Care*.1994;17(suppl 1):22–27.

153. Solberg LI, Reger LA, Pearson TL, Cherney LM, O'Connor PJ, Freeman SL, Bishop DB. Using continuous quality improvement to improve diabetes care in populations: The IDEAL model. *J Qual Improvement*. 1997; 23(11):581–592.

154. Bishop D, O'Connor P, Clark C. Project IDEAL: Innovative partnerships to improve diabetes care. Paper presented at: The HMO Group and CDC Diabetes Symposium, Atlanta, Ga: September 1996.

155. National Diabetes Education Program (NDEP): A joint program supported by the National Institutes of Health and Centers for Disease Control and

Prevention. Planning the National Diabetes Education Program: Executive Summary. June 1997.

156. Wong FL. The National Diabetes Education Program. Paper presented at:12th National Conference on Chronic Disease Prevention and Control: Prevention Opportunities for the 21st Century, December 1997; Washington, DC.

157. US Dept of Health and Human Services. *Prevention Report: Reducing Diabetes Morbidity and Mortality.* Washington, DC: US Public Health Service; September 1991.

158. Heath GW, Leonard BE, Wilson RH, Kendrick JS, Powell KE. Community-based exercise intervention: Zuni Diabetes Project. *Diabetes Care.* 1987;10: 579–583.

159. Heath GW et al. Community-based exercise and weight control: Diabetes risk reduction and glycemic control in Zuni Indians. *Am J Clin Nutr.* 1994; 53(suppl 6):1642S–1646S.

160. Macaulay AC, Paradis G, Potvin L, et al. The Kahnawake schools diabetes prevention project: Intervention, evaluation, and baseline results of a diabetes primary prevention program with a Native community in Canada. *Prev Med.* 1997;26:779–790.

161. Bishop DB, Kollmeyer AL, Bluhm JH, Roesler JS, Stone SA, Perry CL. A comparison of American Indian, African American, and White early elementary school children on diet and physical activity measures. Paper presented at: the Eighteenth Annual Scientific Sessions of the Society of Behavioral Medicine, April 1997; San Francisco, Calif.

162. Kollmeyer A, Bishop D, Perry C, Bluhm J, Stone S. WOLF-A school based primary prevention of diabetes project for urban American Indian youth. Paper presented at: Annual Meeting of the American Public Health Association; November 1997; Indianapolis, Indiana.

163. Wagner EH. Population-based management of diabetes care. *Patient Educ Couns.* 1995;26(1-3):225–230.

164. Michigan Diabetes Research and Training Center. *Diabetes in Communities, II.* Ann Arbor, Mich: University of Michigan; 1992.

165. Stepien CJ, Bowbeer MA, Hiss RG. Screening for diabetic retinopathy in communities. *Diabetes Educ.* 1992;18:115-120.

166. NIDDK. *Diabetes Overview.* NIH Publication No. 96-3873. October 1995.

167. Peters AL, Legorreta AP, Ossorio RC, Davidson MB. Quality of

outpatient care provided to diabetes patients: An HMO experience. *Diabetes Care.* 1996;19:601–606.

168. Miller KL, Hirsch IB. Physicians' practices in screening for the development of diabetic retinopathy and the use of glycosylated hemoglobin levels. *Diabetes Care* 1994;17:1495–1497.

169. Marrero DG. Current effectiveness of diabetes health care in the U.S. *Diabetes Rev.* 1994;2:292–309.

170. Kenny SJ, Smith PJ, Goldschmid MG, Newman JM, Herman WH. Survey of physician practice behaviors related to diabetes mellitus in the U.S. *Diabetes Care.* 1993;16:1507–1510.

171. Hiss RG, Anderson RM, Hess GE, Stepien CJ, Davis WK. Community diabetes care: A 10-year perspective. *Diabetes Care.* 1994;17:1124–1134.

172. American Diabetes Association: Clinical practice recommendations 1998. *Diabetes Care.* 1998;21(suppl 1).

173. Nathan DM, Singer DE, Schaffran R, Latkin M, McKitrick C. Glycemic control in diabetes mellitus: have changes in therapy made a difference? *Am J Med.* 1996;100(2):157–163

174. Eastman RC, Harris M, Garfield SA, Kotsanos J. Model of complications of NIDDM. II.

Analysis of the health benefits and cost-effectiveness of treating NIDDM with the goal of normoglycemia. *Diabetes Care.* 1997;20(5):735–744.

175. Kaplan RM, Atkins CJ, Wilson DK. The cost-utility of diet and exercise interventions in non-insulin-dependent diabetes mellitus. *Health Promotion.* 1988;2:331–340.

176. Harris MI. Classification, diagnostic criteria, and screening for diabetes. In: Harris MI, Cowie CC, Stern MP et al., eds. *Diabetes in America.* 2nd ed. National Institutes of Health, National Institute of Diabetes and Digestive and Kidney Diseases; 1995;2:15–36.

177. Vinicor F. Features of macrovascular disease of diabetes. In: Haire-Joshu D, ed. *Management of Diabetes Mellitus: Perspectives of Care Across the Life Span,* 2nd ed. St. Louis, Mo: Mosby,1996.

178. Stern MP. Do non-insulin-dependent diabetes mellitus and cardiovascular disease share common antecedents? *Ann Intern Med.* 1996;124(1 Pt 2):110–116.

179. Wishner KL. Diabetes mellitus: its impact on women. *Int J Fertil Menopausal Stud.* 1996;41(2):177–186.

180. Lasker RD. The Diabetes Control and Complications Trial: putting prevention into practice

under health care reform. *Diabetes Rev.* 1994;2(4):350–358.

181. Vinicor F. Barriers to the translation of the Diabetes Control and Complications Trial. *Diabetes Rev.* 1994;2(4):371–383.

182. Thompson CJ, Cummings JFR, Chalmers J, Gould C, Newton RW. How have patients reacted to the implications of the DCCT? *Diabetes Care.* 1996;19(8):876–879.

183. Lorenz RA, Bubb J, Davis D, et al. Changing behavior: practical lessons from the Diabetes Control and Complications Trial. *Diabetes Care.* 1996;19(6):648–652.

184. U.K. Prospective Diabetes Study Group. U.K. Prospective Diabetes Study 16: Overview of 6 years' therapy of type II diabetes: a progressive disease. *Diabetes.* 1995;44;1249–1258.

185. Greenfield S, Kaplan SH, Silliman RA, et al. The uses of outcomes research for medical effectiveness, quality of care, and reimbursement in type II diabetes. *Diabetes Care.* 1994; 17(suppl 1):32–39.

186. Quickel KE Jr. Managed care and diabetes, with special attention to the issue of who should provide care. *Trans Am Clin Climatol Assoc.* 1996;108: 184–195.

187. Peters AL. Commentary. *Diabetes Spectrum* 1996;9(3):175.

188. Sidorov J, Harris R. The integrated approach to diabetes mellitus: the impact of clinical information systems, consumerism, and managed care. *Diabetes Spectrum* 1996;9(3):158–163.

189. O'Connor PJ, Lasch S, Keogh C, Cherney L, Morben P. Continuous quality improvement can improve glycemic control for HMO patients with diabetes. *Arch Fam Med* 1996;5(9):502–506.

190. Minnesota Dept of Health. *Diabetes and Quality Improvement: A Guide for Primary Care.* Minneapolis, Minn: Minnesota Dept of Health;, 1995.

191. American Diabetes Association Consensus Statement. The pharmacological treatment of hyperglycemia in NIDDM. *Diabetes Care.* 1995;18:1510–1518.

192. O'Rahilly S. Science, medicine, and the future. Non-insulin dependent diabetes mellitus: the gathering storm. *BMJ.* 1997; 314(7085):955–959.

193. The U. K. Prospective Diabetes Study Group. Prospective diabetes study 16: overview of 6 years' therapy of type II diabetes: a progressive disease. *Diabetes.* 1995;44:1249-1258.

194. Larsen JL, Stratta RJ. Pancreas transplantation: a treatment

option for insulin-dependent diabetes mellitus. *Diabetes Metab.* 1996;22(2):139–146.

195. Harris MI. Medical care for patients with diabetes. Epidemiologic aspects. *Ann Intern Med.* 1996;124:117-122.

196. Curhan GC, Willett WC, Rimm EB, Spiegelman D, Ascherio AL, Stampfer MJ. Birth weight and adult hypertension, diabetes mellitus, and obesity in US men. *Circulation.* 1996;94(12):3246–3250.

SUGGESTED READING

American Diabetes Association: Clinical practice recommendations 1998. *Diabetes Care.* 1998;21(suppl 1). Available at: http:// www.niddk.nih.gov/. Accessed August 30, 1998.

Centers for Disease Control and Prevention. *Take Charge of Your Diabetes.* 2nd ed. Atlanta, Ga: Dept. of Health and Human Services, 1997. Available at: http://www. cdc.gov/nccdphp/ddt/. Accessed August 30, 1998.

Centers for Disease Control. *Diabetes: A Serious Public Health Problem: At-A-Glance 1996.* Atlanta, Ga; 1996. Available at: http://www.cdc.gov/nccdphp/ddt/. Accessed August 30, 1998.

National Institutes of Health. *Diabetes in African Americans.* Washington, DC; March 1997. NIH Publication 97-3266. Available at: http://www.niddk. nih.gov/DIAA/afam.htm. Accessed August 30, 1998.

National Diabetes Data Group. *Diabetes in America,* 2nd ed. Washington, DC: National Institutes of Health, National Institute of Diabetes and Digestive and Kidney Diseases; 1995. NIH publication 95-1468. Available at: http://diabetes-in-america.s-3.com/ Accessed September 23, 1998

National Institutes of Health. *Diabetes in Hispanic Americans.* Washington, DC; April 1997. NIH publication 97-3266. Available at: http://www.niddk.nih.gov/ HISPAN/hispan.htm. Accessed August 30, 1998.

The Expert Committee on the Diagnosis and Classification of Diabetes Mellitus. Report of the Expert Committee on the Diagnosis and Classification of Diabetes Mellitus. *Diabetes Care.* 1997;20(7):1183—1197. Available at: http://www.diabetes.org/. Accessed August 30, 1998.

National Diabetes Fact Sheet. http:// www.cdc.gov/nccdphp/ddt/ facts.htm. Accessed August 30, 1998.

RESOURCES

American Association of Diabetes
Educators
444 N. Michigan Ave., Suite 1240
Chicago, IL 60611
(800) 338-3633 or (312) 644-2233
http://www.diabetesnet.com/
aade.html

American Diabetes Association
1660 Duke Street
Alexandria, VA 22314
(800)-DIABETES (800-342-2383)
http://www.diabetes.org

Division of Diabetes Translation
National Center for Chronic Disease
Prevention and Health Promo-
tion
Centers for Disease Control and
Prevention
4770 Buford Highway NE, Mailstop
K-10
Atlanta, GA 30341-3724
Tel: (770) 448-5015 Fax: (770) 488-
5966
http://www.cdc.gov/diabetes

Juvenile Diabetes Foundation
International
120 Wall Street
New York, NY 10005-4001
(212) 785-9500
http://www.jdfcure.com

National Diabetes Information
Clearinghouse
1 Information Way
Bethesda, MD 20892-3560
Tel: (301) 654-3327 Fax: (301) 907-
8906
E-mail: ndic@aerie.com
http://www.aerie.com/nihdb/ndic/
dmdbase.html

National Institute of Diabetes and
Digestive and Kidney Diseases
of the National Institutes of Health
http://www.niddk.nih.gov

15

ARTHRITIS AND OTHER MUSCULOSKELETAL DISEASES

ICD-9 274, 710-739

Arthritis and musculoskeletal diseases are the most common causes of physical disability in the United States.[1] Arthritis was second only to sinusitis as the most common chronic condition reported in the 1989–1991 National Health Interview Survey (NHIS). According to the NHIS data, 15% of the US population reported having arthritis. By applying this prevalence to 1990 population figures, an estimated 37.9 million individuals are affected.[2] Females are affected more often than males, and prevalence rises with increasing age (Figure 15.1).[3]

According to 1989–1991 NHIS data on the epidemiology of arthritis and self-reported disability, 49.5% of all interviewees aged 65 and over reported having arthritis or rheumatism.[2] Disability, which is defined as some difficulty in performing one or more activities of daily living or instrumental activities of daily living

Jean C. Scott, DrPH, RN
Marc C. Hochberg, MD, MPH

such as dressing or eating, was present in 43% of interviewees. Groups with higher rates of arthritis and disability included elderly people; females; Blacks and Hispanics; people with little education; people with low incomes; people who are widowed, separated, or divorced; people living alone or with a nonspouse; and people living in regions of the United States other than the Northeast. Verbrugge and colleagues noted that people with other chronic diseases or illnesses (ie, comorbidity) and people who were either underweight (body mass index [BMI] <20 kg/m^2) or severely overweight (BMI ≥30 kg/m^2) were also more likely to have arthritis resulting in disability.[4]

Musculoskeletal diseases such as arthritis are a heavy economic burden in the United States. The total cost to the US economy (including in-patient and out-patient care, nursing home care, medications, and lost productivity) in 1988 of arthritis has been estimated at $54.6 billion. Overall costs of fractures added $20 billion to this

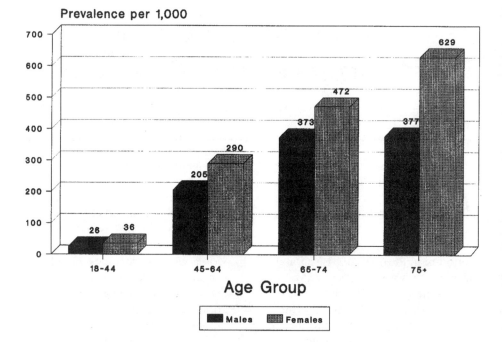

Prevalence per 1,000

Figure 15.1—Prevalence of self-reported arthritis by age and sex, National Health Interview Survey, 1990.[4]

amount.[5] The National Hospital Discharge Survey estimates that hospitalizations for arthritis and related disorders accounted for 2.9 million days of hospital care in 1988. Data from the 1984–1986 NHIS indicated that more than 16 million persons reported having some musculoskeletal condition, resulting in more than 122 million physician visits and 4 million hospitalizations. [6, 7] The use of such health services is greatly increased among people who have another chronic condition (Table 15.1).[7] Overall, 62% of the survey's respon-

dents who had musculoskeletal conditions had at least some limitation in their activities, and 22% were limited in activities of daily living. By comparison, of the overall US population, 14% had some limitation in their activities and 13% were limited in activities of daily living.[7]

More than 100 diseases make up the spectrum of arthritis and musculoskeletal disorders. Most of these diseases are uncommon, are of unknown cause, and allow little opportunity for primary or secondary prevention in the general population.[8]

Table 15.1—Average Annual Per Capita Medical Care Use and Prevalence of Activity Limitation among Persons with Musculoskeletal Conditions by Presence of Comorbid Disease, United States, 1984-86

	Persons with Musculoskeletal Conditions	
	Comorbidity[a] Present	No Comobidity Present
Physician visits/subject	9.6	4.5
Hospitalizations/subject	0.3	0.1
Length of hospital stays (days)/subject	8.2	6.7
Proportion with activity limitation	72%	39%
Proportion with limitation in activities of daily living	27%	8%

Note: Adapted from Yelin and Felts.[7]
[a]Comorbidity indicates another chronic disease or illness.

However, two disorders, osteoarthritis and osteoporosis, make up the vast majority of the disability and economic costs and are subject to primary and secondary prevention initiatives. The remainder of this chapter reviews the epidemiology of these conditions as well as the opportunities for their prevention and control. In addition, shorter descriptions are provided for two other common types of arthritis: rheumatoid arthritis and gout.

OSTEOARTHRITIS

ICD-9 715

SIGNIFICANCE

The prevalence of osteoarthritis has been estimated in two national studies: the National Health Examination Survey (NHES) and the first National Health and Nutrition Examination Survey (NHANES-I), conducted from 1971 to 1975. The case definitions were based on x-ray changes in the hands and feet in NHES and on x-ray changes in knees and hips in NHANES-I. NHANES-I is the only national survey that has included x-ray data for the knees and hips. A physician's clinical diagnosis was also available in NHANES-I. Overall, about one-third of adults aged 25 to 74 years had x-ray evidence of osteoarthritis involving at least one site. Specifically, 33% had x-ray changes of definite osteoarthritis of the hands, 21% of the feet, and 4% of the knee.[9] Among people aged 55 to 74, corresponding rates were about 70% for the hands, 40% for the feet, 10% for the knees, and 3% for the hips.

Overall, a clinical diagnosis of osteoarthritis—that is, based on both x-ray findings and patient symptoms—was made by the examining physician in 12% of examinees aged 25 to 74 years in NHANES-I.[9]

PATHOPHYSIOLOGY

Osteoarthritis, also known as degenerative joint disease, is defined as a "heterogeneous group of conditions that lead to joint symptoms and signs that are associated with defective integrity of articular (joint) cartilage, in addition to related changes in the underlying bone and at joint margins."[10] The pathophysiologic basis of osteoarthritis is a biomechanical alteration in the properties of articular cartilage that affects the joint and surrounding tissue. These biomechanical alterations lead to loss of cartilage in areas of increased load, thickening of underlying bone, formation of spurs or marginal osteophytes (evidence of repair), and a variable degree of inflammation. The clinical features of osteoarthritis, including pain, tenderness, swelling, and decreased function, result from these biomechanical and morphologic alterations.[11]

DESCRIPTIVE EPIDEMIOLOGY

High-Risk Groups

The incidence of osteoarthritis increases with advancing age.[12]

Prevalence of osteoarthritis, as well as the proportion of cases with moderate or severe disease, also increases with age at least through ages 65 to 74 years.[12] These findings are consistent with observations of excess mortality in elderly subjects with symptomatic osteoarthritis.[13]

Osteoarthritis is more common among males than among females under age 45 and more common among females than among males over age 54.[9] Clinically, patterns of joint involvement also demonstrate sex differences, with females having on average more joints involved and more frequent complaints of morning stiffness and joint swelling. Among adults in the United States, knee osteoarthritis is more common among Blacks than among Whites.[14] No racial differences have been noted for hip osteoarthritis.[15]

Other groups at higher risk of osteoarthritis include (1) people with a genetic predisposition, especially females with the syndrome of bony nodes, usually in the joints of the fingers; (2) people with congenital or developmental disease of bones and joints, such as congenital hip subluxation and ipsilateral hip osteoarthritis; (3) people with prior inflammatory joint disease, such as gout or rheumatoid arthritis; and (4) people with metabolic diseases such as hyperparathyroidism, hypothyroidism, and chrondocalcinosis.

Geographic Distribution

Data from national surveys suggest that arthritis and associated disabilities are most prevalent in the South and least prevalent in the Northeast.[6] Possible explanations for these patterns include a lower socioeconomic status and greater proportion of population employed in manual labor in the South. No specific studies have been conducted to determine reasons for these regional variations, however.

Time Trends

No data are available on time trends in the prevalence of osteoarthritis in the United States. The National Center for Health Statistics has finished data collection for NHANES-III, which includes the collection of data on x-rays of the hands and knees. When these data become available, they may be useful in comparing the prevalence of osteoarthritis with the prevalence based on earlier national surveys.

Risk factors for the development of osteoarthritis have been the subject of many studies. Results will only be summarized here, and readers are referred to the bibliography for more detailed reviews and citations to original studies.

Magnitude of Risk Factors

The major modifiable risk factors for osteoarthritis are joint trauma, obesity, and repetitive joint usage (Table 15.2).[16] A history of joint trauma is the strongest risk factor for unilateral osteoarthritis at either the knee[17] or the hip.[15]

Obesity has been convincingly demonstrated to have a causal role in osteoarthritis of the knee. In cross-sectional studies, obesity as measured by body mass index is a strong risk factor for both unilateral and bilateral knee osteoarthritis in both sexes.[14, 17] Furthermore, in longitudinal studies, obesity predicts the development of knee osteoarthritis in

Table 15.2—Modifiable Risk Factors for Osteoarthritis,[a] United States

Magnitude	Risk Factor
Strong (relative risk[b] >4)	Joint trauma
Moderate (relative risk 2–4)	Repetitive occupational usage
	Obesity
Weak (relative risk <2)	None

[a]Risk factors differ in their magnitude based on the site of osteoarthritis involved.
[b]Relative risk is defined in Table 2.4, page 51.

both sexes.[18] Weight loss decreases the risk of developing symptomatic knee osteoarthritis in women.[19] Data regarding the association of obesity with both hand and hip osteoarthritis, however, are inconsistent.[15, 16, 20, 21]

Repetitive joint use, largely the result of occupational demands, is also associated with osteoarthritis. Numerous studies have demonstrated an excess of site-specific osteoarthritis in occupational groups with repetitive use of specific joints. Occupations requiring knee-bending have been associated with knee osteoarthritis in both retrospective and prospective studies.[14, 18] Farming has been associated with hip osteoarthritis in several retrospective studies.[21, 22] However, avocational activities, including running and other sports activities, have not been associated with the development of osteoarthritis among people who have not had joint injuries.

In the studies of socioeconomic factors associated with osteoarthritis, having less than 12 years of formal education and having a low family income were each associated with a clinical diagnosis of osteoarthritis;[7]

however, neither factor was associated with the presence of knee or hip osteoarthritis diagnosed on the basis of x-ray criteria.[14, 15, 23]

Population-Attributable Risk

Although attributable risk estimates are not available for multiple sites of osteoarthritis, estimates for osteoarthritis of the knee are available (Table 15.3).[18] These estimates indicate that repetitive occupational joint-bending and obesity account for large portions of knee osteoarthritis.

PREVENTION AND CONTROL MEASURES

Prevention

Epidemiologic considerations in the primary prevention of osteoarthritis have been reviewed elsewhere.[16] On the basis of current knowledge of risk factors, avoiding joint trauma, preventing obesity, and modifying occupational-related joint stress through ergonomic approaches can all be recommended for the prevention of osteoarthritis. National recommendations include reducing obesity (BMI >27.8 for men and

Table 15.3—Proportion of Osteoarthritis of the Knees[a] Attributed to Various Modifiable Risk Factors, United States

Factor	Best Estimate (%)	Range (%)
Obesity	19	13.5–24
Occupational knee bending	13.5	6–21

[a]Adapted from Felson;[18] population attributable risk is defined in Table 2.4, page 51.

>27.3 for women) to a prevalence of no more than 20% among adults and 15% among adolescents and reducing the number of nonfatal unintentional injuries, especially those that are work related. Reduction of weight has been shown to reduce pain in symptomatic osteoarthritis of the knee.[19]

Screening and Early Detection

Screening and early detection of osteoarthritis are not feasible at present.

Treatment, Rehabilitation, and Recovery

Multidisciplinary treatment of osteoarthritis is required. This involves the use of analgesics and/or nonsteroidal anti-inflammatory drugs to control symptoms of pain and stiffness; physical therapy to maintain and improve joint range of motion and muscle strength; and occupational therapy to maximize the patient's independent ability to perform activities of daily living including dressing, feeding, bathing, toileting, and grooming. Surgery, especially total joint replacement, is indicated in patients with severe pain and/or limitation of physical activities who have failed to respond to medical therapy; indeed, osteoarthritis is the most common indication for elective total hip replacement among Medicare recipients aged 65 and over.[24]

Increasing evidence indicates that people with arthritis are less physically active and less fit than their peers.[25] They can benefit significantly from conditioning exercise programs to improve both cardiovascular and musculoskeletal fitness without disease exacerbation or joint damage.[26]

EXAMPLES OF PUBLIC HEALTH INTERVENTIONS

Several states, including Maryland, Michigan, Missouri, and Ohio, have set up task forces on arthritis to document the extent of the impact of arthritis and musculoskeletal diseases on their populations. One such program, the Missouri Arthritis Program,[27] consists of a state arthritis advisory board and seven regional arthritis centers that provide education programs for patients, the community, and nonarthritis specialists who treat arthritis patients. The education programs provide patients with information on the causes and types of arthritis, the nature and types of available treatments, sources of long-term care, exercise and self-management classes, and sources of additional information about arthritis.[27, 28]

The Arthritis Self-Help Course was designed in 1979 by the Stanford University Arthritis Center[29] and was adopted by the Arthritis Foundation for national dissemination in 1982.

Studies involving more than 2500 participants have indicated that applying the Arthritis Self-Help Course results in increased knowledge about arthritis, improved healthy behaviors (exercise, adherence, self-care), psychosocial well-being, and health status, as well as decreased health care utilization.[29]

AREAS OF FUTURE RESEARCH AND DEMONSTRATION

If the Missouri program proves to be effective in improving the quality of life for arthritis patients, then the establishment of similar programs in other states should be pursued. According to a 1990 survey of state health departments, only four states have developed objectives for statewide arthritis prevention programs.[30] Although arthritis and musculoskeletal diseases are the major causes of disability among older Americans, statewide programs for arthritis control are not a high priority in most states.

RHEUMATOID ARTHRITIS

ICD-9 714

SIGNIFICANCE

Rheumatoid arthritis is an autoimmune disease involving chronic inflammation. The inflammation begins in the synovial membranes of the joints and spreads to other joint tissues. Outgrowths of the inflamed tissue may invade and damage the cartilage in the joints and erode bone, leading to joint deformities. The usual clinical symptoms include stiffness, pain, and swelling of multiple joints, commonly the small joints of the hands and wrists. Although it primarily affects the joints, rheumatoid arthritis can also affect the connective tissue throughout the body and can cause disease in a variety of organs, including the lungs, the heart, and the eyes.

According to the NHES data, the prevalence of definite rheumatoid arthritis is almost 1.0% among adults aged 18 years and older.[9] A similar prevalence estimate (0.8%) was found from physical examinations done by physicians in NHANES-I.[9]

DESCRIPTIVE EPIDEMIOLOGY

In general, the prevalence of rheumatoid arthritis increases with age in both sexes. In addition, prevalence rates are two to three times greater among females than among males. No striking differences in morbidity rates have been noted between Blacks and Whites. Several Native American tribes, however, have a particularly high prevalence of rheumatoid arthritis, including the Yakima of central Washington State and the Mille-Lac Band of Chippewa in Minnesota. Asians, including

Japanese and Chinese, appear to have lower prevalence rates than do Whites.[31] The reasons for these differences are unknown, but they may relate to both genetic and environmental factors.

RISK FACTORS

Although the causes of rheumatoid arthritis are unknown, genetic factors play an important role in a person's predisposition to rheumatoid arthritis. The disease exhibits familial aggregation and a higher concordance rate in monozygotic (identical) twins than in dizygotic (fraternal) twins.[32] In addition, the susceptibility to rheumatoid arthritis appears to be inherited as an autosomal dominant trait in multicase families. Studies have demonstrated a strong association between the Class II major histocompatibility antigen (HLA-DR4) and rheumatoid arthritis. In Whites, the relative risk for this association exceeds 5.0. This association also crosses ethnic and racial boundaries, with just a few exceptions, such as the Yakima of Washington State, Asian Indians, Greeks, and Israeli Jews. In Whites who lack HLA-DR4 and in these other racial and ethnic groups, an association exists between rheumatoid arthritis and HLA-DR1. The role of other MHC genes in disease susceptibility has been suggested by several studies but is not established.[31, 32]

A protective effect of the use of oral contraceptives on the development of rheumatoid arthritis has been suggested by a number of studies.[32] However, a recent meta-analysis has failed to support this observation; it concludes that there may be some evidence for protection for severe forms of rheumatoid arthritis.[33]

Rheumatoid arthritis is associated with excess mortality. Causes of death that are more frequent in rheumatoid arthritis patients include respiratory and infectious diseases and gastrointestinal disorders. Although the proportionate mortality from cancer is reduced in rheumatoid arthritis, the actual incidence of and mortality from non-Hodgkin's lymphoma is higher for these patients than for the general population. Some of the excess mortality caused by gastrointestinal disorders may be related to the complications of therapy for the arthritis. Low socioeconomic status, as measured by education level, is also associated with increased mortality and excess disability.

PREVENTION AND CONTROL MEASURES

No screening or primary prevention measures are available at present. Treatment of rheumatoid arthritis is similar to that for osteoarthritis. In addition, patients with rheumatoid arthritis are usually treated with second-line antirheumatic drugs such as hydroxychloroquine, gold compounds, methotrexate, penicillamine, azathioprine, and other immunosuppressive agents.

Because of the excess mortality from respiratory and infectious diseases among patients with rheumatoid arthritis, the single most important public health intervention available is immunization with pneumococcal vaccine and an annual influenza vaccine.

Growing evidence shows that participation in conditioning levels of regular, moderate physical activity improves health status, emotional well being, and physical fitness without aggravation of rhematoid arthritis.[25]

GOUT

ICD-9 274

SIGNIFICANCE

Gout is a metabolic disease characterized by recurrent attacks of acute arthritis, an increase in serum uric acid concentration (hyperuricemia), and deposition of sodium urate monohydrate crystals in and around joints. Because gout is relatively easy to diagnose, most reports of prevalence are based on self-reported physician diagnosis—that is, the patient's response to the question, "Have you been told by a physician that you have gout?" Concerns about the validity of such data have been raised, however. It has been suggested that the classification criteria proposed by the American Rheumatism Association be used for case validation in epidemiologic studies.[9]

DESCRIPTIVE EPIDEMIOLOGY

The most recent estimates of the prevalence of gout in the United States are based on patients' responses to the question, "Have you had gout within the last year?" in the 1986 NHIS.[9] The prevalence rates were 13.5 per 1000 for men and 6.4 per 1000 for women. Prevalence rates increased sharply with age for both sexes and were greater among Blacks than among Whites over age 45. Based on comparable data from the 1969 NHIS, the prevalence rate of gout has increased as much as fourfold in both sexes over a 17-year period.[9] The increase in gout prevalence is the result of (1) a temporal increase in mean serum uric acid levels among men; (2) increased use of drugs known to produce secondary hyperuricemia, especially diuretics used by women; and (3) longer survival by people with gout. Also, part of the apparent increase may be artifactual and attributable to the incorrect diagnosis of individuals with joint pain and hyperuricemia who do not actually have gout. The most recent estimates of the annual incidence of gout in adults from the

Framingham Study were 3.2 per 1000 for White men and 0.5 per 1000 for White women.[34]

RISK FACTORS

In addition to having hyperuricemia and being male, other risk factors for gout include high blood pressure, obesity, consumption of alcohol (especially moonshine), renal disease, occupational and environmental lead exposure, and a family history of gout.[35, 36] Numerous family studies suggest a multifactorial inheritance, and environmental factors probably contribute significantly to the familial aggregation.

PREVENTION AND CONTROL MEASURES

The prevention of gout in people with asymptomatic hyperuricemia should include lifestyle modifications such as weight reduction, dietary changes, moderating or eliminating alcohol intake, and control of hypertension (without the use of diuretics) and hyperlipidemia. In addition, because of the known association of occupational lead exposure with gout, prevention efforts should also reduce such exposure in high-risk professions such as painting, plumbing, shipbuilding, and steel work.

Hyperuricemia is a known necessary risk factor for the development of gout and can be readily identified in normal people through automated multichannel analysis of serum specimens. The decision as to when to treat people with asymptomatic hyperuricemia is controversial. Several practical arguments against routine treatment include poor patient compliance, high costs, and adverse drug reactions. Furthermore, acute gout attacks are easily, inexpensively, and effectively treated with short courses of nonsteroidal anti-inflammatory drugs.

Medical treatment of gout is at the stage where recurrent attacks of arthritis may be prevented through long-term use of colchicine and through reversal of hyperuricemia with agents that either increase uric acid excretion or inhibit its production. The control strategies for gout should be employed in conjunction with treatment of associated conditions such as hypertension and hyperlipidemia.

OSTEOPOROSIS

ICD-9 733

SIGNIFICANCE

Osteoporosis is a major public health problem in countries with aging populations. An estimated 20 million people in the United States are affected, and approximately 1.3 million related fractures occur each year.[37] About 281 000 of these are hip fractures,[38] costing more than $8.7 billion a year for acute and chronic care.[5] The National Nursing Home Survey reported 66 300 admissions for hip fracture in 1985.

PATHOPHYSIOLOGY

Osteoporosis can be defined as a bone disorder in which the reduction of bone tissue per unit volume of anatomic bone compromises the skeleton to the extent that fractures occur with minimal or trivial trauma.[39] The clinical manifestations may include fractures of the spine, hip, wrist, or other areas of the skeleton. Traditionally, fractures of the hip among older adults, especially when they occur in association with minimal or moderate trauma, have been considered to be related to osteoporosis. Many epidemiologic studies use fracture as a surrogate measure of osteoporosis because of lack of access to technology to measure bone density. Therefore, the epidemiology of osteoporosis is a combination of both the epidemiology of low bone density and the epidemiology of fracture.

DESCRIPTIVE EPIDEMIOLOGY

High-Risk Groups

Although osteoporosis is usually considered a woman's disease, both men and women lose bone mass with aging. Peak bone mass is higher in men than in women, so the loss for men proceeds from a higher baseline. In NHANES-III, where bone density of the hip was measured as part of the examination men had higher bone density than women in every racial group reported (Figure 15.2).[37] In addition, women experience an accelerated rate of bone loss after menopause. Not surprisingly, age-specific incidence rates for hip fracture are higher among women than among men through the ninth decade (Figure 15.3).[39]

In Western populations, Blacks have higher bone density and fewer hip fractures than Whites (Figures 15.2 and 15.3). Age-specific incidence rates of hip fracture are about twice as high among White women as they are among Black women,[40] and most studies indicate a higher risk for hip fractures among White men than among Black men. Mexican-American populations have lower hip fracture rates than Whites but slightly higher rates than Blacks.[41] Bone density is lower in Asians than in Whites, but Asians may experience a lower incidence of hip fracture.[42]

Twin and family studies suggest that genetic factors may explain as much as 75% of the variation in age-specific bone density in the population. Genetics may play the largest role in attainment of peak bone mass and probably has a lesser role in the rate of bone loss with aging or after

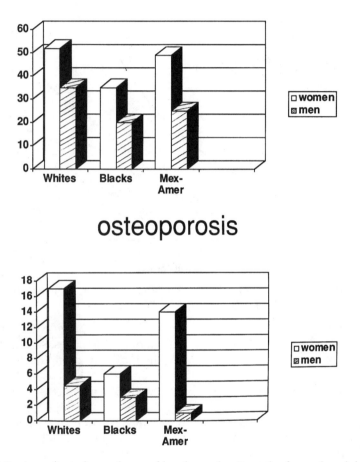

Figure 15.2—Age-adjusted prevalence of low bone density at the femoral neck by sex and race/ethnicity, ages 50 years and older, United States, 1988–1994 (NHANES-III). Adapted from Looker et al.[38]

menopause. The search for single gene effects on bone density is an active area of investigation. Allelic variations of the vitamin D receptor are associated with bone density in some, but not all populations studied. Other candidate genes, such as estrogen receptor genes and genes for collagen, may also play important roles in the regulation of bone

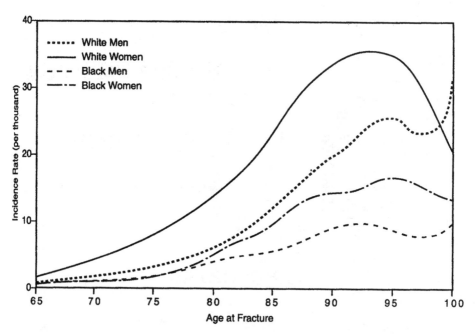

Figure 15.3—Annual age-specific incidence of hip fracture among the elderly by sex and race, United States, 1984–1987[40]

density, either alone or through an interaction with lifestyle factors.[43–46]

The rate of bone loss in women increases during natural and surgically induced menopause. Women who undergo early surgical menopause and do not receive exogenous estrogens are at an increased risk of hip fracture.[47] In addition, women who undergo a relatively early natural menopause appear to be at some increased risk of fracture.[48]

Geographic Distribution

Currently, no reports of large national or international population studies of bone density have been published to provide data on geographic differences, so differences in the incidence of hip fracture have been used as a proxy measure. Internationally, the highest rates of hip fracture are found in the Scandanavian countries, followed by the United States and western Europe.[49]

Jacobsen and colleagues studied regional variations in hip fracture incidence among White women in the United States.[50] By calculating age-specific rates of hip fracture at the county level, they identified a north-south gradient of increasing hip fracture occurrence, with a cluster of high incidence in the Southeast. The explanation for this phenomenon is unclear.

Time Trends

No population studies measuring bone density over time have been conducted, but time trends in fracture rates have been studied. The results of a study of US hospital discharge rates for hip fracture, based on data collected in the National Hospital Discharge Survey, indicate that the age-, race-, and sex-adjusted rates increased slightly from 28.9 per 10 000 in 1970 to 30.9 per 10 000 in 1983.[51] The increase was most pronounced in the 65- to 74-year age group, which experienced an increase of 16.5%. In Rochester, Minnesota, the Mayo Clinic database gives evidence of a rise of 53% in age-adjusted hip fracture rates between 1940 and 1980.[49] Several

studies suggest that recent increases may affect men differentially.[52]

RISK FACTORS

A number of conditions and lifestyle factors are associated with osteoporosis and osteoporotic fractures (Table 15.4). (See the Suggested Readings for more detailed reviews and original citations.)

Magnitude of Risk Factors

Prolonged periods of immobility result in substantial risk for osteoporosis.(see Table 15.4) In addition, thin women have lower bone density and are at a higher risk of hip fracture than are heavy women.[53] This protective effect of obesity may be related to an increased amount of biologically available estrogen after menopause in women with more adipose cells.

Table 15.4—Modifiable Risk Factors for Osteoporosis, United States

Magnitude	Risk Factor
Strong (relative risk[a] >4)	Immobility
Moderate (relative risk 2–4)	Thin body build
	Heavy alcohol use
	Chronic use of corticosteroids
	Lack of use of estrogen replacements[b]
Weak (relative risk <2)	Cigarette smoking
	Physical inactivity
	Low calcium intake

[a] Relative risk is defined in Table 2.4, page 51.
[b] Postmenopausal estrogen replacement therapy reduces risk.

Heavier women may also achieve a higher peak bone mass in early adulthood and may benefit from increased stimulus to bone through the increased bearing of weight.[54]

Alcoholism also has been implicated as a risk factor for osteoporosis.[55] The effect of consuming modest amounts of alcohol, however, does not appear to have a negative effect on bone.

Strong evidence indicates that bone mass is decreased and fracture rates are increased among patients treated over the long-term with corticosteroids, although the effect of underlying disease often confounds the relationship.[56]

Estrogen replacement therapy, started at the time of menopause (surgical or natural), seems to retard or prevent bone loss and reduce fracture risk for as long as the estrogen is taken.[57] Benefit to bone has been demonstrated with both oral and transdermal routes of administration.[52] Once a woman stops using estrogen, bone loss occurs at a rate similar to that among untreated menopausal women, and the risk of fracture increases.

The results of some studies indicate that cigarette smokers tend to have lower bone density than nonsmokers, but it is unclear whether smoking precludes the attainment of peak bone mass or accelerates the loss of bone after menopause.[58] Cigarette smoking has

also been associated with an increased risk of hip and wrist fractures.[53] Most evidence suggests that these effects are estrogen ediated.[59]

Vigorous exercise by mathletes increases bone mass above that of control subjects.[60] It is not known how long this increment in bone mass lasts after exercise stops; thus, it remains unclear whether a person can achieve lifetime protection from decreases in bone mass associated with aging by exercising early in life.[61] Prolonged or lifelong exercise programs do seem to reduce bone loss[62] and exercise may have other effects that decrease the risk of falls, such as improvements in balance, reaction time, strength, and flexibility.[63] This reduced risk of falling may, in turn, reduce the risk of fracture.

Calcium consumption in childhood, adolescence, and early adulthood seems to enhance peak bone mass.[64] Also, evidence from clinical trials supports that calcium supplementation reduces bone loss in postmenopausal women.[65] However, the role of calcium in hip fracture prevention is not entirely clear. Observational studies have had conflicting results and the clinical trial evidence of hip fracture protection in a group of nursing home patients was complicated by the use of both calcium and vitamin D_3 in the treatment group.[66]

Several studies have suggested an association between caffeine intake and hip fracture, and some evidence indicates that caffeine intake correlates negatively with bone density.[67] However, these studies did not adequately examine other lifestyle differences among people with high caffeine intake, so other factors may account for the bone density and fracture risk differences. Studies indicating higher bone mass in vegetarians also have not adjusted for other differences in lifestyle or diet.[68]

Calcium balance is positively affected by thiazide diuretics even in individuals with osteoporosis. These drugs have been associated with increased bone density, but the effect of thiazides on fracture rates has not been consistent. The protective effect may be primarily among long-term users.[69]

Population-Attributable Risk

Elimination of risk factors, especially those that are more prevalent, has the potential to reduce the occurrence of low bone density and hip fracture. Table 15.5 presents calculations of population-attributable risk for hip fractures. Because of the lack of definitive studies, attributable risk estimates for osteoporosis are not available.

PREVENTION AND CONTROL MEASURES

Prevention

The prevention of osteoporosis must focus on optimizing the attainment of peak bone mass and on slowing the rate of bone loss with aging. Measures aimed at affecting peak bone mass must begin in childhood and adolescence. These include maintaining a good diet with an adequate intake of calcium and an active lifestyle, with an emphasis on weight-bearing physical activities. Young women, in particular, should be discouraged from smoking cigarettes or drinking excessive amounts of alcohol. The ideal of extreme thinness also should be discouraged.

Table 15.5—Proportion of Hip Fractures[a] Attributed to Various Modifiable Risk Factors, United States

Factor	Best Estimate (%)	Range (%)
Nonuse of estrogen replacements	19	6–31
Thin body build	18	10.5–26
Cigarette smoking	10	4–16

Note: Adapted from Paganini-Hill et al.[70,71] Population attributable risk is defined in Table 2.4, page 51.

To slow bone loss, clinicians should consider prescribing hormone replacement therapy or another bone-preserving medication (such as a bisphosphonate or a selective estrogen receptor modulator) beginning at menopause. Again, vigorous weight-bearing exercise and adequate calcium intake should be encouraged, and smoking and heavy alcohol consumption should be discouraged.

Clinicians also should consider ways of addressing the risk factors for falling. An environmental assessment to help older men and women "fall-proof" their living areas is helpful. This may include ensuring optimal lighting, installing appropriate and graspable hand rails on stairs and in the bathroom, checking throw rugs and extension cords, and placing "soft" corners on cabinets and furniture to minimize injuries if falls occur. In addition, attention to appropriate footwear to prevent tripping is important.

Screening and Early Detection

Screening for low bone density remains somewhat controversial. There is evidence indicating that bone density measurements predict future fractures and that the level of risk can be stratified on the basis of these measurements. However, unresolved issues remain, such as the acceptability and effectiveness of screening, access to screening facilities, predictive value of measurements using some of the

new bone density and bone ultrasound instruments, and issues involving the cost of screening. The National Osteoporosis Foundation suggests the following indications for measurement of bone mass among specific population subgroups: (1) in estrogen-deficient women, to aid in decisions about hormone replacement therapy; (2) in patients with vertebral fracture or osteopenia on x-ray, to aid in decisions about further diagnostic evaluation and therapy; (3) in patients receiving long-term glucocorticoid therapy, to diagnose low bone mass and aid in decisions about therapy; and (4) in patients with asymptomatic primary hyperparathyroidism, to identify those at risk of severe skeletal disease and to aid in decisions about surgical intervention. Screening-related issues are discussed in more detail elsewhere.[72, 73]

Treatment, Rehabilitation, and Recovery

Secondary prevention involves the treatment of low bone density and the prevention of fractures. Currently, three medications (estrogen, calcitonin, and alendronate) which act to slow bone loss, are approved for treatment of osteoporosis. No currently approved drug will increase bone density once it is lost.

Prompt treatment of fractures and aggressive rehabilitation afterward, even among elderly patients, could greatly decrease long-term morbidity.

Public health nursing services, physical therapy services, and support services in the home often enable recovering fracture patients to stay in their own homes.

EXAMPLES OF PUBLIC HEALTH INTERVENTIONS

Both the National Osteoporosis Foundation and the Arthritis Foundation produce written information and informational programs to educate professional and lay audiences about osteoporosis. A model program is the exercise/education program "Stronger Body—Stronger Bones!" sponsored jointly by the University of Michigan Multipurpose Arthritis Center, the Michigan Chapter of the Arthritis Foundation, and the Michigan Department of Public Health.[74] It includes an exercise class, educational materials, and a customized home exercise program that features a videotape, audiotape, and exercise manual.

In addition, the US Consumer Product Safety Commission produces a home safety inventory checklist for older Americans that allows them to rate the safety of their homes and gives them helpful ideas to minimize falls.

AREAS OF FUTURE RESEARCH AND DEMONSTRATION

Research on osteoporosis has focused on preventing or slowing bone loss in perimenopausal women and on preventing fractures in older women. However, bone density is profoundly influenced by habits in adolescence and young adulthood. A better understanding of the factors that influence the attainment of peak bone mass in younger women will be vital to future prevention efforts. Factors that may influence risk—such as dieting practices in adolescence, age at menarche, regularity of menses, athletic activities, pregnancy, and lactation—have not been studied in sufficient detail.

For older women who are trying to slow bone loss associated with aging, additional data on some of the known risk factors would be helpful. For example, although we know that weight-bearing activity is the best type of exercise for bone health, the optimal type and schedule of exercise is unclear. Factors such as the use of carbonated beverages and the use of caffeine have not been widely studied. Further, although alcoholism has a negative effect on bone, the effect of moderate use of alcohol is not entirely clear.

REFERENCES

1. Kelsey JL, Hochberg MC. Epidemiology of chronic musculoskeletal disorders. *Ann Rev Public Health*. 1988;9:379–401.
2. Centers for Disease Control. Arthritis prevalence and activity

limitations—United States, 1990. MMWR. 1994; 43: 433–438.

3. Adams PF, Benson V. Current estimates from the National Health Interview Survey. *Vital Health Stat.* (Series 10, No. 181) 1991; DHHS publication PHS 92-1509.

4. Verbrugge LM, Gates DM, Ike RW. Risk factors for disability among US adults with arthritis. *J Clin Epidemiol.* 1991;44:167–182.

5. Praemer, A, Furner, S, Rice, DP. *Musculoskeletal Conditions in the United States.* Park Ridge, Illinois, American Academy of Orthopaedic Surgeons; 1992.

6. Hochberg MC, Ardey SL, Diamond EL. The association of self-reported arthritis with disability: data from the 1984 National Health Interview Survey Supplement on Aging (SOA). *Arthritis Rheum.* 1989;32(suppl 4):S101.

7. Yelin EH, Felts WR. A summary of the impact of musculoskeletal conditions in the United States. *Arthritis Rheum.* 1990;33:750–755.

8. Hochberg MC. Arthritis and connective tissue diseases. In: Thoene J, ed. *Physician's Guide to Rare Diseases.* Montvale, NJ: Dowden Publishing Co; 1992: 907–959.

9. Lawrence RC, Hochberg MC, Kelsey JL, et al. Estimates of the prevalence of selected arthritic and musculoskeletal diseases in the United States. *J Rheumatol.* 1989;16:427–441.

10. Altman RD, Asch E, Bloch DA, et al. Development of criteria for the classification and reporting of osteoarthritis: classification of osteoarthritis of the knee. *Arthritis Rheum.* 1986;29:1039–1049.

11. Hochberg MC. Osteoarthritis. In: Stobo JD, Hellmann DB, Ladenson PW, Petty BG, Traill TA, eds. *Principles and Practice of Medicine.* 23rd ed. Norwalk, Conn: Appleton & Lange; 1993.

12. Hochberg MC. Epidemiology of osteoarthritis: current concepts and new insights. *J Rheumatol.* 1991;18(suppl 27):4–6.

13. Hochberg MC, Lawrence RC, Everett DF, Cornoni-Huntley J. Epidemiologic associations of pain in osteoarthritis of the knee. *Semin Arthritis Rheum.* 1989; 18:4–9.

14. Anderson JJ, Felson DT. Factors associated with osteoarthritis of the knee in the First National Health and Nutrition Examination Survey (NHANES-I): evidence for an association with overweight, race, and physical demands of work. *Am J Epidemiol.* 1988;128: 179–189.

15. Tepper S, Hochberg MC. Factors associated with hip osteoarthritis: data from the National Health and Nutrition Examination Survey (NHANES-I). *Am J Epidemiol.* 1993;137: 1081–1088.

16. Hochberg MC. Epidemiologic considerations in the primary prevention of osteoarthritis. *J Rheumatol.* 1991;18: 1438–1440.

17. Davis MA, Ettinger WH, Neuhaus JM. Obesity and osteoarthritis of the knee: evidence from the National Health and Nutrition Examination Survey (NHANES I). *Semin Arthritis Rheum.* 1990;20: 34–41.

18. Felson DT. The epidemiology of knee osteoarthritis: results from the Framingham Osteoarthritis Study. *Semin Arthritis Rheum.* 1990;20 (suppl 1):42–50.

19. Felson DT, Zhang Y, Anthony JM, Nalmark A, Anderson JJ. Weight loss reduces the risk of symptomatic knee osteoarthritis in women: the Framingham Study. *Ann Intern Med.* 1992; 116: 535–539.

20. Hochberg MC, Lethbridge-Cejku M, Plato CC, Wigley FM, Tobin JD. Factors associated with osteoarthritis of the hand in males: data from the Baltimore Longitudinal Study of Aging. *Am J Epidemiol.* 1991;134:1121–1127.

21. Scott JC, Hochberg MC. Epidemiologic insights into the pathogenesis of hip osteoarthritis. In: Hadler NM, ed. *Clinical Concepts in Regional Musculoskeletal Illness.* Orlando, Fla: Grune & Stratton; 1987:89–107.

22. Croft P, Coggon D, Cruddas M, Cooper C. Osteoarthritis of the hip: an occupational disease in farmers. *Br Med J* 1992;304:1269–1272.

23. Hannan, MT, Anderson, JJ, Pincus, T, Felson, DT. Educational attainment and osteoarthritis: differential associations with radiographic changes and symptom reporting. *J Clin Epidemiol* 1992;45:139–147.

24. Whittle J, Steinberg EP, Anderson GF, Herbert R, Hochberg MC. Incidence of and indications for total hip replacement among elderly Americans. Arthritis Rheum. 1990;33:S139. Abstract.

25. Centers for Disease Control and Prevention. Prevalence of leisure-time physical activity among persons with arthritis and other rheumatic conditions—United States, 1990–1991. *MMWR.* 1997;46:389–393.

26. Minor MA, Lane NE. Recreational exercise in arthritis. *Rheum Dis Clin North Am.* 1996;22:563–577.

27. Sharp GC, Singsen BH, Hazelwood SE, Hall PJ, Oliver CL, Smith C. The Missouri Arthritis Program: legislation, implementation, and funding of a regional centers program. *Missouri Med.* 1988;85:79–83.

28. Dubbert ML, Sharp GC, Kay DR, Sylvester JL, Brownson RC. Implications of a statewide survey of arthritis in Missouri. *Missouri Med.* 1990;87:145–148.

29. Lorig K, Holman H. Arthritis self-management studies: a twelve

year review. *Health Educ Q.* 1993;20:17–28.

30. Brownson R, Taylor J, Bright F, et al. Chronic disease prevention and control activities--United States, 1989. *MMWR.* 1991;40: 697–700.

31. Alarcon, GS. Epidemiology of rheumatoid arthritis. *Rheum Dis Clin N Am.* 1995; 21: 589–604.

32. Silman, AJ. Epidemiology of rheumatoid arthritis. *APMIS.* 1994; 102: 721–728.

33. Pladevall-Villa, M, Delclos, GL, Varas, C, Guyer, H, Brugues-Tarradellas, J, Anglada-Arisa, A. Controversy of oral contraceptives and risk of rheumatoid arthritis: meta-analysis of conflicting studies and review of conflicting meta-analyses with special emphasis on analysis of heterogeneity. *Am J Epidemiol.* 1996; 144:1–14.

34. Abbott RD, Brand FN, Kannel WB, Castelli WP. Gout and coronary heart disease the Framingham Study. *J Clin Epidemiol.* 1988;41:237–242.

35. Roubenoff, R, Klag, MJ, Mead, LA, Liang, K-Y, Seidler, AJ, Hochberg, MC. Incidence and risk factors for gout in white men. *JAMA.* 1991; 266: 3004–3007.

36. Hochberg, MC, Thomas, J, Thomas, DJ, Mead, L, Levine, DM, Klag, MJ. Racial differences in the incidence of gout. *Arth Rheum.* 1995; 38: 628–632.

37. Barth RW, Lane JM. Osteoporosis. *Orthop Clin North Am.* 1988;19:845–858.

38. Looker, AC, Orwoll, ES, Johnston, et al. Prevalence of low femoral bone density in older US adults from NHANES III. *J Bone Miner Res.* 1997; 12: 1761–1768.

39. Lindsay R. Osteoporosis. *Clin Geriatr Med.* 1988;4:411–430.

40. Jacobsen SJ, Goldberg J, Miles TP, et al. Hip fracture among the old and very old: a population-based study of 745,435 cases. *Am J Public Health.* 1990;80:871–873.

41. Bauer RL. Ethnic differences in hip fracture: a reduced incidence in Mexican Americans. *Am J Epidemiol.* 1988;127:145–149.

42. Yano K, Heilbrun LK, Wasnich RD, et al. The relationship between diet and bone mineral content of multiple skeletal sites in elderly Japanese-American men and women living in Hawaii. *Am J Clin Nutr.* 1985;42: 877–888.

43. Salamone, LM, Glynn, NW, Black, DM, et al. Determinants of premenopausal bone mineral density: the interplay of genetic and lifestyle factors. *J Bone Miner Res.* 1996; 11:1557–1565.

44. Khoury, MJ. Genetic and epidemiologic approaches to the search for gene–environment interaction: the case of os-

teoporosis. *Am J Epidemiol.* 1998;147: 1–2.

45. Nguyen, TV, Howard, GM, Kelly, PJ, Eisman, JA. Bone mass, lean mass, and fat mass: same genes or same environment? *Am J Epidemiol.* 1998;147: 3–16.

46. Hopper, JL, Green, RM, Nowson CA, et al. Genetic, common environment, and individual specific components of variance for bone mineral density in 10- to 26-year-old females: a twin study. *Am J Epidemiol.* 1998; 147:17–29.

47. Kreiger N, Kelsey JL, Holford TR, et al. An epidemiologic study of hip fracture in postmenopausal women. *Am J Epidemiol.* 1982; 116:141–148.

48. Gardsell P, Johnell O, Nilsson BE. The impact of menopausal age on future fragility fracture risk. *J Bone Miner Res.* 1991 ;6:429–433.

49. Melton LJ, O'Fallon WM, Riggs BL. Secular trends in the incidence of hip fractures. *Calcif Tissue Int.* 1987;41: 57–64.

50. Jacobsen SJ, Goldberg J, Miles TP, et al. Regional variation in the incidence of hip fracture. *JAMA.* 1990;264: 500–502.

51. Rodriguez JG, Sattin RW, Waxweiler RJ. Incidence of hip fractures, United States, 1970–83. *Am J Prev Med.* 1989;5:175–181.

52. Cumming, RG, Nevitt, MC, Cummings, SR. Epidemiology of hip fractures. *Epidemiol Rev.* 1997; 19: 244–257.

53. Williams AR, Weiss NS, Ure CL, et al. Effect of weight, smoking, and estrogen use on the risk of hip and forearm fractures in postmenopausal women. *Obstet Gynecol.* 1982;60: 695–699.

54. Cummings SR, Kelsey JL, Nevitt MC, et al. The epidemiology of osteoporosis and osteoporotic fractures. *Epidemiol Rev.* 1985;7: 178–208.

55. Diamond T, Steil D, Lunzer M, et al. Ethanol reduces bone formation and may cause osteoporosis. *Am J Med.* 1989;86:282–288.

56. Reid IR. Steroid osteoporosis. *Calcif Tissue Int.* 1989;45:63–67.

57. Grady, D, Rubin, SM, Petitti, DB, et al. Hormone therapy to prevent disease and prolong life in postmenopausal women. *Ann Intern Med.* 1992;117:1016–1037.

58. Slemenda CW, Hui SL, Longcope C, et al. Cigarette smoking, obesity, and bone mass. *J Bone Miner Res.* 1989;4:737–741.

59. Barrett-Connor, E. Smoking and endogenous sex hormones in men and women. In: Wald, NJ, Baron, J, eds. *Smoking and Hormone-Related Disorders.* New York, NY: Oxford University Press Inc; 1990:183–196.

60. Talmage RV, Stinnett SS, Landwehr JT, et al. Age-related loss of bone mineral density in

non-athletic and athletic women. *Bone Miner.* 1986;1:115–125.

61. Sinaki M, Wahner HW, Offord KP, et al. Efficacy of nonloading exercises in prevention of vertebral bone loss in postmenopausal women: a controlled trial. *Mayo Clin Proc.* 1989;64:762–769.

62. Brewer V, Meyer BM, Keele MS, et al. Role of exercise in prevention of involutional bone loss. *Med Sci Sports Exerc.* 1983;15:445–449.

63. Smith EL, Gilligan C. Physical activity effects on bone metabolism. *Calcif Tissue Int.* 1991;49:S50–S54.

64. Heaney RP. Lifelong calcium intake and prevention of bone fragility in the aged. *Calcif Tissue Int.* 1991;49: S42–S45.

65. Cumming, RG. Calcium intake and bone mass: a quantitative review of the evidence. *Calcif Tissue Int.* 1990; 47: 194–201.

66. Chapuy, MC, Arlot, ME, Duboef, F, et al. Vitamin D and calcium to prevent hip fractures in elderly women. *N Engl J Med.* 1992;327:1637–1642

67. Kiel DP, Felson DT, Anderson JJ, et al. Hip fracture and the use of estrogens in postmenopausal women. The Framingham Study. *N Engl J Med.* 1987;317:1169–1174.

68. Marsh AG, Sanchez TV, Mikelson O, et al. Cortical bone density of adult lacto-ovo-vegetarian and omnivorous women. *J Am Diet Assoc.* 1980;76:148–151.

69. Jones, G, Nguyen, T, Sambrook, PN, et al. Thiazide diuretics and fractures: can meta-analysis help? *J Bone Miner Res* 1995;10:106–111.

70. Paganini-Hill A, Ross RK, Gerkins VR, et al. Menopausal estrogen therapy and hip fractures. *Ann Intern Med.* 1981;95:28–31.

71. Paganini-Hill A, Chao A, Ross RK, et al. Exercise and other factors in the prevention of hip fracture: the Leisure World Study. *Epidemiology.* 1991;2:16–25.

72. Johnston CC, Melton LJ. Bone density measurement and the management of osteoporosis. In: Favus MJ, ed. *Primer on the Metabolic Bone Diseases and Disorders of Mineral Metabolism.* Kelseyville, Calif: American Society for Bone and Mineral Research; 1990: 93–100.

73. Cummings SR, Black D. Should peri-menopausal women be screened for osteoporosis? *Ann Intern Med.* 1986;104:817–823.

74. University of Michigan. *Stronger Body—Stronger Bones!* Ann Arbor, Mich: University of Michigan; 1991.

SUGGESTED READING

Alarcon, GS. Epidemiology of rheumatoid arthritis. *Rheum Dis Clin N Am..* 1995;21:589–604.

Cooper, C. The crippling consequences of fractures and their impact on quality of life. *Am J Med.* 1997;103(2A):S12–S19.

Cumming, RG, Nevitt, MC, Cummings, SR. Epidemiology of hip fractures. *Epidemiol Rev.* 1997;19: 244–257.

Felson DT. Epidemiology of hip and knee osteoarthritis. *Epidemiol Rev.* 1988;10:1–28.

Kelsey JL, Hochberg MC. Musculoskeletal disorders. In: Last JM, Wallace RB, eds. *Maxcy-Rosenau-Last Textbook of Public Health and Preventive Medicine.* 13th ed. Norwalk, Conn: Appleton & Lange; 1992:913–928.

Scott, JC. Epidemiology of osteoporosis. *J Clin Rheumatol* 1997;3:S9–S13.

Silman AJ, Hochberg MC. *Epidemiology of Rheumatic Diseases.* New York, NY: Oxford University Press Inc; 1993.

Silman, AJ. Epidemiology of rheumatoid arthritis. *APMIS.* 1994;102: 721–728.

RESOURCES

National Arthritis Foundation
PO Box 19000
Atlanta, GA 30326
(800) 283-7800

National Arthritis, Musculoskeletal, and Skin Disease Information Clearinghouse
9000 Rockville Pike
Box AMS
Bethesda, MD 20892
(301) 495-4484

National Osteoporosis Foundation
2100 M Street, NW
Suite 602
Washington, DC 20037
(202) 223-2226

National Institute on Aging
Public Information Office
Office of Planning, Analysis, and Communication
Federal Building, Room 6C12
Bethesda, MD 20892
(301) 496-1752

16

CHRONIC NEUROLOGIC DISORDERS

ICD-9 290.4, 331.0, 332.0, 335.2, 340, 345.0-345.9, 346.0-346.9, 354.0, 357.0,
358.0, 722.1-722.2, 722.52, 722.6, 724.02, 724.2-724.6, 800-801, 803-804 [EXCEPT .0 AND .5],
806.0-806.9, 846.0, 847.2, 850-854, 952.0-952.9

N eurologic disorders impose a considerable burden on society in terms of disability, lost productivity, and direct health care costs. Despite the prominence of neurologic disorders as an important cause of death and disability, national prevalence estimates of the frequency of these disorders are scarce. Estimates of incidence and prevalence are often obtained from community-based studies and extrapolated to the nation as a whole. Tables 16.1 and 16.2 summarize major types and estimates of the burden (incidence and prevalence) of neurologic disorders.[1] The neurologic disorders are classified into three broad categories: classic neurologic diseases, unintentional injuries, and intermittent disorders. To the extent possible, this chapter includes discussion of whether efforts at primary, secondary, or tertiary prevention would yield public health benefit for these disorders.

Gary M. Franklin, MD, MPH
Lorene M. Nelson, PhD

However, because little is known about the causes of the classic neurologic diseases, including Alzheimer's disease, Parkinson's disease, and multiple sclerosis, efforts at primary prevention are not possible. By contrast, most severe brain and spinal cord injuries are preventable. These unintentional injuries are among the six top state health agency chronic disease priorities.[2] Intermittent disorders, such as epilepsy, low back pain, and headache, impose a considerable burden of disability despite their relatively benign nature, and these disorders are often preventable or treatable.

In the United States, the direct annual cost of providing health care to people with chronic neurologic disorders exceeds $140 billion (Table 16.2). Indirect costs related to lost productivity exceed the direct burden related to health care. For example, chronic pain (eg, backache, headache) results in the loss of an estimated 400 million workdays per year in the United States.[3]

Table 16.1—Types of Chronic Neurologic Disorders

Category	Disorder
Classic neurologic diseases	
Dementia	Alzheimer's
	Multi-infarct
Neurodegenerative disorders	Parkinson's disease
	Amyotrophic lateral sclerosis
Neuroimmunologic disorders	Multiple sclerosis
	Guillain-Barrè syndrome
Unintentional injury	Head injury
	Spinal cord injury
	Carpal tunnel syndrome
	Back injury
Intermittent disorders	Epilepsy
	Headache

The classic neurologic diseases typically have a long latency prior to clinical recognition. For example, the mean age at which multiple sclerosis is diagnosed is approximately 33 years, but epidemiologic evidence suggests that the etiologic event occurs prior to age 15. The pandemic of influenza in 1918 through 1919 caused an increase in Parkinson's disease in the ensuing 3 decades caused by a postinfectious process.

The general etiologic model for the classic neurologic disorders may be explained by a convergence of genetic susceptibility and environmental factors, most of which are not clearly known. A more specific subtheory, that of abiotrophy, adds aging of the nervous system as an interactive factor for the neurodegenerative disorders and Alzheimer's dementia.[4] This theory holds that specific neuronal cell populations are depleted after an environmental insult and that subsequent cell death related to aging results in clinically evident disease.

The diagnosis of Alzheimer's disease and neurodegenerative disorders such as Parkinson's disease and amyotrophic lateral sclerosis occurs only when neuronal cell death has progressed to the point of clinical recognition. Such cell loss may exceed 50% to 80% before clinical diagnosis can occur. New imaging technologies such as magnetic resonance imaging and positron emission tomography may be used to detect lesser degrees of cell loss prior to clinical detection. Application of these technologies holds some promise for secondary prevention.

Table 16.2—Population Burden of Chronic Neurologic Disorders, United States

Disorder	Average Annual Incidence Per 100 000 Persons	Estimated Prevalence Per 100 000 Persons	Current Ability for 1, 2, 3 Prevention	Estimated Annual Cost
Dementia, including Alzheimer's disease	50	250	3°	$90 billion
Parkinson's disease, other neurodegenerative disorders	20	200	3°	—[a]
Multiple sclerosis, other neuroimmunologic disorders	6	173[b]	3°	$2.5 billion
Brain injury and persistent postconcussion syndrome	200	880	1°, 2°, 3°	$25 billion
Spinal cord injury	3	50	1°, 3	$5 billion
Carpal tunnel syndrome and other peripheral nerve injury	100	—[b]	1°, 2°, 3	—
Spinal pain and vertebrogenic disorders	300	800	1°, 2°, 3	$20 billion
Epilepsy (not including febrile or single seizures)	50	650	1°, 2°, 3	—
Severe headache, including migraine	450	3 500	1°, 2°, 3	—

Note: Adapted from Kurtzke.[1]
[a] Unavailable.
[b] More recent estimate than that cited by Kurtzke.[1]

The classic neurologic diseases typically progress until disability or death. A smaller proportion of cases remain benign and do not progress with the same certainty to disability or death. Comparisons of benign and progressive cases may yield clues to factors that predict progression or that may be altered for tertiary prevention.

Disorders related to unintentional injury include those secondary to acute injury of the central nervous system (CNS) (eg, brain and spinal cord injury) as well as chronic, repetitive injury to the peripheral nerves (eg, carpal tunnel syndrome) or musculoskeletal system (eg, back injury). Acute injury of the brain or spinal cord causes an abrupt onset of neurologic deficit. Although early mortality is high in the most severe cases, most patients survive the acute hospitalization and either remain stable or improve neurologically over time. Premature death may occur from later complications related to the injured nervous system.

The initial bout of a repetitive injury typically is subacute in onset, and for the most part such injuries heal rapidly. For example, 80% of workers with occupational back injury return to work within 6 weeks. Approximately 10% of workers, however, develop progressive and long-term disability in the context of workers' compensation, with huge indirect costs in loss of productivity.

This progressive disability may be related to reinjury but is commonly inexplicable in biologic terms. The largest public health impact for unintentional injury will be in primary prevention of the injury, secondary prevention to reduce the severity of the injury, and tertiary prevention to maximize recovery through successful rehabilitation and prevention of complications.

The intermittent disorders such as epilepsy and headache may occur very infrequently, or they may occur so frequently as to render a patient disabled. The hallmark of these disorders is that each episode has a finite beginning and end. With a few exceptions, there is little evidence of disturbance between acute episodes. Disability occurs with increasing frequency or severity of episodes. Primary prevention may be possible for epilepsy because, except for congenital and genetic varieties not covered here, the principal etiologies relate to other preventable conditions, such as cerebral trauma or stroke. Although headaches are generally benign, their etiology is unclear. Secondary and tertiary prevention, by adequate medical treatment and other preventive measures, is available for all of the intermittent disorders.

Neurologic diseases have not received the same intensive degree of epidemiologic investigation as have other chronic conditions such as cancer and cardiovascular disease. With neurologic diseases, the evidence is weak regarding a causal relationship for most exposures; therefore, attributable risks are not reported in this chapter, except those for brain injury.

This chapter provides relatively brief reviews of 12 different chronic neurologic conditions and diseases under the three major categories of classic neurologic diseases, unintentional injuries, and intermittent disorders.

CLASSIC NEUROLOGIC DISEASES: ALZHEIMER'S DISEASE
ICD-9 331.0

SIGNIFICANCE

Alzheimer's disease is the principal dementing disorder of adults, accounting for approximately 50% to 60% of all known cases of dementia in people over 50 years of age.[5] The hallmark symptoms of Alzheimer's disease are progressive loss of memory and other cognitive functions. The disorder is characterized by loss of neurons in the medial temporal and frontal cortices, with neuropathologic features of neurofibrillary tangles, senile plaques, and ß-amyloid deposits. These pathologic findings at autopsy correlate well with the degree of

cognitive loss[6] and serve as a gold standard for cases diagnosed by clinical criteria.[7] Associated selective loss of neurotransmission as measured by a decrement in activity of the brain enzyme choline acetyl transferase is a biochemical hallmark of the disorder.[8]

DESCRIPTIVE EPIDEMIOLOGY

Both the incidence and prevalence of Alzheimer's disease rise with each decade after age 50. Incidence rates increase from 0.2% per year at age 70 to 0.5% per year at age 85. Prevalence rates increase from 0.2% in the 65- to 74-year age group to 0.7% in the 75- to 84-year group and to 3% or higher in the 85-year and older age group.[5] The earlier definitions of cases diagnosed before age 65 as "presenile"' and after 65 as "senile" types of Alzheimer's disease are no longer supportable on epidemiologic or neuropathologic grounds.

Studies report modestly higher prevalence rates in women (1.6:1), and one community-based study in the United States demonstrated higher prevalence rates among Blacks than among Whites.[9] No clear time trends have been demonstrated for incidence. Increasing prevalence in some communities might be explained by longer survival related to better access to medical care. Although an inverse relationship between education level and the incidence or progression of Alzheimer's disease has been widely reported,[5] higher levels of education, or its correlates, may simply confer more compensatory reserve, thus delaying the onset of disease.[10] A similar association of greater educational attainment and less cognitive decline has been described for other disorders causing such decline (eg, HIV/AIDS, coronary artery bypass patients).[11]

RISK FACTORS

Many studies have demonstrated a familial occurrence of Alzheimer's disease in the absence of a clearly autosomal pattern of inheritance. The cumulative incidence among relatives of Alzheimer probands may approach 50% by the eighth decade.[12] Less than 5% of Alzheimer's patients exhibit evidence of fully penetrant, autosomal dominant inheritance; genetics studies suggest these patients' kindreds are genetically heterogeneous, with at least three gene mutations implicated.[13] However, studies of twins have shown no difference in concordance between monozygotic (identical) and dizygotic (fraternal) pairs. These findings suggest that a genetic predisposition may interact with other environmental influences to cause Alzheimer's disease. Both familial and sporadic cases have shown a strong association with the presence of the E-4 allele of the apolipoprotein E (APOE) gene.[13] While presence of this allele has been associated with increased ß-amyloid deposition in susceptible brain regions,[14] the biological basis of the APOE association is not yet clear.

Patients with Down's syndrome are at an increased risk of developing Alzheimer changes in their brains when they live beyond 40 years of age. A common genetic link between Down's syndrome and Alzheimer's disease in terms of pathogenesis may exist but is not well defined.

A history of head injury with loss of consciousness has been associated with an increased risk of Alzheimer's disease (Table 16.3). A particular variety of dementing illness, dementia pugilistica, has been described in boxers. The presence of the APOE E-4 allele may add to risk of Alzheimer's in traumatically brain injured patients.[15] Very young (15 to 19 years) and very old ($\geq$40 years) maternal age have been associated with an increased risk in a small number of studies. Aluminum has drawn particular attention because of its ability to cause Alzheimer-type pathological changes in experimental animals, however, brain aluminum concentration is not elevated in Alzheimer brain, nor does it correlate with neuropathologic changes.[16]

A modest association of Alzheimer's with a history of treated depression

Table 16.3—Modifiable Risk Factors for Alzheimer's Disease, United States

Magnitude	Risk Factor
Strong (relative risk[a] >4)	None
Moderate (relative risk 2–4)	Down's syndrome
Weak (relative risk <2)	Head injury with loss of consciousness, including boxing
	Maternal age (<20 years; ≥40 years)
Possible	Organic solvents

[a]Defined in Table 2.4, page 51.

has been found.[17] Smoking has shown a consistent negative association, with relative risks averaging 0.64,[18] similar to that described for Parkinson's disease. Weak and inconsistent associations with organic solvent exposure have been seen.

PREVENTION AND CONTROL MEASURES

There are no known preventive measures, and no currently available treatments significantly alter the course of Alzheimer's disease. The most promising treatment—the replacement or enhancement of declining cholinergic neurotransmitter stores—has shown some efficacy in recent randomized, controlled clinical trials.[19, 20] This avenue of investigation is ongoing, with current trials focusing on patients at early stages of disease.

Epidemiologic studies of Alzheimer's disease have identified head or limb trauma as risk factors. This association with trauma deserves further study, with an attempt to determine if the finding could be influenced by recall bias on the part of the neurologically impaired patient or by some third factor that might explain the association.

Other areas of future investigation include incident case-control and cohort studies that closely scrutinize associations with environmental toxicant, dietary, or occupational exposures. Toxicant exposures with chronic adverse effects on central cholinergic neurotransmission would have a theoretical basis for investigation. Further studies of the relationship between Alzheimer's disease and Down's syndrome are also warranted.

Future analytic studies of risk factors for sporadic and familial Alzheimer's disease should adjust for age, sex, education, smoking and, if possible, APOE E-4 allele status. The ability to detect other putative environmental risk factors would be seriously impaired in the absence of such adjustment.[21] Prospective studies, studies using neuropathologic endpoints (such as ß-amyloid deposition), and phenotopic differentiation are areas ripe for epidemiologic research.

MULTI-INFARCT DEMENTIA

ICD-9 290.4

SIGNIFICANCE

Multi-infarct dementia is a stepwise progression of cognitive loss punctuated by multiple episodes of strokelike events. These events may be subclinical if the areas of cerebral infarction are small or located in relatively quiescent areas of the brain. Multiple underlying etiologies are likely, since either small or large vessels may be principally involved.

DESCRIPTIVE EPIDEMIOLOGY

Multi-infarct dementia accounts for up to 12% to 20% of all dementia in the elderly.[5] No population-based incidence or prevalence rates are available, and no standard case definition is in use.

RISK FACTORS

Hypertension and multifocal cerebrovascular disease probably account for the majority of cases of multi-infarct dementia.[22] Prospective studies of an incident stroke cohort would yield information on other contributing factors.

PREVENTION AND CONTROL MEASURES

Reducing the risk factors for stroke (eg, hypertension) may have a beneficial impact on reducing the incidence of multi-infarct dementia.

It is likely that early detection of multi-infarct dementia could be accomplished by using a valid case definition that includes (1) neuropsychologic tests sensitive enough to detect early stages of both cortical and subcortical dementia, and (2) brain and vascular imaging tests that demonstrate a strong correlation between brain lesion burden and cerebrovascular disease.

Early medical treatment of hypertension and appropriate medical or surgical intervention for cerebrovascular disease may be effective in preventing further cognitive decline in multi-infarct dementia.

PARKINSON'S DISEASE

ICD-9 332.0

SIGNIFICANCE

Parkinson's disease is a common adult-onset neurodegenerative disorder, second in frequency only to Alzheimer's disease, with an average annual incidence of 20/100 000.[23] The pathologic hallmark of Parkinson's disease is the loss of melanin-containing neurons in the substantia nigra with a corresponding reduction in dopamine and other neurotransmitters in the region. Parkinson's disease has a gradually progressive course characterized by resting tremor, muscular rigidity, postural instability, and a slowness in the initiation and execution of movement (bradykinesia). The disease course is progressive and often severely limits functional abilities, posing a significant burden for affected individuals and their family members.

DESCRIPTIVE EPIDEMIOLOGY

The diagnosis of Parkinson's disease is usually assigned on the basis of a clinical examination. No standardized case definition is in wide use. Population-based studies in the United States report average annual incidence rates for Parkinson's disease of approximately 20 per 100 000.[23] Repeated studies of the Rochester, Minnesota, population show no evidence of temporal changes in the incidence of Parkinson's disease. The onset of Parkinson's disease is usually after age 50, with age-specific incidence rates reaching a peak between ages 75 and 84. In most studies, the age-adjusted incidence and prevalence of Parkinson's disease is higher among men than among women. Most hospital-based studies have indicated that Parkinson's disease is more common among Caucasians than among Blacks, although a door-to-door prevalence survey in Copiah County, Mississippi, revealed similar prevalence ratios for Caucasians and Blacks.[24]

RISK FACTORS

Some Parkinsonism syndromes share clinical and pathologic features with idiopathic Parkinson's disease, and information on the causes of these disorders may lead to speculation about etiology of idiopathic Parkinson's disease. Earlier in this century, Parkinsonism occurred as a sequela to an epidemic of encephalitis in 1919. Although this syndrome gave evidence that a viral agent can cause selective destruction of neurons in the substantia nigra, no subsequent studies have identified a viral cause for idiopathic Parkinson's disease. In 1983, Langston and his colleagues[25] reported four cases of Parkinson's disease that developed rapidly over a course of days in young IV drug users who had injected a synthetic heroin-like compound contaminated with 1-methyl-4-phenyl-1,2,3,6-tetrahydropyridine (MPTP). The symptoms in these cases were irreversible and clinically indistinguishable from Parkinson's disease.

With the exception of MPTP-induced Parkinsonism, no other toxicant exposure has been shown to produce the classical pathologic features of idiopathic Parkinson's disease; however, epidemiologic studies have identified other environmental factors that may be associated with disease risk. Epidemiologic studies identified two broad categories of exposure—factors associated with rural living and certain occupations—as possible risk factors for Parkinson's disease. The rural-associated factors include rural residence, farm work, well-water drinking, and occupational exposure to insecticides or herbicides (Table 16.4). Attempts to identify a specific agricultural chemical or herbicide have been inconclusive. In other studies, nonfarm occupations were associated with an increased risk for PD, including fire fighting, welding, and employment in chemical, pharmaceutical manufacturing or printing industries.[25]6

The role of genetic susceptibility in the pathogenesis of PD is controversial. Twin studies have found no difference in concordance between monozygotic and dizygotic twins, and, although 10% of patients with Parkinson's disease have one or more affected relatives, many investigators have attributed this to shared environment rather than heritability. Genetic susceptibility to environmental neurotoxicants may be an important etiologic factor in Parkinson's disease. Support for this hypothesis comes from two studies associating the presence of a mutant variety of a specific cytochrome P450 enzyme with a twofold increased risk of Parkinson's disease.[27, 28] Further evidence for a genetic contribution to PD was provided by the recent study of a large Italian kindred with autosomal dominant PD; linkage with genetic markers on chromosome 4q21-q23 was identified.[29]

Recent studies have indicated a possible protective role for high vitamin E intake.[30] A significant

Table 16.4—Modifiable Risk Factors for Parkinson's Disease, United States

Magnitude	Risk Factor
Strong (relative risk[a] >4)	None
Moderate (relative risk 2–4)	Rural living
Weak (relative risk <2)	Well water drinking
	Agricultural chemicals
	Industrial chemicals
Possible	Dietary antioxidants (vitamins E and C)[b]
	Cigarette smoking[a]

[a]Defined in Table 2.4, page 51.
[b]Some studies have suggested a protective effect.

inverse association of cigarette smoking with Parkinson's disease has been consistently observed in epidemiologic studies,[31] and, although several biological hypotheses have been proposed to explain this association, none is definitively proven.

PREVENTION AND CONTROL MEASURES

Although no treatment is effective in halting the neuronal degeneration that underlies Parkinson's disease, a patient's functional status can be improved with symptomatic therapy and rehabilitation. Very few studies have focused on prognostic factors in Parkinson's disease, except in relation to responsiveness to levodopa therapy. Dopamine repletion (eg, with levodopa) and dopamine agonists (eg, with bromocriptine) are used to improve bradykinesia and postural imbalance. Although pharmacologic therapy is very effective early in the course of Parkinson's disease, treatment with dopamine agonists eventually becomes less effective with longer-duration therapy and can be associated with dyskinetic or psychiatric side effects. Recent clinical trials have shown encouraging results with deprenyl (an MAO-B inhibitor) and vitamin E (an antioxidant).

The role of environmental toxicants in Parkinson's disease deserves further study,[30] with attention to the presence of genetically defective enzymes that can impair their detoxification. More research is also needed on the role of dietary factors. Future research progress will be enhanced by the collaboration of epidemiologists, clinicians, and laboratory scientists.

AMYOTROPHIC LATERAL SCLEROSIS
ICD-9 335.2

SIGNIFICANCE

Amyotrophic lateral sclerosis (ALS), also known as Lou Gehrig's disease, is a fatal motor neuron disease that causes rapidly progressive muscle weakness and death within 2 to 3 years of onset. Selective neuronal death occurs in two populations of motor neurons: lower motor neurons in the spinal cord that innervate skeletal muscles and upper motor neurons in the corticospinal tract and prefrontal motor cortex that descend and synapse on the lower motor neurons.

DESCRIPTIVE EPIDEMIOLOGY

Three forms of ALS are recognized: classic sporadic ALS, classic familial ALS, and a variant of ALS present in the western Pacific. In the 1950s, ALS was reported to occur in epidemic proportions in several areas of the western Pacific

(Guam, Kii Peninsula, New Guinea), with annual incidence rates of 50 per 100 000.[33] Since then, the incidence of ALS in the western Pacific has diminished considerably. Although not easily distinguishable from sporadic ALS on a clinical basis, the western Pacific variant of ALS has some distinct pathologic characteristics and is further differentiated by its co-occurrence with Parkinsonism and/or dementia in some individuals. Because of its neurotoxic properties, a traditional food source from the cycad tree (the cycad nut) is a suspect toxicant for the western Pacific variants of ALS.[34]

Apart from the foci of ALS in the western Pacific, the incidence rate of ALS around the world is fairly uniform.[35, 36] Annual incidence rates are close to 1 per 100 000 in developed countries (range 0.5 to 2.4 per 100 000) and somewhat lower in developing countries, perhaps because of underdiagnosis or a younger population. Age-specific incidence rates of ALS rise with advancing age and peak in the sixth decade of life. The incidence of ALS is higher among men than women (male:female ratio from 1.2:1 to 2.5:1) and is twice as high for Caucasians as it is for other racial groups. Most surveys show a temporal increase in ALS incidence rates in recent decades.

RISK FACTORS

Other than age and gender, the only indisputable risk factor for ALS is genetic susceptibility, with the classic familial form of ALS comprising 7% to 10% of cases. Some families display a pattern consistent with autosomal dominant inheritance of a disease gene. Genetic linkage has been observed between familial ALS and mutant forms of the gene that code for the enzyme Cu/Zn superoxide dismutase (SOD1), an endogenous free radical scavenger. Mutations of the SOD1 gene occur in 15% to 20% of familial cases,[37] providing evidence that free radical toxicity may contribute to the pathogenesis of familial ALS.

Epidemiologic studies have identified hard physical labor or vigorous physical activity as risk factors for ALS, with an apparent twofold increase in the risk of ALS associated with vigorous physical or athletic activities (Table 16.5). Other studies have identified physical trauma and limb injury as risk factors for ALS but have failed to adjust for physical activity level, a factor that could predispose an individual to traumatic injury.[38] Some studies have suggested that the increased risk for skeletal fractures is highest in the years immediately preceding the onset of ALS. This raises the possibility that the presence of subclinical disease may have increased the risk of fracture.

Table 16.5—Modifiable Risk Factors for Amyotrophic Lateral Sclerosis, United States

Magnitude	Risk Factor
Strong (relative risk[a] >4)	None
Moderate (relative risk 2–4)	Vigorous physical activity
	Physical trauma, limb injury
Weak (relative risk <2)	Certain occupations[b]
Possible	Viruses

[a]Defined in Table 2.4, page 51.
[b]Includes work in agriculture, the leather industry, and plastics manufacturing, as well as jobs with exposure to heavy metals, solvents, and electrical shock.

Several epidemiologic studies have identified excesses of ALS cases among workers in agriculture, leather, and plastics manufacturing. Other studies have reported an association between ALS and occupational exposure to heavy metals (lead, mercury), organic solvents, and electrical shock (Table 16.5); however, other studies have failed to identify these associations. Hypotheses under active investigation by laboratory researchers include a possible immunologic basis for ALS, a viral cause, a defect in DNA cell repair capacity, and a defect in the metabolism or transport of glutamate in the central nervous system.

PREVENTION AND CONTROL MEASURES

Median survival with ALS is 2 years from disease onset, but the duration of the disease can range from several months to several years. Prognostic studies have indicated that later age at onset and onset with predominantly bulbar symptoms may be associated with shortened survival. A recent controlled trial demonstrated that the antiglutamate drug riluzole is effective for slowing the progression of ALS,[39] and trials with other glutamate antagonists and neural growth factors are underway.

As with Parkinson's disease, the role of environmental toxicants and dietary antioxidants in ALS deserves further study. Neurodegenerative disorders such as ALS, Parkinson's disease, and Alzheimer's disease may be pathologically or etiologically related, and future studies to investigate the aggregation of these disorders in families are warranted.

MULTIPLE SCLEROSIS

ICD-9 340

SIGNIFICANCE

Multiple sclerosis (MS) is characterized by plaques or lesions of the myelin sheath, a white fatty substance that serves as insulating material around neurons in the central nervous system. The symptoms of MS are highly variable but frequently include impaired vision, weakness, tremor, impaired balance, disturbances of sensation, and bowel or bladder difficulties. A standardized case definition for MS has been widely used in clinical trials.[40] The presence of two relatively distinct clinical courses—the relapsing-remitting course and the chronic-progressive course—have led some investigators to speculate that MS may be more than one disease entity. Others conclude that MS is a single disease entity because a large proportion of patients with relapsing-remitting disease eventually develop a progressive disease course.

DESCRIPTIVE EPIDEMIOLOGY

Multiple sclerosis is the most prevalent chronic neurologic disease affecting adults between the ages of 20 and 50, with average age of onset in the early 30s.[41] As a group, patients with MS live to 75% of life expectancy, with median survival of 30 years following disease onset. MS is more common among women than among men (1.7:1 ratio), more common among Caucasians than among other races, and more common among individuals in upper socioeconomic groups.

Periodic surveillance of MS is carried out in Rochester, Minnesota, where case ascertainment is thorough because of the record linkage system of the Mayo Clinic. The prevalence for MS during 1985 was 173 per 100 000. The annual incidence was 6.3 per 100 000.[42] The prevalence of MS has increased in recent decades, most likely due to earlier diagnosis and longer survival. Repeated studies of the Rochester, Minnesota, population also suggest that the incidence of disease may be increasing. This cannot be explained solely on the basis of diagnostic advances.[42]

RISK FACTORS

MS prevalence and mortality rates have consistently been shown to increase with increasing distance from the equator.[41] Northern United States, Canada, northern Europe, southern Australia, and New Zealand have high prevalence rates (over 30 per 100 000), whereas southern United States, southern Europe, and northern Australia have medium frequency rates (5 to 25 per

100 000). Areas with a low percentage of Caucasians, such as Africa and Asia, have low prevalence rates (less than 5 per 100 000). The geographic distribution of MS may be related to a variation in susceptibility according to race or ethnicity, a variation in the availability of medical care, or environmental factors correlated with latitude or climate. Migration studies indicate that adolescence may be a critical age for acquiring MS. Individuals migrating from high-risk to low-risk areas before age 15 appear to acquire the lower risk of the adopted residence, whereas individuals migrating as adults retain the high risk of the area from which they migrated.[43]

Support for the role of genetic factors in the occurrence of MS comes from evidence for familial aggregation, lower susceptibility among races other than Caucasians, and the high occurrence of certain HLA haplotypes among MS cases. Between 5% and 15% of patients with MS will have one or more relatives with the disease. The strongest evidence for a genetic component in MS comes from a twin study in Canada, in which 28% of monozygotic (maternal) twins were concordant for MS, but only 2.5% of dizygotic (fraternal) twins were concordant.[44] Recent genetic linkage studies have identified regions on several chromosomes that are associated with disease risk, suggest-

ing that two or more genes may interact to confer genetic susceptibility to MS.[45] Although genetic factors may be operative in MS, they cannot fully account for the geographic distribution of MS, because the gradient in MS risk with latitude is similar for most ethnic groups. MS most likely results from the interaction between an infectious or environmental agent(s) and a genetically determined immunologic response to such an agent(s).

Because the prevalence of MS varies significantly with latitude, epidemiologic and laboratory studies have largely focused on the potential role of infectious agents in MS. The most widely held theory of MS etiology is that a genetically susceptible individual is exposed to a virus in childhood that remains latent for many years before initiating the onset of symptoms, either by direct reinfection or through an immunologic mechanism. The measles and canine distemper viruses have received the most attention as potential infectious agents in MS, but epidemiologic studies have consistently failed to yield any clues about the specific infectious agents that may be involved. Some studies have observed that measles antibody titers were higher among patients with MS than among control subjects, with the risk of MS increasing when measles infection occurred later than usual in childhood. Several studies have reported that patients with MS were more frequently exposed to infectious diseases during childhood than were control subjects; however, these studies may be compromised by the potential for recall bias on the part of patients with MS and the difficulty in establishing the age at which infections occurred. An epidemic of MS in the Faroe Islands following World War II appeared to coincide with the introduction of British troops, a finding compatible with the introduction of an infectious agent.[41]

The myelin sheath is largely composed of lipids, leading some researchers to focus on the possible role of dietary fat intake. However, studies have failed to demonstrate an association between dietary fat and MS. The suggestion that trauma or stress are risk factors for MS is highly controversial. More likely, trauma or stress could trigger disease exacerbation in patients with MS. Some investigators have suggested that autoimmune disorders such as diabetes mellitus, rheumatoid arthritis, and autoimmune thyroid disease occur with greater frequency among patients with MS and their family members, but these findings await replication.

PREVENTION AND CONTROL MEASURES

The clinical management of MS is largely comprised of therapy to alleviate its symptoms and rehabilitation techniques to improve the functional capacity of patients. Treatment with some steroids such as prednisone, or ACTH may shorten acute exacerbations of MS but have no proven influence on the subsequent course of the disease. The exception is high dose intravenous methylprednisolone (Solumedrol) which has been demonstrated to reduce the likelihood that optic neuritis (ie, demyelinating lesions of the optic nerve) progresses to multiple sclerosis.[46] Two new classes of agents have recently been demonstrated to have therapeutic benefit in MS. Recombinant interferon beta has been shown to reduce the frequency of exacerbations and the accumulation of brain lesions among patients with the relapsing-remitting form of MS.[47,48] A second new type of agent, copolymer 1, also has been shown to reduce relapse rate[49] Other agents that merit further investigation include cyclophosphamide and low-dose oral methotrexate.

To foster prevention efforts, studies are needed to explore the possible role of hormonal factors in the etiology of MS as well as the possible interaction between genetic susceptibility and exposure to infectious or environmental agents. As with insulin-dependent diabetes mellitus, further investigations should emphasize the search for agents that have antigenic determinants in common with components of the myelin sheath.

GUILLAIN-BARRÉ SYNDROME

ICD-9 357.0

SIGNIFICANCE

Guillain-Barré syndrome is an acute demyelinating polyneuropathy characterized by muscle weakness that often progresses over days or weeks but is reversed in the majority of patients. The prevailing belief is that Guillain-Barré syndrome is caused by a nonspecific immune response directed at the myelin of peripheral nerves following the triggering influence of a recent viral infection or other exogenous agent. A standardized case definition for Guillain-Barré syndrome has been widely applied.[50]

DESCRIPTIVE EPIDEMIOLOGY

Studies of Guillain-Barré syndrome in geographically defined populations have reported crude annual incidence rates ranging from 0.6 to 1.9 per 100 000.[51] Incidence rates rise with advancing age, are higher for men than for women, and are reported to be higher among Whites than among Blacks. No geographic or seasonal clustering of Guillain-Barré syndrome has been observed, nor have any strong temporal trends in disease incidence been reported.

RISK FACTORS

Antecedent infection is considered a strong risk factor for Guillain-Barré syndrome. Several case-control studies have reported that patients with Guillain-Barré syndrome were more likely than control subjects to have had an upper respiratory infection or mild gastrointestinal illness within 2 to 4 weeks prior to the onset of weakness. Epstein-Barr virus and cytomegalovirus have received the most attention as potential infectious agents in Guillain-Barré syndrome. The reported association of the Guillain-Barré syndrome with the A/New Jersey (swine flu) strain of the influenza vaccine used in 1976 and 1977 ignited public concern regarding the safety of immunization programs in general. Schonberger and colleagues[52] reported an increased risk of Guillain-Barré syndrome among swine flu vaccine recipients, with an estimated attributable risk of one excess case of Guillain-Barré syndrome for every 100 000 vaccines administered. This association was the subject of much controversy until a group of investigators recently restudied the association between Guillain-Barré syndrome and swine flu vaccine in two states.[53] The relative risk of Guillain-

Barré syndrome during the 6-week period following vaccination was 7.1, a finding comparable to the relative risk of 7.6 reported in the original study. Subsequent studies indicated that swine flu vaccine administered after 1977 was not associated with a rise in Guillain-Barré syndrome cases, raising the possibility that the earlier A/New Jersey vaccine stimulated a different immunologic reaction than did the more recent vaccines.

PREVENTION AND CONTROL MEASURES

Although the majority of patients with Guillain-Barré syndrome achieve complete neurologic recovery, 7% to 22% are left with some neurologic disability, and 2% do not survive. Treatment consists of supportive ventilation during the acute phase and physical therapy during the recovery phase. Plasmapheresis or intravenous immune globulin are of value if patients are treated early in the course of hospitalization.[54]

UNINTENTIONAL INJURIES:

BRAIN INJURY

ICD 9- 800-801, 803-804 [EXCEPT .0 AND .5], 850-854

SIGNIFICANCE

Brain injuries are a significant cause of mortality and morbidity in the United States. Death from brain injury accounts for approximately 44% of all deaths related to injury.[55] Severe brain injuries result in contusion or hemorrhage in the brain. They are often related to prolonged hospitalization and are associated with neurologic and cognitive deficits that may cause severe, permanent functional impairment.

At least 50% of all brain injuries are mild.[56] Mild brain injuries, secondary to concussion of the brain, are usually associated with some period of loss of consciousness or amnesia for the event. Identifying these patients may be difficult because many do not require hospitalization. Among those that are hospitalized, other multiple injuries may be predominant, and the mild brain injury may not be well documented.

DESCRIPTIVE EPIDEMIOLOGY

Overall incidence of brain injury in the United States from population-based studies is approximately 0.2% per year, with somewhat higher rates reported for northern Europe (0.2% to 0.4% per year).[55] Incidence rates for males are two to three times higher than those for females. Incidence rates generally peak in the 15- to 24-year age group, with smaller secondary peaks among children and people over age 65.

Population-based prevalence studies for brain injury are difficult to perform because past patients are not followed up. Two national hospital discharge surveys have found discrepant prevalence rates (0.12%, 0.44%),[56, 57] most likely because of differences in case definition and case finding methodologies. The prevalent sex ratio (male:female = 1.7:1) is lower than the incident sex ratio, perhaps suggesting greater severity or worse survival for males.

RISK FACTORS

Estimates of population-attributable risk illustrate the preventability of brain injury (Table 16.6). The most common risk factors for unintentional brain injury include transport-related injuries, falls, and sports or recreation injuries. Transport-related injuries include those to occupants of cars and trucks, as well as to bicyclists, motorcyclists, and

Table 16.6—Proportion of Unintentional Brain Injury[a] Attributed to Various Modifiable Risk Factors, United States

Factor	Range (%)
Transportation-related	40–50
Fall-related	25–30
Sports/recreation-related	5–10

Note: Adapted from Kraus[55]; population-attributable risk is defined in Table 2.4, page 51.

pedestrians. Alcohol consumption is an interactive risk factor for transport-related occurrence of brain injury. Work-related brain injuries probably account for 5% to 10% of all brain injuries. Workers in logging, roofing, construction, trucking, garbage collection, and dairy farming are at increased risk of brain injury.[58]

PREVENTION AND CONTROL MEASURES

Brain injury and other unintentional injuries have great potential for primary, secondary, and tertiary prevention. CNS trauma can be reduced by preventing vehicle crashes through better roadway and vehicle design, educating operators and pedestrians, and preventing drinking and driving. Safety programs, such as prevention of falls, should be targeted to industries with high rates of head injury. Use of bicycle helmets may reduce brain injury risk by 69% to 74%.[59] Specific recommendations on bicycle helmet use have recently been published by the Centers for Disease Control and Prevention.[60]

Morbidity from crashes can be reduced by increased use of passenger restraints and helmets as well as improved vehicle and roadway design and by assuring excellence in emergency medical services, both on the scene and at the hospital. The nature and extent of the injury, time to reach a hospital, and the presence of a trauma center are factors that can affect the early outcome of severe brain injury. Standard assessment of initial severity (Glasgow Coma Scale), outcome at hospital discharge (Glasgow Outcome Scale), and case fatality rates are important measures related to outcome.

Repeated concussions, particularly in contact sports, may lead to cumulative neuropsychologic deficits. Guidelines for the management of concussion in sports, including the timing of reentry, have recently been published.[61]

The outcome of severe brain injury is important in relation to loss of productivity and medical costs. It is important to assure that the appropriate rehabilitation services are available to maintain and restore the injured person's function and self-reliance. A large number of post-acute head injury programs have arisen in the past decade, many of which are hospital or treatment center based. They are extraordinarily expensive, yet little outcome data related to their efficacy in tertiary prevention are available. Undertreatment of patients with inadequate health insurance coverage may also be a problem.

A minority of patients with mild brain injury may have persistent symptoms including insomnia, positional vertigo, and inattention. Other patients with mild closed head injury may not have been hospital-ized, may not have had documented brain injury (concussion), and may have less specific symptoms.

SPINAL CORD INJURY

ICD-9 806.0-806.9, 952.0-952.9

SIGNIFICANCE

Severe spinal cord injury, although a much rarer event than brain injury, may cause permanent paralysis. Cervical spinal cord injuries result in varying degrees of quadriparesis, whereas injuries in the thoracic and upper lumbar regions of the spinal cord result in varying degrees of paraparesis. As with brain injury, data on minor or transient spinal cord dysfunction are lacking.

DESCRIPTIVE EPIDEMIOLOGY

Annual incidence estimates for spinal cord injury range from 15 to 50 per million persons, and the peak age of occurrence is 15 through 24 years.[55] The estimated annual number of spinal cord injury cases in the United States has ranged from 111 000[62] to 200 000,[63] with a twofold to threefold increase in such cases between 1950 and 1980.[62]

RISK FACTORS

Strong risk factors are similar to those for brain injury: transport-related injury (approximately 50% of spinal cord injuries), falls (15%), recreational injury (15%), and work-related injury (15%). Most spinal cord injuries in persons <65 years of age are caused by falls.[69] Diving accidents are an important subset of recreational injury.

PREVENTION AND CONTROL MEASURES

Primary prevention of spinal cord injuries could reduce much of their burden. The strategies addressed earlier for brain injury also apply here.

Outcome depends on the degree of transection or damage to the spinal cord and the location of the lesion. Short-term survival is especially reduced after cervical cord transection. Survival is reduced among people who survive for 30 days after spinal cord injury and who experience pulmonary, cardiovascular, or renal complications. Recent research suggests that high doses of methylprednisolone in the first 8 hours is associated with improved neurologic function 6 months after injury.[65]

After recovery, patients with spinal cord injury require ongoing rehabilitation and the development of self-care skills to minimize common complications such as skin ulcers, urinary tract infections, and blood clots caused by prolonged inactivity.

CARPAL TUNNEL SYNDROME

ICD-9 354.0

SIGNIFICANCE

Carpal tunnel syndrome is the entrapment of the median nerve in the wrist as it passes under the transverse carpal ligament; it is the most common entrapment syndrome of the peripheral nerves. Tingling or burning pain in the affected hand, especially at night, and an abnormal delay in median nerve conduction at the wrist are the clinical hallmarks. Consensus criteria for the identification of carpal tunnel syndrome in epidemiologic studies have been recently developed.[66]

DESCRIPTIVE EPIDEMIOLOGY

Carpal tunnel syndrome reporting has increased dramatically since 1975, primarily as a result of increased recognition of the disorder. In Rochester, Minnesota, the average annual incidence between 1961 and 1980 was reported to be 1 per 1000, with a mean age of 51 years and a 3:1 female: male ratio.[67] Annual incidence was higher in a strictly work-related population (1.8 per 1000), where mean age (38.4 years) and female:male ratio (1.2:1) differed from the Rochester study.[68]

RISK FACTORS

A strong risk factor for carpal tunnel syndrome is direct trauma to the median nerve at the wrist (eg, fracture, crush injury). Moderate risk factors include underlying neuropathy from another cause, such as diabetes, hypothyroidism, or congenital neuropathies, or any occupation or hobby requiring repetitive, forceful, or awkward hand or wrist movements (Table 16.7).[69] The occupations most commonly associated with high rates of reported workers' compensation claims include food processing and canning, roofing, carpentry, production sewing, and mill work. Other moderate risk factors include the use of hand-held vibrating tools and obesity.[70] These risk factors may have multiplicative effects.

Weak risks are reported in those industries commonly associated with continuous typing or use of video display terminals.[68] Symptoms of carpal tunnel syndrome frequently accompany pregnancy, but the symptoms dissipate postpartum. A previously suspected but unproven association is with pyridoxine insufficiency.

PREVENTION AND CONTROL MEASURES

Primary prevention of carpal tunnel syndrome can be accomplished by enhancing worker safety programs, reducing hazardous exposures in the workplace, and helping to establish surveillance programs for carpal tunnel syndrome. Because of the huge burden in terms of costs and disability in the workplace, many industries are using screening tools to identify workers who may be at risk for developing carpal tunnel syndrome. The use of such tools raises serious ethical and legal issues. In addition, the examinations and psychophysical measures used in such screening programs have not been well validated.

Table 16.7—Modifiable Risk Factors for Carpal Tunnel Syndrome, United States

Magnitude	Risk Factor
Strong (relative risk[a] >4)	Fracture, crush injury
Moderate (relative risk 2–4)	Underlying neuropathy
	Repetitive, forceful, or awkward hand or wrist movements
	Hand-held vibrating tools
	Obesity
Weak (relative risk <2)	Continuous typing or video display terminal use
Possible	Pyridoxine (vitamin B6) insufficiency

[a]Defined in Table 2.4, page 51.

Nevertheless, the development of a reliable and specific marker of early or preclinical carpal tunnel syndrome would be useful in early detection and treatment programs.

Disability and workers' compensation costs related to carpal tunnel syndrome have increased dramatically in the past decade. In spite of its relatively benign nature, carpal tunnel syndrome independently predicts a longer duration of disability than do other work-related injuries.[71] Moreover, such disability is much more likely to occur in situations that require compensation for the worker. Although surgical decompression allows most patients with carpal tunnel syndrome to achieve pain relief and return to work, some cannot do so. Significant efforts at job modification are indicated for workplaces with high rates of occurrence.

LOW BACK PAIN

ICD-9 722.1-722.2, 722.52, 722.6,
724.02, 724.2-724.6, 846.0, 847.2

SIGNIFICANCE

Low back pain has become enormously expensive, with annual direct and indirect costs of between $15 and $25 billion. Most low back pain is attributable to muscular sprain, strain, or spasm; ligamentous injury; or abnormalities of the vertebral bones, discs, or facet joints.

Most often, no objective correlate (by examination or diagnostic test) of low back pain is available. Sciatica, or compression of the lumbar nerve root(s) by a disc or bone, may accompany acute low back pain.

DESCRIPTIVE EPIDEMIOLOGY

The most frequently reported population-based rates of low back pain are from industrial populations. Up to 2% of all workers in the United States report disabling back pain each year.[72] In general, incidence rates in the United States are equal for men and women, and these rates peak in the 20- to 40-year age group; however, incidence rates for women exceed those for men in the over-65 age group. Reported rates of low back pain are higher in lower socioeconomic classes. More recent birth cohorts are associated with increased reporting of low back pain.[73]

RISK FACTORS

Moderate risk factors for low back pain include prolonged driving, materials handling, and lifting that exceeds strength capability.[74] Examples of high-risk occupations include trucking and warehousing, farm work, lumber and mill work, mining, and construction. Premature menopause has also been reported to have a moderate association with low back pain.[75] Risks specific to intervertebral disc herniation (related to sciatica) include repetitive lifting of heavy objects in a forward bent-and-twisted position and exposure to vehicular or machine-related vibration.[76] Smoking is a weak risk factor for reported back pain or herniated intervertebral disc. No clear association with low back pain or sciatica has been found for scoliosis of less than 60° or for anthropometric measures such as height or weight, unequal leg length, or measures of spinal flexibility.

PREVENTION AND CONTROL MEASURES

Future analytic studies should differentiate acute from chronic low back pain.[77] Retrospective studies of incident acute pain cases and prospective studies of previously asymptomatic persons[78] would add substantial value to the extant risk factor literature.

Improved ergonomic or engineering design of the workplace and vehicles, including improved lifting techniques and conditioning for those who must lift, may prevent back injuries. People with known, recurrent back pain or prior back surgery may prevent recurrence or worsening of back pain with improved conditioning and selected low back exercises. Ninety percent of patients recover from acute low back pain within 6 weeks. The

remainder are at risk for going on to longer-term, and sometimes permanent, disability. This 10% of workers accounts for 80% of the cost among back injury claims.[79] The evolution of increasing disability from a lumbar sprain to total and permanent disability is more clearly related to administrative, legal, psychosocial, and economic factors than to the biology or severity of the original injury. The use of inappropriate medical procedures may also contribute to this evolving disability. Lumbar fusion, for example, a very invasive and expensive procedure, is rarely indicated in the treatment of chronic low back pain in workers' compensation.[80]

INTERMITTENT DISORDERS: EPILEPSY
ICD-9 345.0-345.9

SIGNIFICANCE

Epilepsy is the repeated occurrence of seizures in patients who have not been provoked to have such seizures. Seizures are the physical manifestation of an abnormal electrical discharge of cerebral neurons, which is often documentable by electroencephalography. Isolated seizures with provocation may occur in anyone with cerebral hypoxia or in young children with fever. Such events probably account for 50% to 75% of all people who have ever had a seizure, with the remaining 25% to 50% having epilepsy.

DESCRIPTIVE EPIDEMIOLOGY

Classifying the various forms of epilepsy is extremely complex, and case definitions for epidemiologic purposes are generally not comparable between studies.[81] Annual age-adjusted incidence rates for epilepsy are in the range of 29 to 53 per 100 000.[82] The highest age-specific incidence rates are for young children and older adults, with approximately 50% of all epilepsy beginning in childhood or early adolescence. Incidence rates are consistently slightly higher for males. Blacks and people in a low socio-economic class had higher incidence rates of epilepsy in one study.[83] Secular trends reveal decreasing incidence among children and increasing incidence among older adults.[82] The most commonly reported prevalence rates for epilepsy are 4 to 8 per 1000.

RISK FACTORS

Strong risk factors for the development of epilepsy include cerebral hypoxia, congenital malformations, and structural brain abnormalities in the newborn; mental retardation, cerebral palsy, and CNS infections (eg, bacterial meningitis and viral encephalitis) in children; moderate to severe brain injury, especially in 15- to 35-year-old males; cerebrovascular and Alzheimer's disease in the elderly; and brain tumors and neurosurgical procedures (especially shunts) in any age group (Table 16.8). Moderate risk factors for epilepsy include a family history of epilepsy in a sibling, parent (especially mother), or first-degree relative; multiple sclerosis; and chronic alcohol or heroin abuse. Suspected risk factors include a history of asthma and advancing age. Factors with no clear independent risk for epilepsy include childhood febrile convulsions or adverse perinatal events in the absence of cerebral palsy, pertussis immunization, mild brain injury, or aseptic meningitis.

PREVENTION AND CONTROL MEASURES

Future epidemiologic studies of epilepsy should focus on genetic influences, particularly in those types of epilepsy whose cause is unknown. Special methodologic precautions should be taken in interpreting data on familial risk and lifetime prevalence.[84]

Prevention of known underlying causes of epilepsy is most likely for hypoxia in newborns, CNS infection in children, cerebrovascular disease in older adults, brain injury, and alcohol or heroin abuse. Adequate use of antiepileptic medications may

Table 16.8—Modifiable Risk Factors for Epilepsy, United States

Magnitude/Group	Risk Factor
Strong (relative risk[a] >4)	
Newborns	Anoxia
	Congenital malformation
	Structural brain abnormality
Children	Mental retardation
	Cerebral palsy
	Central nervous system infection
Adults	Moderate to severe brain injury
Elderly	Cerebrovascular disease
All age groups	Neurosurgical procedures
Moderate (relative risk 2–4)	
Adults	Chronic alcohol or heroin use
Weak (relative risk <2)	None
Possible	Pertussis immunization
	Mild brain injury

[a]Defined in Table 2.4, page 51.

prevent recurrent seizures or premature death in the majority of patients with epilepsy. At least 70% of patients with a single isolated seizure have no recurrence and should not be considered to have epilepsy.[85] Most people with treated epilepsy (70% to 80%) become seizure-free with medication, and up to 70% of children in this category remain seizure-free even after medication is withdrawn.[86] Patients who have recurrent seizures and who have undergone treatment for 5 years and children with mental retardation or cerebral palsy are the least likely to achieve ultimate remission.

Tertiary prevention of status epilepticus,[87] and of sudden unexplained death in treated persons with epilepsy,[88] should be the focus of future prospective studies.

HEADACHE: MIGRAINE
ICD-9 346.0–346.9

MUSCLE CONTRACTION HEADACHE
ICD-9 307.81

SIGNIFICANCE

Up to 80% of women and 65% of men in the United States report a history of headache. A national ambulatory medical care survey found that more than 10 million visits to physicians' offices over 2 years were accounted for by head-ache.[89] The principal public health impacts of headache are related to restricted activity because of frequent or severe headaches; disability related to chronic, severe headaches; and the associated medical and disability costs.

Several major attempts at classifying headache types have occurred since 1962.[90] None of these systems has resulted in uniform case definitions that could be easily incorporated into epidemiologic studies.[91, 92] In ambulatory practice, the two principal headache types are migraine, or vascular headaches, and muscle contraction headaches. A reasonable case definition for severe migraine has recently been reported in one of the few population-based studies of this disorder.[93] A clear distinction between these two headache types is critical for epidemiologic purposes and has been demonstrated by cluster analysis.[94]

DESCRIPTIVE EPIDEMIOLOGY

Average annual incidence of severe headache has been estimated at 0.45%.[1] The peak incidence of migraine occurs in the 10- to 20-year age group, and peak prevalence occurs in the 35- to 40-year age group.[95] Migraine often presents in childhood, and new onset of migraine after age 40 is rare. First onset of migraine after age 50 may be an exaggerated vasomotor response associated with variant angina[96] or a harbinger of cerebrovascular disease. The risk of migraine among men and women is approximately equal until puberty but is two to four times higher in women after that time. Migraine prevalence was nearly twice as high among people with low incomes (<$10 000) as among higher-income (≥$30 000) groups in one study.[97] The proportion of persons in the general population classified as migraine, headaches without migraine, or nonheadachers varies by sex (males: 7.8%, 76.1%, and 16.1% respectively; females: 24.9%, 65.8%, and 9.4% respectively).[98] The majority of nonmigraine headaches are of muscle contraction variety.

RISK FACTORS

Factors repeatedly described in the clinical literature as being important in the occurrence of migraine include hormonal factors such as menstruation, dietary factors (eg, red wine, chocolate, nitrites), family history, seasonal variation, let-down from stress, allergy, and cigarette smoking. However, their roles as risk factors have not been clearly substantiated in well-designed epidemiologic studies. Many of these factors may simply be triggers for individual headaches rather than etiologic factors. The following risk factors for migraine have little support in either the clinical or epidemiologic literature: hypertension, personality, intelligence, marital status, and epilepsy. Strong risk factors for muscle contraction headache include stress and depression.[99]

PREVENTION AND CONTROL MEASURES

Future epidemiologic studies should focus on genetic risks and risk factors for specific headache subtypes.[100]

Chronic stress is a major contributor to the etiology of muscle contraction headache. Adequate prevention measures reduce or eliminate stressful exposures. Frequent migraine headaches can be successfully aborted with prophylactic medications including propranolol, ergonovine, or cyproheptadine. Disabling muscle contraction headaches are best treated with stress management and psychophysiologic techniques such as electromyogram biofeedback. Disabling headaches may result from inadequate efforts at secondary prevention. Such patients may require intermittent relief with analgesic medications; however, prolonged chronic use of such medications, particularly in conjunction with sedative/hypnotics, may lead to increased disability. For all chronic headaches, the patient's increased participation in the process—for example, by keeping a detailed daily log of headaches—can be both diagnostic and therapeutic.

REFERENCES

1. Kurtzke JF. Neuroepidemiology. *Ann Neurol.* 1984;16:265–277.
2. Association of State and Territorial Chronic Disease Program Directors. *Reducing the Burden of Chronic Disease: Needs of the States. Executive Summary.* Washington, DC: Public Health Foundation; 1991.
3. National Advisory Neurological Disorders and Stroke Council. Implementation Plan. *Decade of the Brain.* Washington, DC: National Institute of Neurological Disorders and Stroke; 1990.
4. Calne DB, Eisen A, McGeer E, Spencer P. Alzheimer's disease, Parkinson's disease and motor-neurone disease: abiotrophic interaction between aging and environment? *Lancet.* 1986;2:1067–1070.
5. Graves AB, Kukull WA. The epidemiology of dementia. In: Morris JC, ed. *Handbook of Dementing Illnesses.* New York, NY: Marcel Dekker; 1992;23–69.
6. Joachim CL, Morris JH, Selkoe DD. Clinically diagnosed Alzheimer's disease: autopsy results in 150 cases. *Ann Neurol.* 1987;22:724–729.

7. McKhann G, Drachman D, Folstein M, Katzman R, Price D, Stedlan EM. Clinical diagnosis of Alzheimer's disease: report of the NINCDS-ADRDA Work Group under the auspices of the Department of Health and Human Services Task Force on Alzheimer's disease. *Neurology.* 1984;34:939–944.

8. Perry EK, Tomlinson BE, Blessed G, Bergmann K, Gibson PH, Perry RH. Correlation of cholinergic abnormalities with senile plaques and mental test scores in senile dementia. *Br Med J.* 1978;2:1457–1489.

9. Schoenberg BS, Anderson DW, Haerer AF. Severe dementia: prevalence and clinical features in a biracial US population. *Arch Neurol.* 1985;42:740–743.

10. Stern Y, Alexander GE, Prohovnik I, Mayeux R. Inverse relationship between education and parietotemporal perfusion deficit in Alzheimer's disease. *Ann Neurol.* 1992;32:371–375.

11. Albert MS. How does education affect cognitive function? *Ann Epidemiol.* 1995;5:76–78.

12. Breitner JC, Silverman JM, Mohs RC, Davis KL. Familial aggregation in Alzheimer's disease: comparison of risk among relatives of early- and late-onset cases, and among male and female relatives in successive generations. *Neurol.* 1988;38:207–212.

13. Lendon CL, Ashall F, Goate AM. Exploring the etiology of Alzheimer disease using molecular genetics. *JAMA.* 1997;277: 825–831.

14. Polvikoski T, Sulkava R, Haltia M, et al. Dementia, and cortical deposition of beta-amyloid protein. *N Engl J Med.* 1995;333: 1242–1247.

15. Mayeux R, Ottman R, Maestre G, et al. Synergistic effects of traumatic head injury and apolipoprotein-epsilon 4 in patients with Alzheimer's disease. *Neurology.* 1995;45:555–557.

16. Bjertness E, Candy JM, Torvik A, et al. Content of brain aluminum is not elevated in Alzheimer disease. *Alzheimer Dis Assoc Disord.* 1996;10:171–174.

17. Speck CE, Kukull WA, Brenner DE, et al. History of depression as a risk factor for Alzheimer's disease. *Epidemiology.* 1995;6: 366–369.

18. Lee PN. Smoking and Alzheimer's disease: a review of the epidemiological evidence. *Neuroepidemiology.* 1994;13:131–144.

19. Davis KL, Thal LJ, Gamzu ER, et al. A double-blind, placebo-controlled multicenter study of tacrine for Alheimer's disease. The Tacrine Collaborative Study Group. *N Engl J Med.* 1992; 327:1253–1259.

20. Knapp JM, Knopman DS, Solomon PR, Pendlebury WW,

Davis CS, Gracon SI. A 30-week randomized controlled trial of high dose tacrine in patients with Alzheimer's disease. The Tacrine Study Group. *JAMA.* 1994;271:985–991.

21. Breitner JC, Welsh KA. Genes and recent developments in the epidemiology of Alzheimer's disease and related dementia. *Epidemiol Rev.* 1995;17:39–47.

22. H'ebert R, Brayne C. Epidemiology of vascular dementia. *Neuroepidemiology.* 1995;14:240–257.

23. Rajput AH, Offord KP, Beard CM, Kurland LT. Epidemiology of parkinsonism: incidence, classification and mortality. *Ann Neurol.* 1984;16: 278–282.

24. Schoenberg BS, Anderson DW, Haerer AF. Prevalence of Parkinson's disease in the biracial population of Copiah County, Mississippi. *Neurology.* 1985;35:841–845.

25. Langston JW, Ballard P, Tetrud JW, Irwin I. Chronic parkinsonism in humans due to a product of meperidine analog synthesis. *Science.* 1983;219;979–980.

26. Tanner CM, Chen B, Wang W, et al. Environmental factors and Parkinson's disease: a case-control study in China. *Neurology.* 1989;39:660–664.

27. Armstrong M, Daly AK, Cholerton S, et al. Mutant debrisoquine hydroxylation genes in Parkinson's disease. *Lancet.* 1992;339:1017–1018.

28. Smith CAD, Gough AC, Leigh PN, et al. Debrisoquine hydroxylase gene polymorphism and susceptibility to Parkinson's disease. *Lancet.* 1992;339: 1375–1377.

29. Polymeropoulous MH, Higgins JJ, Golbe LI, et al. Mapping of a gene for Parkinson's disease to chromosome 4q21-q23. *Science.* 1996;274:1197–1199.

30. Golbe LI, Farrel T. Case-control study of early-adult dietary factors in Parkinson's disease. *Arch Neurol.* 1988;45:1350–1353.

31. Baron JA. Cigarette smoking and Parkinson's disease. *Neurology.* 1986;36:1490–1496.

32. Tanner CM, Langston JW. Do environmental toxins cause Parkinson's disease? A critical review. *Neurology.* 1990;40:17–30.

33. Bobowick AR, Brody JA. Epidemiology of motor neuron diseases. *N Engl J Med.* 1973; 288:1047-1055.

34. Spencer PS, Nunn PB, Hugon J, et al. Guam ALS-Parkinson-dementia linked to plant neurotoxin. *Science.* 1987;237:717–722.

35. Kurtzke JF. Epidemiology of amyotrophic lateral sclerosis. *Adv Neurol.* 1982;36:281–302.

36. Mulder DW, Kurland LT. Motor neuron disease: epidemiologic

studies. In: Cosi V, Kato AC, Parlette W, Pinelli P, eds. ALS: *Therapeutic, Psychologic and Research Aspects.* New York, NY: Plenum Press; 1987:325–332.

37. Rosen DR, Siddique T, Patterson D, et al. Mutations in Cu/Zn superoxide dismutase gene are associated with familial amyotrophic lateral sclerosis. *Nature.* 1993;362:59–62.

38. Kondo K, Tsubaki T. Case-control studies of motor neuron disease. Association with mechanical injuries. *Arch Neurol.* 1981;38:220–226.

39. Bensimon G, Lacomblez L, Meininger V. A controlled trial of riluzole in amyotrophic lateral sclerosis. ALS/Riluzole Study Group. *N Engl J Med.* 1994; 330:585–591.

40. Poser CM, Paty DW, Scheinberg L, et al. New diagnostic criteria for multiple sclerosis: guidelines for research protocols. *Ann Neurol.* 1983;13:227–231.

41. Kurtzke JF. Epidemiologic contributions to multiple sclerosis: an overview. *Neurology.* 1980;30:61–79.

42. Wynn DR, Rodriguez M, O'Fallon WM, Kurland LT. A reappraisal of the epidemiology of multiple sclerosis in Olmsted County, Minnesota. *Neurology.* 1990;40:780–786.

43. Alter M, Kahana E, Lowewenson R. Migration and risk of multiple sclerosis. *Neurology.* 1978;28: 1089–1093.

44. Ebers GC, Bulman D, Sadovnick AD, et al. A population-based study of multiple sclerosis in twins. *N Engl J Med.* 1986;64: 808–817.

45. Bell JI, Lathrop GM. Multiple loci for multiple sclerosis. *Nature Genet.* 1996;13:377–378.

46. Beck RW, Clear PA, Trobe JD, et al. The effect of corticosteroids for acute optic neuritis on the subsequent development of multiple sclerosis. The Optic Neuritis Study Group. *N Engl J Med.* 1993;329:1764-1769.

47. The IFNB Multiple Sclerosis Study Group. Interferon beta-1b is effective in relapsing-remitting multiple sclerosis. I. Clinical results of a multicenter, randomized, double-blind, placebo controlled trial. *Neurology.* 1993;43:655–661.

48. Jacobs LD, Cookfair DL, Rudick RA, et al. Intramuscular interferon beta-1a for disease progression in relapsing multiple sclerosis. The Multiple Sclerosis Collaborative Research Group (MSCRG). *Ann Neurol.* 1996;39: 285–294.

49. Johnson KP, Brooks JA, Cohen JA, et al. Copolymer 1 reduces relapse rate and improves disability in relapsing-remitting multiple sclerosis: results of a phase III multicenter, double-

blind, placebo-controlled trial. *Neurology.* 1995;45:1268–1276.

50. Asbury AK, Arnason BGW, Karp HR, McFarlin DE. Criteria for diagnosis of Guillain-Barré syndrome. *Ann Neurol.* 1978; 3:565–566.

51. Alter M. The epidemiology of Guillain-Barré syndrome. *Ann Neurol.* 1990;27(suppl):S7–S12.

52. Schonberger LB, Hurwitz ES, Katina P, Holman RC, Bregman DJ. Guillain-Barré syndrome: its epidemiology and associations with influenza vaccine. *Ann Neurol.* 1981;9(suppl):31–38.

53. Safranek TJ, Lawrence DN, Kurland LT, et al. Reassessment of the association between Guillain-Barré syndrome and the receipt of the swine influenza vaccine in 1976–1977: results of a two state study. *Am J Epidemiol.* 1991;133:940–951.

54. van der Mech'e FG, Schmitz PI. A randomized trial comparing intravenous immune globulin and plasma exchange in Guillain-Barré syndrome. Dutch Guillan-Barré Study Group [see comments]. *N Engl J Med.* 1992;326:1123–1129.

55. Kraus JF. Epidemiologic features of injuries to the central nervous system. In: Anderson DW, ed. *Neuroepidemiology: A Tribute to Bruce Schoenberg.* Boston, Mass: CRC Press; 1991:333–357.

56. Graham D. Detailed diagnoses and procedures for patients discharged from short-stay hospitals, United States, 1986. *Vital Health Stat* 1988;13. DHHS publication PHS 88-1756. 1988.

57. Kalsbeek WD, McLaurin RL, Harris BSH, Miller JD. The National Head and Spinal Cord Injury Survey: major findings. *J Neurosurg.* 1980;53:S19–S31.

58. Franklin GM, Heyer NJ. Occupational morbid brain injury in Washington State, 1988-1990. *Am J Public Health.* 1994;84:1106–1109.

59. Thompson DC, Rivara FP, Thompson RS. Effectiveness of bicycle safety helmets in preventing head injuries. A case-control study. *JAMA.* 1996;276:1968–1973.

60. Injury-control recommendations: bicycle helmets. National Center for Injury Prevention and Control, Centers for Disease Control and Prevention. *MMWR.* 1995;44:1–17.

61. Practice Parameter: the management of concussion in sports (summary statement). Report of the Quality Standards Subcommittee. *Neurology.* 1997;48:581–585.

62. Griffin M, O'Fallon W, Opitz J, Kurland L. Mortality, survival and prevalence: traumatic spinal cord injury in Olmstead County, Minnesota, 1935–1981. *J Chronic Dis.* 1985;38: 643–653.

63. DeVivo MJ, Fine PR, Maetz HM, Stover SL. Prevalence of spinal

cord injury: a reestimation employing life table techniques. *Arch Neurol.* 1980;37:707–708.

64. Trends in traumatic spinal cord injury—New York, 1982–1988. *MMWR.* 1991;40:535–537; 543.

65. Bracken MV, Shepard MJ, Collins WF, et al. A randomized, controlled trial of methylprednisolone or naloxone in the treatment of acute spinal cord injury. Results of the Second National Acute Spinal Cord Injury Study. *N Engl J Med.* 1990;322: 1405–1411.

66. Rempel D, Evanoff B, Amadio P, et al. Consensus criteria for the classification of carpal tunnel syndrome in epidemiologic studies. *Am J Public Health.* In press.

67. Stevens JC, Sun J, Beard CM, O'Fallon WM, Kurland LT. Carpal tunnel syndrome in Rochester, Minnesota, 1961 to 1986. *Neurology.* 1988;38: 134–138.

68. Franklin GM, Haug J, Heyer N, et al. Occupational carpal tunnel syndrome in Washington State, 1984-1988. *Am J Public Health.* 1991;81:741–746.

69. Silverstein BA, Furie LJ, Armstrong TJ. Occupational factors and carpal tunnel syndrome. *Am J Ind Med.* 1987;11: 343–358.

70. Wieslander G, Norback D, Gothe C-J, Juhlin L. Carpal tunnel syndrome and exposure to vibration, repetitive wrist movements, and heavy manual work: a case-referent study. *Br J Ind Med.* 1989;46:43–47.

71. Cheadle A, Franklin GM, Wolfhagen C, Savarino J, Liu PY, Salley MS, Weaver M. Factors influencing duration of work-related disability: a population-based study from Washington State. *Am J Public Health.* 1994;84:190–196.

72. Deyo RA, Tsui-Wu YJ. Descriptive epidemiology of low back pain and its related medical care in the US. *Spine.* 1987;12:264–268.

73. Walsh K, Varnes N, Osmond C, Styles R, Coggon D. Occupational causes of low back pain. *Scand J Work Environ Health.* 1989;15:54–59.

74. Snook SH. Low back pain in industry. In: White AA, Gordon SL, eds. Symposium on Idiopathic Low Back Pain. St. Louis, Mo: Mosby; 1982:23–38.

75. Adera T, Deyo RA, Donatell RJ. Premature menopause and low back pain. A population-based study. *Ann Epidemiol.* 1994;4: 416–422.

76. Kelsey JL, Golden AL, Mundt DJ. Low back pain/prolapsed lumbar intervertebral disc. *Rheum Dis Clin North Am.* 1990;16:699–716.

77. Carey TS, Evans AT, Hadler NM, et al. Acute severe low back pain. A population-based study

of prevalence and care-seeking. *Spine.* 1996;21:339–344.

78. Nuwayhid IA, Steward W, Johnson JV. Work activities and the onset of first-time low back pain among New York City fire fighters. *Am J Epidemiol.* 1993; 137:539–548.

79. Spengler DM, Bigos SJ, Martin NA, Zeh J, Fisher L, Nachemson A. Back injuries in industry: a retrospective study. I. Overview and cost analysis. *Spine.* 1986;11: 241–245.

80. Franklin GM, McKeefrey S, Haug J, Picciano J. Outcome of lumbar fusion in Washington State workers' compensation. *Spine.* 1994;19:1897–1904.

81. Commission on Classification and Terminology of the International League Against Epilepsy. Proposal for revised classification of epilepsies and epileptic syndromes. *Epilepsia.* 1989;30:389–399.

82. Hauser WA, Hasdorfer DC. Epidemiology of epilepsy. In: Anderson DW, ed. *Neuroepidemiology: A Tribute to Bruce Schoenberg.* Boston, Mass: CRC Press; 1991:98–119.

83. Shamansky SL, Glaser GH. Socioeconomic characteristics of childhood seizure disorders in the New Haven area: an epidemiologic study. *Epilepsia.* 1979;20:457–474.

84. Ottman R, Lee JH, Hauser WA, Risch N. Birth cohort and familial risk of epilepsy: the effect of deminished recall in studies of lifetime prevalence. *Am J Epidemiol.* 1995;141:235–241.

85. Hauser WA, Rich SS, Annegers JP, Anderson VL. Seizure recurrence after a first unprovoked seizure: an extended follow up. *Neurology.* 1990;40:1163–1170.

86. Shinnar S, Vining EPG, Mellits ED, et al. Discontinuing antiepileptic medication in children with epilepsy after two years without seizures: a prospective study. *N Engl J Med.* 1985;313: 976–980.

87. DeLorenzo RJ, Pellock JM, Towne AR, Boggs JG. Epidemiology of status epilepticus. *J Clin Neurophysiol.* 1995;12:316–325.

88. Tennis P, Cole TB, Annegera JF, Lesstma JE, McNutt M, Rajput A. Cohort study of incidence of sudden unexplained death in persons with seizure disorder treated with antiepileptic drugs in Saskatchewan, Canada. *Epilepsia.* 1995;36:29–36.

89. Cypress BK. Patients' reasons for visiting physicians. National Ambulatory Medical Care Survey: United States, 1977-78. *Vital Health Stat* 1981;13. DHHS publication PHS 82-1717.

90. Ziegler DK. Epidemiology of migraine. In: Anderson DW, ed. *Neuroepidemiology: A Tribute to Bruce Schoenberg.* Boston, Mass: CRC Press; 1991:167–192.

91. Mortimer MJ, Kay J, Jaron A. Epidemiology of headache and childhood migraine in an urban general practice using Ad Hoc, Vahlquist and IHS criteria. *Dev Med Child Neurol.* 1992;34:1095–1101.

92. Merikangas KR, Whitaker AE, Angst J. Validation of diagnostic criteria for migraine in the Zurich longitudinal cohort study. *Cephalalgia.* 1993;13:47–53.

93. Stewart WF, Linet MS, Celentano DD, VanNatta M, Ziegler D. Age- and sex-specific rates of migraine with and without visual aura. *Am J Epidemiol.* 1991;134:1111–1120.

94. Diehr P, Diehr G, Koepsell T, et al. Cluster analysis to determine headache types. *J Chronic Dis.* 1982;35:623–633.

95. Linet MS, Stewart WF. Migraine headache: epidemiology perspectives. *Epidemiol Rev.* 1984; 6:107–139.

96. Miller D, Waters DD, Warnica W, Szladcis J, Kreeft J, Theroux P. Is variant angina the coronary manifestation of a generalized vasospastic disorder? *N Engl J Med.* 1981;304:763–766.

97. Stewart WF, Lipton RB, Celentano DD, Reed ML. Prevalence of migraine headache in the United States relative to age, income, race and other socio-demographic factors. *JAMA.* 1992;267:64–69.

98. O'Brien B, Goeree R, Streiner D. Prevalence of migraine headache in Canada: a population-based survey. *Int J Epidemiol.* 1994;23: 1020–1026.

99. Goldstein M, Chen TC. The epidemiology of disabling headache. *Adv Neurol.* 1982;33: 377–390.

100. Italian Cooperative Study Group on the Epidemiology of Cluster Headache (ICECH). Case-control study on the epidemiology of cluster headache. I: Etiological factors and associated conditions. *Neuroepidmiology.* 1995; 14:123–127.

SUGGESTED READING

Anderson DW, ed. *Neuroepidemiology: A Tribute to Bruce Schoenberg.* Boston, Mass: CRC Press; 1991.

Gorelick PB, Alter M, eds. *Handbook of Neuroepidemiology.* New York, NY: Marcel Dekker; 1994.

Koprowski CD, Longstreth WT Jr, Cebul RD. Clinical neuroepidemiology: III. Decision. *Arch Neurol.* 1989;46:223–229.

Kurtzke JF. The current neurologic burden of illness and injury in the United States. *Neurology.* 1982;32:1207–1214.

Longstreth WT Jr, Koepsell TD, van Belle G. Clinical neuroepidemiology: I. Diagnosis. *Arch Neurol.* 1987;44:1091–1099.

Longstreth WT Jr, Koepsell TD, van Belle G. Clinical neuroepidemiology: II. Outcome. *Arch Neurol.* 1987;44:1196–1202.

National Advisory Neurological Disorders and Stroke Council. *Implementation Plan. Decade of the Brain.* Washington, DC: National Institute of Neurological Disorders and Stroke; 1990.

Subcommittee on Brain and Behavioral Sciences. *Decade of the Brain, 1990–2000. Maximizing Human Potential.* Washington, DC: National Technical Information Service; 1991. Publication PB91-133769.

RESOURCES

Alzheimer's Association
919 N Michigan Avenue, Suite 1000
Chicago, IL 60611-1676
(800) 272-3900
(312) 355-8700

Alzheimer's Disease Education and Referral Center (ADEAR)
PO Box 8250
Silver Spring, MD 20907-8250
(800) 438-4380
e-mail: adear@alzheimers.org

The Alzheimer's Foundation (AF)
8177 South Harvard
M/C-114
Tulsa, OK 74137
(918) 481-6031

American Parkinson Disease Association
1250 Hyland Boulevard—Suite 4B
Staten Island, NY 10305
(718) 981-8001
e-mail: apda@admin.con2.com

National Parkinson Foundation, Inc.
1501 NW 9th Ave
Bob Hope Road
Miami, FL 33136-1494
(800) 327-4545

Parkinson's Action Network
822 College Avenue—Suite C
Santa Rosa, CA 95404
(800) 850-4726
e-mail: Parkactnet@aol.com

Parkinson's Disease Foundation (PDF)
William Black Medical Building
710 West 168th Street
New York, NY 10032
(212) 923-4700

United Parkinson Foundation (UPF)
833 West Washington Boulevard
Chicago, IL 60607
(312) 733-1893

Muscular Dystrophy Association
3300 East Sunrise Drive
Tucson, AZ 85718
(602) 529-2000
e-mail: mda@mdausa.org

National Multiple Sclerosis Society
733 3rd Avenue
New York, NY 10017-3288
(800) 344-4867 (FIGHT MS)
(212) 986-3240
e-mail: info@nmss.org

Brain Injury Association, Inc.
1776 Massachusetts Ave. NW
Suite 100
Washington, DC 20036

Paralyzed Veterans of America
Spinal Cord Research Foundation
801 18th Street, NW
Washington, DC 20006
(800) 424-8200
(202) 872-1300

Epilepsy Foundation of America
4351 Garden City Drive
Landover, MD 20785-4951
(800) EFA-1000
(301) 459-3700

National Headache Foundation
428 W. Saint James Place, 2nd floor
Chicago, IL 60614-2750
(800) 843-2256
(312) 388-6399

INDEX

Acute anticoagulation therapy, 322
Administrative data collection systems
  function of, 64–65
  strengths and weaknesses of, 59
Adolescents. *See also* Children
  alcohol use and, 154, 167
  cholesterol reduction in, 288–289
  diabetes in, 421
  physical activity and, 198–199, 207
  tobacco use and, 124–126, 128–129,
    131–133, 135
African Americans
  alcohol use and, 156–157
  Alzheimer's disease and, 495
  arthritis and, 465, 468
  asthma and, 380, 381
  cancer and, 335–337, 343, 347, 351,
    355–356, 363, 364
  cardiovascular disease and, 297, 301,
    302
  cystic fibrosis and, 392
  diabetes and, 427–429, 441–442
  diet and, 229
  epilepsy and, 515
  high blood pressure and, 264, 267
  mortality rates and, 16–17
  osteoporosis and, 476
  Parkinson's disease and, 499
  stroke and, 316–318, 323
  tobacco use and, 124, 128
Age factors. *See also* Elderly individuals
  alcohol use and, 154–155
  Alzheimer's disease and, 495, 496

amyotrophic lateral sclerosis and,
    502
  arthritis and, 465–468
  cancer and, 32, 34–35, 335, 343, 351
  cardiovascular disease and, 297, 300
  cholesterol levels and, 281, 288–289
  diabetes and, 421–422, 428
  epilepsy and, 515
  gout and, 474
  headaches and, 517
  multi-infarct dementia and, 498
  osteoarthritis and, 468
  osteoporosis and, 475–479, 483
  Parkinson's disease and, 499
  physical inactivity and, 197
  stroke and, 316
Age-adjusted rates, 35
Agency for Health Care Policy and
    Research (AHCPR), 137
Age-specific rates, 35
Alaska Natives
  alcohol use and, 158–159
  cystic fibrosis and, 392
  stroke and, 317
  tobacco use and, 124
Alcohol Dependence Scale (ADS), 173
Alcohol Misuse Prevention Study (AMPS),
    170
Alcohol use
  adolescents and, 154, 167
  cancer and, 364
  as cause of death, 8, 149
  cholesterol levels and, 284